DENTAL OFFICE MANAGEMENT

SECOND EDITION

CYNTHIA LAMKIN RDA, RDH

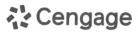

Australia • Brazil • Canada • Mexico • Singapore • United Kingdom • United States

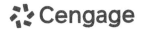

Dental Office Management, **Second Edition**
Cynthia Lamkin

Vice President, Careers & Computing: Dawn Gerrain

Director of Learning Solutions: Steve Helba

Acquisitions Editor: Jadin Kavanaugh

Director, Development-Career and Computing: Marah Bellegarde

Product Development Manager: Juliet Steiner

Senior Content Developer: Darcy M. Scelsi

Editorial Assistant: Nicole Manikas

Brand Manager: Michele McTighe

Market Development Manager: Erica Glisson

Senior Production Director: Wendy Troeger

Production Manager: Andrew Crouth

Art and Cover Direction, Production Management, and Composition: PreMediaGlobal

Cover Image: iStockphoto.com/Yunus Arakon

Interior Design Images:
Skill Building: shutterstock/Aleksandr Bryliaev

Challenge Your Understanding: shutterstock/VLADGRIN

For product information and technology assistance, contact us at
**Cengage Customer & Sales Support, 1-800-354-9706
or support.cengage.com.**

For permission to use material from this text or product, submit all requests online at **www.copyright.com**.

Library of Congress Control Number: 2013953091

Book Only ISBN-13: 978-1-285-08944-7
Package ISBN-13: 978-1-133-28311-9

Cengage
200 Pier 4 Boulevard
Boston, MA 02210
USA

Cengage is a leading provider of customized learning solutions with employees residing in nearly 40 different countries and sales in more than 125 countries around the world. Find your local representative at: **www.cengage.com.**

To learn more about Cengage platforms and services, register or access your online learning solution, or purchase materials for your course, visit **www.cengage.com.**

Printed in the United States of America
Print Number: 07   Print Year: 2022

TABLE OF CONTENTS

SECTION TWO   Practice Communications   89

Dental Office Management was written to satisfy the need expressed by dental professionals for a comprehensive, detailed, and up-to-date text for dental office managers. Dental assistants have often gravitated into the role of the office manager and this text specifically addresses the skills they need for a successful administrative career. Because of the increased complexity of dental practice management, a growing number of individuals with business or marketing backgrounds are using their education and experience in dental practices. This text will enable them to expand their understanding of dentistry.

In recognition of the increasing responsibilities delegated to the dental office manager, *Dental Office Management* aims to enable the dental assistant pursuing a dental management career or the business manager seeking a dental career to respond to the needs of a state-of-the-art dental practice. Topics included for the dental office manager are government trends and regulations, insurance coding and billing, financial tracking of production and expenditures, an emphasis on marketing including online marketing of the practice, practice management software, and scheduling to maximize production.

Because practice management software has become a necessity in contemporary dental offices, this text includes Dentrix G4 Learning Edition software and comprehensive step-by-step instructions for its use. This in-depth study of a popular software package should enable students to confidently transfer those skills to other dental practice management systems.

Organization of the Text

This text is divided into six sections: The Business of Dentistry, Practice Communications, Clinical Records Management, Business and Financial Records Management, Dental Office Employment, and The Use of Practice Management Software. The chapters within each section contain instructional objectives and key terms that appear in bold in the text.

You will also note that cross-referencing of topics is used throughout this text. This feature enables students to adequately prepare when comprehension of information from another chapter is required before proceeding, or for additional or expanded information on a specific topic.

At the end of each chapter students will find the sections *Exploring the Web*, *Skill Building* exercises, and a *Challenge Your Understanding* post-test. The *Exploring the Web* encourages the student to explore material outside of this text by using trustworthy websites. The skill building exercises are designed for the student to use critical thinking, problem solving, and role-playing using the information presented in each chapter. These exercises help the student work through practical problem-solving situations commonly encountered in the life of a dental office manager. The post-test is designed for quick assessment of information learned in the chapter through multiple choice and true/false questions.

An attempt has been made to reduce gender bias in the preparation of the text and references throughout the text are given as he or she or dental office manager. Although the profession is currently dominated by women, it is a challenging career for anyone interested in the business of dentistry regardless of gender.

New to this Edition

Chapter 1

- New chapter focusing on the goals and responsibilities of the dental office manager in a progressive dental practice
- Update on credentials available to office managers
- Includes content regarding Dental Practice Philosophy and Mission Statements from Chapter 1 of the first edition
- Ideas for making a dental practice more environmentally friendly are spread throughout this second edition

Chapter 2

- Formerly Chapter 1
- An updated look at the dental team including educational requirements and responsibilities
- Introduces new specialties and looks at possible future specialties

Chapter 3

- Formerly Chapter 2
- Expanded discussion of the legal practice of dentistry
- Updates on importance of office manuals in supervising staff. Addition of information regarding HIPAA

Chapter 4

- Formerly Chapter 3
- Updated and expanded information on hazard communication plans
- Updates to regulations and the office managers role in keeping the dental team safe

Chapter 5

- Formerly Chapter 4
- Current thoughts regarding creating a comfortable patient environment
- Consideration of a comfortable environment as a marketing tool

Chapter 6

- Formerly Chapter 5
- Current trends in marketing the dental practice through websites and social networking
- Includes discussing importance of referrals and methods of tracking practice growth

Chapter 7

- Formerly Chapter 6
- Includes discussion of digital communication such as email

Chapter 8

- Formerly Chapter 7
- Includes discussion of newer technologies such as hands-free phone systems and digital technologies
- Outdated equipment has been deleted

Chapter 9

- Formerly Chapter 8
- Updated illustrations

Chapter 10

- Formerly Chapter 9
- Updates and new figures

Chapter 11

- Formerly Chapter 10
- Includes discussion of electronic records
- Includes discussion of digital radiography

Chapter 12

- Formerly Chapter 11
- Increasing efficiency with the use of computers and digital technologies

Chapter 13

- Formerly Chapter 12
- Includes updates to CDT codes and third-party payments
- Updated ADA insurance claim form that includes HIPAA-mandated ICD codes

Chapter 14

- Formerly Chapter 13
- Managing online banking

Chapter 15

- Formerly Chapter 14
- Cost containment by using expert ordering techniques

Chapter 16

- Formerly Chapter 15
- Updated resume ideas
- Where to look for jobs in an online world

Chapter 17

- New chapter on hiring a cohesive dental team
- Creating an employment plan
- Making the most of a working interview

Chapters 18 through 24

- New section that provides practice and an overview of the use of dental practice management software
- The Dentrix G4 Learning Edition CD is provided with the text and used as a tutorial throughout these chapters
- Step-by-step instruction and numerous practice activities are provided

Teaching and Learning Package

CourseMate

CourseMate complements your textbook with several robust and noteworthy components:

- An interactive eBook, with highlighting, note taking, and search capabilities
- Interactive and engaging learning tools including, flashcards, quizzes, games, PowerPoint presentations, and much more
- Engagement Tracker, a first-of-its-kind tool that monitors student participation and retention in the course

To access CourseMate content:

- Go to www.cengagebrain.com.
- For an Internet access code (Order # 978-1-1332-8316-4)
- For a Print access code (Order # 978-1-1332-8315-7)

Instructor Companion Website

An Instructor Companion Website is available to facilitate classroom preparation, presentation, and testing. This content can be accessed through your Instructor SSO account.

To set up your account:

- Go to www.cengagebrain.com/login.
- Choose **Create a New Faculty Account.**
- Next you will need to select your **Institution.**
- Complete your personal **Account Information.**
- Accept the **License Agreement.**
- Choose **Register.**
- Your account will be pending validation — you will receive an email notification when the validation process is complete.
- If you are unable to find your Institution; complete an **Account Request Form.**

Once your account is set up or if you already have an account:

- Go to www.cengagebrain.com/login.
- Enter your email address and password and select **Sign In.**
- Search for your book by author, title, or ISBN.
- Select the book and click **Continue.**
- You will receive a list of available resources for the title you selected.
- Choose the resources you would like and click **Add to My Bookshelf.**

Components available on the Instructor Companion site include a(n):

- The Instructor's Manual to accompany the text. This resource includes teaching strategies and lesson plans correlated to each chapter.
- Instructor presentations in Power Point™ that coordinate with each chapter. These are fully customizable to accommodate the needs of your course materials.
- Computerized Testbank that contains multiple choice questions correlating to each chapter. The testbank is also fully customizable
- Image Library that contains many of the images from the text. These images can be used in the Instructor Presentations on PowerPoint™

Acknowledgments

Without the support and encouragement of many wonderful people this book would not have been possible. First, I want to thank to Ellen Dietz who was the author of the first edition of this text. Though she was unable to write the second edition, she provided a foundation to build on. I am grateful to her for sharing her knowledge and expertise.

Throughout my dental career, I have been very fortunate to have worked for wonderful dentists who invested in my continuing education in the office and the classroom. Thank you to Donald J. Meis, DDS, for stressing to me that choosing words carefully is very important. Since that first job I have taken x-rays "for" patients and not "on" them. My sincere gratitude to the doctors of Southdale Dental Associates for investing so much time and effort into creating a fabulous team and allowing me to be part of it. Special thanks to Jerry W. Crawford, DDS, whose commitment to excellence has been an inspiration.

I would also like to thank Darcy Scelsi at Cengage Learning for helping me put my thoughts and experience into words.

Finally thank you to my students who are constantly teaching and inspiring me with their dedication and enthusiasm.

Reviewers of the Second Edition
Michelle Bissonette, CDA, EFDA, BS
Dental Assisting Clinical Director
Indiana University School of Dentistry

Judith A. McCauley, RDH, MA
Department Chair, Associate Professor
Palm Beach State College

Stephanie Joyce Schmidt, CDA, CPFDA, DCT, RDAEF2, FADAA, MS
Pasadena City College

Diana M. Sullivan, LDA, CDA, MS
Program Director
Dakota County Technical College

Tracie E. West
Dental Assisting Instructor
Remington College — Cleveland West

Reviewers of the First Edition
Lori Burch, RDA
Corinthian College
Reseda, California

Robin Caplan, CDA, EFDA, DRT
Medix School
Owings Mills, Maryland

Lana Barnett Edwards, DMD
Lewis and Clark College
Godfrey, Illinois

Darlene Hunziker, CDA, RDA
Eton Technical Institute
Everett, Washington

Barbara Melanson, RDH, MS
Quinsigamond Community College
Worcester, Massachusetts

Fred Rich
Gwinett School of Dental Assisting
Lilburn, Georgia

Debbie Reynon, CDA, RDA
Monterey Peninsula College
Monterey, California

Deanne Shuman, BSDH, MS
Old Dominion University
Norfolk, Virginia

About the Author

Cynthia Lamkin has been employed in the dental field for over 35 years. She graduated from the University of South Dakota with a degree in dental hygiene. In addition to practicing clinical hygiene, she has also worked in dental office administration and treatment coordination. Her career includes family dentistry, and specialty practices of periodontics, endodontics, pediatric dentistry, and orthodontics. Cynthia has both Registered Dental Assistant and Registered Dental Hygienist credentials and is licensed to practice in multiple states.

Currently, Cynthia is a facilitator and course developer for ed2go online continuing education and teaches programs in *Administrative Dental Assisting, Clinical Dental Assisting,* and *Exploring a Career in a Dental Office.*

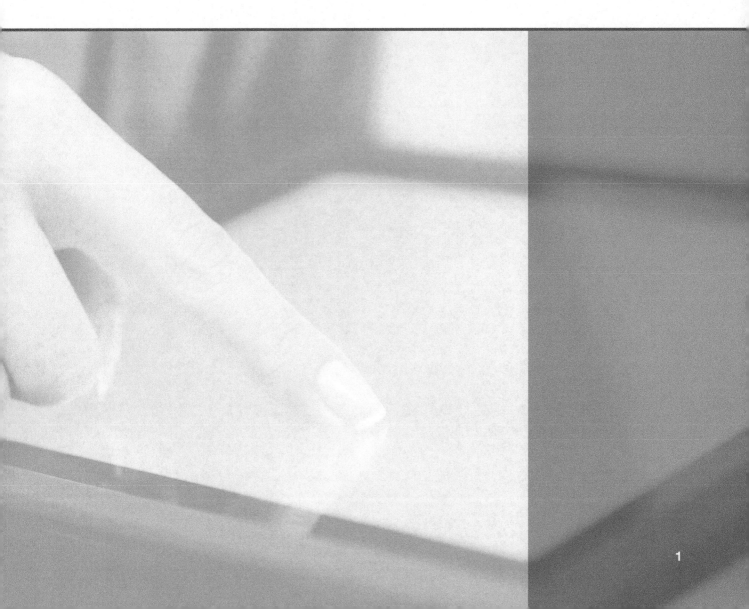

SECTION I

The Business of Dentistry

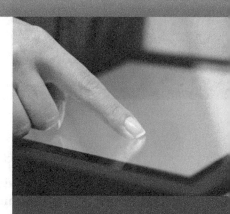

CHAPTER 1

The Dental Office Manager

KEY TERMS

American Association
  of Dental Office
  Managers (AADOM)
continuing education
  (CE)
Dental Assisting National
  Board (DANB)
dental office manager
fellowship
practice mission
  statement
practice philosophy
recall
recare

LEARNING OBJECTIVES

Upon completion of this chapter, the reader should be able to:

1. List the responsibilities of the dental office manager.
2. Describe educational requirements for the dental office manager.

3. Describe the importance of the practice's philosophy, mission statement, and goals from the point of view of the dental office manager.
4. Discuss the importance of continuing education for the dental office manager.
5. List the professional organizations and formal credentials available to the dental office manager.

The Dental Office Manager

The **dental office manager** is in charge of all business aspects associated with running the practice (Figure 1-1). Depending upon the size of the office, he or she may also act as receptionist, appointment scheduler, and billing clerk. In larger practices, the office manager may supervise administrative (front office) staff as well as clinical (chairside) dental assistants. The dental office manager may

- have a business background or degree;
- have specific training in dental office administration or clinical dental assisting; or
- be trained on the job.

Although some office managers are former clinical assistants who are familiar with the clinical aspects of the practice, such as terminology, inventory control, and personnel requirements of the dentist, an increasing number of

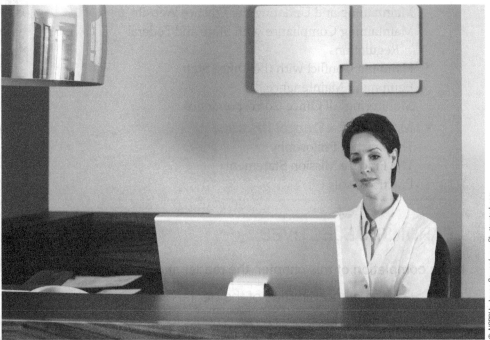

© AISPIX by Image Source/www.Shutterstock.com

FIGURE 1-1 The dental office manager handles the business of practicing dentistry.

office managers have business degrees and are qualified to run the complex business aspects of the practice.

The demands of the business of dentistry have grown beyond making appointments and sending recall cards. A successful practice includes marketing the practice; leveraging social media; managing human resources; an understanding of time management; knowledge of complicated insurance plans and benefits, and accounting; and possessing advanced computer skills. Regardless of whether the office manager is moving from a business background to dental care or from dental care to business, he or she will need extensive on-the-job training and continuing education (CE) to run an efficient dental practice.

Continuing education for the dental office manager and administrative staff refers to programs whose content relates directly to dental practice management or the art and science of oral health and treatment of dental disease. Continuing education is measured in units commonly called continuing education units (CEUs) with each course having a unit value. CEUs are available in the classroom or online courses from a variety of sources, including local dental societies, colleges, universities, technical schools, independent providers, and companies that sell dental supplies. Excellent continuing education can often be very inexpensive because of sponsorship from dental suppliers.

Career Credentials

The professional organization dedicated to dental office management is the American Association of Dental Office Managers (AADOM). This is an organization of professional office managers, practice administrators, patient coordinators, insurance and financial coordinators, and treatment coordinators of general and specialized dental practices. It is the largest association for dental managers and administrative staff, and its mission is to provide members with networking, resources, and education to help them achieve the highest level of professional development.

There is no state licensure or registration for an office manager but there is professional credentialing available through AADOM.

In today's, increasingly complex and highly specialized workforce, credentials are important. Credentials are professional distinctions that show you are qualified and competent to work in the field. Earning a credential can improve visibility and create opportunities with potential employers. For dental office managers, AADOM offers a fellowship as a professional credential.

The requirements for an AADOM fellowship are the following:

- Attendance of at least One AADOM Annual Conference within the past 3 years (current year does not satisfy this requirement)
- 3 years minimum Dental Office Management experience or CDPMA[1] designation

---

[1]The Certified Dental Practice Management Administrator (CDPMA) was a credential offered by the Dental Assisting National Board (DANB), which is no longer available. It was discontinued because the testing did not address the vast changes in the field of dental office management. Individuals who have earned the CDPMA can continue to use it but the testing for new candidates has been discontinued. The DANB is recognized by the American Dental Association (ADA) and offers credentials for clinical dental assistants through education, testing, and clinical experience.

- Letter of recommendation from current or former employer (dental practice)
- Member in good standing of AADOM
- Member agrees to adhere to AADOM's Code of Conduct
- Passing Level of the Dale Foundation's Accounts Receivable Module[2]
- Passing Level of the DALE Foundation's Human Resources Fundamentals Module[2]
- Passing Level of the DALE Foundation's Financial Reporting for the Dental Office[2]
- 15 AADOM-approved CE hours within a two-year period
- Completion of the Fellowship Application Form and submission of application fee.

Upon approval of Fellowship Status, candidates will earn the designation of FAADOM, Fellow of the American Association of Dental Office Managers.

Responsibilities of the Dental Office Manager

The dental office manager is responsible for making sure all aspects of the office operate efficiently. Tasks may be delegated among office personnel but accountability remains with the office manager.

Scheduling

It is the responsibility of the dental office manager to schedule patients to maximize production and reduce stress for the clinical staff. This is done by careful appointment book management and evaluation of each day's schedule. It requires that the office manager understands the dental procedures being performed and their time requirements. Time must be managed efficiently to provide outstanding patient care while making sure each day meets monetary production goals.

Attracting New Patients to the Practice

A good dental office manager is constantly looking for ways to improve the practice so that there are always new patients and it continues to grow. The patients within a dental practice change frequently; families move to or from an area because of employment opportunities, and patients also leave or join practices as their dental insurance changes. Office managers must track these trends and adapt the practice to them. The office manager must determine where new patients are coming from to understand how to increase the visibility of the practice. New opportunities for marketing the practice must be investigated, at the same time discontinuing what is not working.

Evaluating Practice Goals

By evaluating reports and practice history, the office manager can assist in setting realistic goals for the dental practice. Working closely with the dentist, the dental office manager generally keeps the office on track and monitors

---

[2] These programs are offered through DALE Foundation, the online continuing education provider of the DANB. They do not count toward the 15 hours of required CEUs.

achievement of its goals. Supervision of the business of dentistry by the manager allows the dentist to focus on practicing dentistry.

A dental practice is like any other business and to continue to thrive, the practice must set goals and evaluate whether they are being met. If this isn't done, even small problems can grow out of control quickly. The advances in practice management software such as Dentrix, which we will be working with in Section VI, have made tracking the progress of the business of dentistry much easier. As long as the information is entered into the computer software accurately, it can be organized into a multitude of reports so the office manager is constantly aware of what is happening in the practice. Reports can be run to determine who the new patients are and how they were referred to the practice, as well as who has left the practice or what patients are past due for appointments. Once the office manager gathers the information, areas where improvement is needed can be identified and a goal can be established. For example, in the previous month, there were only two new patients, yet three patients were archived because they had new insurance and four moved from the area. Based on these numbers and the trend, it can easily be understood that it won't be long before the practice is in trouble. The dental team can set a goal of adding eight new patients each month for the next three months. With that goal set, they can discuss ways to achieve it and use reports to track it (Figure 1-2).

Financial Oversight

The dental office manager is responsible for maintaining the financial health of the practice by keeping accounts current. This begins with identifying delinquent accounts and developing an office protocol for dealing with them by sending statements, making phone calls, and/or other written communication. Some of these accounts might be patients that owe the

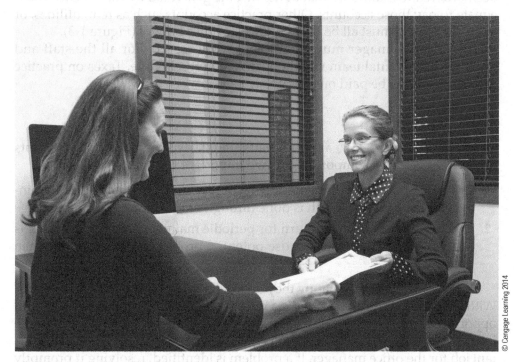

FIGURE 1-2 The practice manager monitors practice goals and makes sure team members are on target for achieving goals.

© Cengage Learning 2014

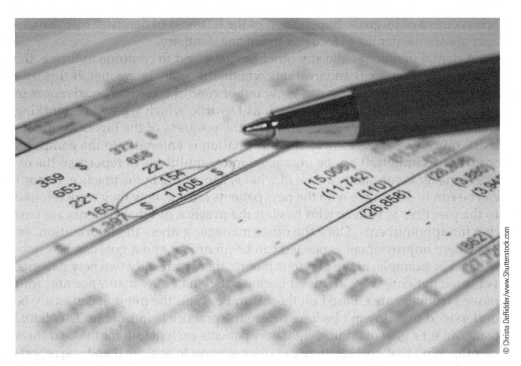

FIGURE 1-3 The office manager monitors and tracks the practice budget.

practice money but also could include insurance companies that are slow in paying claims.

Office accounts payable must be kept current so the practice maintains excellent credit. The office manager needs to monitor the supplies that have been ordered to make sure that at the income generated by the practice is adequate to pay those accounts. Other practice accounts such as rent, utilities, or equipment costs must all be figured into the office budget (Figure 1-3).

The office manager must maintain payroll records for all the staff and make sure the dental team members are paid on schedule. Taxes on practice income must also be paid on a quarterly basis.

Patient Retention

Monitoring recall/recare appointments (regularly scheduled appointments for preventive care) is important for two important reasons:

1. Growth in the practice depends on not only adding patients but also retaining current patients, which is done through recall/recare appointments.

2. Encouraging patients to return for periodic maintenance appointments is healthier for the patient because potential problems are identified when they are small.

When patients are not happy they don't refer friends, family, or co-workers. With the growing number of online review sites giving unhappy patients an opportunity to vent their frustration, one dissatisfied patient can have a huge impact. Listening to patient concerns quickly and with empathy is an important job for the office manager. If a problem is identified, resolving it promptly can keep it from escalating.

Handling Insurance Issues

Many dental offices rely on insurance companies to assist patients with the expense of treatment. It is the job of the office manager to make sure those payments are accounted for correctly and followed up when not received. Offices choosing to become preferred providers for an insurance company must decide if payments for treatment allow the dentist to offer care to patients while maintaining the financial health of the practice (Figure 1-4).

Insurance companies update their payment plans so the office manager needs to be prepared to cope with those changes. If you are dealing with scheduled payments, the office will receive a new payment schedule listing the treatment codes and the amount the insurance company is willing to pay for each procedure. This information must be recorded so that future billing is correct. The office manager must also consult with the dentist regarding whether the practice is financially able to continue working with the insurance company. That decision is based on the amount of the payment versus the cost of doing the procedure. Some insurance companies simply pay a percentage of the dentist's fee but even that must be added to financial records for future billing.

Managing Inventory

Whereas the clinical staff will be making the lists of materials they need, the office manager needs to make sure that supplies are purchased at competitive prices from companies that deliver supplies as promised. When the supplies arrive, there needs to be funds available to pay for them, so the office manager must constantly monitor accounts receivable and accounts payable to make sure that happens.

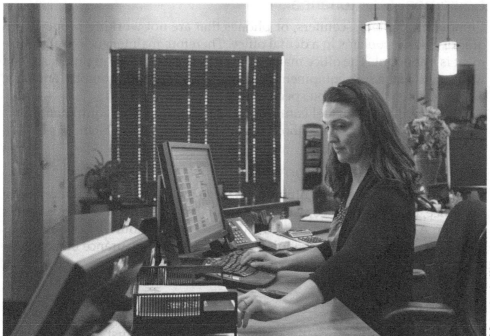

FIGURE 1-4 The office manager must maintain up-to-date information on insurance companies.

Maintaining and Updating the Practice Website

Patients shop online. Even when referred by friends or influenced by their insurance coverage, they will check out the office website or look for online reviews. Dental office managers are responsible for making sure the Website is updated and working properly.

Maintaining Compliance with State and Federal Regulations

The office manager must make sure the office is following guidelines and documenting that compliance. The office manager needs to be aware of any changes in state laws that affect the practice to make sure that all employees are working within the state regulations.

There are state and federal laws that govern the practice of dentistry in every state. Noncompliance can lead to substantial fines or even the loss of the dentist's license to practice. As the person that the dentist trusts to make sure that the office is operating within the law, the office manager needs to make sure that everyone is working within legal boundaries. Some examples might be making sure dental assistants are registered if necessary and that new permits are displayed according to state requirements, providing access to continuing education to meet state or federal requirements, addressing issues of sterilization and patient safety, and assuring all employees understand the importance of patient confidentially.

Handling Conflict with the Office Staff

Few things can destroy employee morale faster than staff who refuse to work together. The office manager needs to be aware of any strong personalities in the office and step in and negotiate compromise when necessary.

Equipment Maintenance

Computers, copiers, scanners, or phones that are not working properly can quickly cause problems in a dental office. Therefore maintenance of all equipment is important. The office manager needs to keep records of purchases and warranties, make sure equipment problems are addressed promptly, and have a reputable repair person on speed dial.

Employees need to feel confident that they can report equipment problems to the office manager without being blamed for the problem.

Monitoring All Office Correspondence

It is the responsibility of the office manager to make sure any mail received in the office, either as hard copy or by electronic mail, is dealt with in a timely fashion. All insurance or personal checks received should be deposited as soon as possible, any bills scheduled for payment, and insurance inquiries answered so claims are paid.

Managing a Dental Practice

To ensure a well-run office, the dental office manager must be familiar with the practice philosophy, practice mission statement, and resulting practice goals. The office manager must also have an understanding of all duties performed in the office by team members.

The Practice Philosophy

The **practice philosophy** is the underlying theme that drives the practice on a daily basis. It includes attitudes, delivery of service, patient satisfaction, and quality of service. The philosophy is the personality of the practice. Not every patient is looking for the same thing from their dental experience, so it's best to be honest and examine your "office" personality, which is probably a reflection of the personality of the "dentist or dentists" practicing in the office. One dentist may feel he or she works best in silence and strives toward "high tech, low touch" dentistry whereas another dentist may be equally competent but loves conversation and laughter and lots of personal interaction. Both of these offices may be very good but their approach to dentistry is very different.

The Practice Mission Statement

The **practice mission statement** is a brief declaration of the practice philosophy, usually formulated into one or two sentences. An example would be, "To provide the highest quality of dental care and service, and to treat each patient as a welcome guest." Many offices include the practice mission statement on their statements, letterhead, newsletter masthead, or other printed communications.

Practice Goals

The primary goal in dental practice is to serve patients. The first priority of the dental team is to treat all patients with courtesy, providing quality dental care with a service-oriented philosophy. To accomplish this goal, all members of the team must work together through a communication system of mutual respect. This begins with full knowledge of each team member's role, job description, and educational background. The practice goals are an extension of the practice philosophy and mission statement.

One of the goals of the dental office may be to practice in an eco-friendly manner. The dental office manager can help the dental practice become more eco-friendly. Promoting environmental health by using technologies and materials that minimize waste and pollution begin in the administrative office. Some ideas to make an office more eco-friendly include the following:

- Recycling cans and plastic water bottles used by staff or brought into the office by patients
- Using shredded documents as packing material or sending them to be recycled
- Always asking yourself "do I really need to print this?" as excess printing leads to wasting paper and ink
- Purchasing products made from recycled materials.

Not only is making the practice more eco-friendly good for the environment but it is also good for the practice. An increasing number of patients are looking for green dental practices. An eco-friendly practice can be part of a marketing campaign to attract patients to the practice.

Every dental practice also has goals beyond serving patients. These goals may range from production goals that secure the financial stability of the practice to community service goals that may or may not be related to dentistry. Goals should be reasonable and attainable, they should be in writing, and everyone on the team should be inspired to reach them by having a reward for the achievement. Often the reward for accomplishing a certain level of a production goal is additional compensation, but it also might be a social activity. Some offices turn their success in the office into an opportunity to serve patients who might have difficulty affording dental work. Other offices might have office goals that when reached allow employees to take time off to volunteer doing something unrelated to dentistry. Attempting to reach a goal should never compromise the primary goal of serving patients.

Obviously there are many things that can't be recycled in the dental office and must be disposed of according to hazardous waste standards. But, determining materials that can be recycled is inexpensive, easy, and can be a worthwhile goal.

WWW Exploring the Web

American Association of Dental Office Managers
   www.dentalmanagers.com

American Dental Association
   www.ada.org

Eco Dentistry Association
   www.ecodentistry.org

Dental Economics, Practice Management Magazine
   www.dentaleconomics.com

Skill Building

1. Plan a trip to a dental office that will allow you to shadow the office manager or administrative staff.

2. Search online for three to five dental office Websites. Evaluate them as a prospective patient might and make a list of things you thought were well done and things that could be improved.

3. Describe how the dental office manager affects the patient experience.

4. Develop a sample practice philosophy or mission statement. Describe how your sample practice could work to follow this philosophy.

5. Develop a sample practice with a different practice philosophy from your practice you described in #4.

6. Compare and contrast your sample practices.

7. List continuing education courses that you feel would be helpful for an office manager.

Challenge Your Understanding

Select the best answer to each of the following questions. Only one answer is correct.

1. To ensure a well-run office, the dental office manager must be familiar with the practice's:
   a. Philosophy and mission statement
   b. Goals
   c. State regulations
   d. All of the above

2. The first priority of the dental practice is to:
   a. Collect all outstanding accounts receivable
   b. Treat all patients with courtesy, providing quality dental care with a service-oriented philosophy.
   c. Set up staff meetings
   d. Define total quality management

3. The dental office manager:
   a. Is in charge of all business aspects associated with running the practice
   b. Must have a business degree
   c. Must be in the office when patients are being seen
   d. Is licensed by the state where he or she works

4. Current credentials for dental office managers are available from:
   a. Dental Assisting National Board (DANB)
   b. American Association of Dental Office Managers (AADOM)
   c. American Dental Association (ADA)
   d. There are no credentials currently available

5. The dental office manager handles conflict between:
   a. Staff members
   b. Patients and the practice
   c. Dentist and staff members
   d. All of the above

6. Responsibilities of the dental office manager include:
   a. Opening and closing the office daily
   b. Writing all office correspondence
   c. Reviewing reports to set realistic goals
   d. Personally making all collection calls

7. To obtain credential, the AADOM fellowship candidate must:
   a. Have one year experience plus be a Certified Dental Assistant
   b. Have three years of experience as a dental office manager
   c. Have five years of experience as a dental office manager
   d. No experience is necessary for candidates with a business degree

8. Insurance plans must be reviewed for:
   a. Updated payment schedules
   b. Number of patients covered
   c. Number of preferred providers
   d. Type of claim form used

9. The practice philosophy includes:
   a. Types of insurance accepted
   b. How the practice deals with conflict
   c. Delegates duties to each staff member
   d. Quality of Service

10. Incorporating green concepts into your dental practice:
    a. Is unsanitary and is against the law
    b. Not worth the effort because all dental waste is a biohazard
    c. May attract eco-friendly patients
    d. Costs the office a significant amount of money

CHAPTER 2

The Dental Team

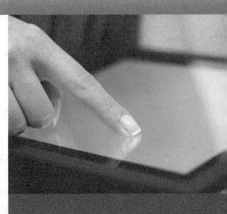

CHAPTER OUTLINES

- **Members of the Dental Team**
  The Dentist
  The Dental Hygienist
  The Clinical Dental Assistant
  The Dental Laboratory Technician
- **Working Together as a Team**
  Staff Meetings
  Morning Meetings
  Office Goals
  Quality Assurance

LEARNING OBJECTIVES

Upon completion of this chapter, the reader should be able to:

1. List and describe the nine recognized dental specialties.
2. List the educational requirements for the dentist, dental hygienist, dental assistant, and dental laboratory technician.
3. Describe the types of certification available to dental assistants.
4. Discuss expanded duties for members of the dental team.
5. List the requirements of licensure for the dentist and hygienist or registration for the dental assistant.

KEY TERMS

Certified Dental Assistant (CDA)
Certified Orthodontic Assistant (COA)
Certified Preventive Functions Dental Assistant (CPFDA)
chairside dental assistant
cosmetic dentistry
dental anesthesiology
dental hygienist
Doctor of Dental Surgery (DDS)
Doctor of Medical Dentistry (DMD)
dentofacial orthopedics
dental laboratory technician
dental public health
endodontics
forensic dentistry
oral maxillofacial surgery
oral and maxillofacial pathology
oral and maxillofacial radiology
orthodontics
pediatric dentistry
periodontics
prosthodontics
Registered Dental Assistant (RDA)
Registered Dental Hygienist (RDH)

6. Describe the importance of staff meetings and the morning meetings as they relate to all dental team members.

7. Define the perception of quality care as it relates to the dentist and the patient, and the responsibilities of the staff associated with providing it.

Members of the Dental Team

The dental team comprises a group of professionals who use their education and clinical training to treat dental disease and promote dental health for their patients. This team includes individuals in both clinical and non-clinical roles. They pursue additional knowledge through continuing education. These continuing education courses may be directly related to improving their practice.

Clinical team members include the dentist, dental hygienist, and dental assistant. The non-clinical team consists of the dental office manager and administrative staff. Every member of the team depends on each other to provide the highest quality of care and a positive patient experience.

The dental team may extend beyond an individual dental practice to include other dental professionals such as when patients are referred to a dental specialist.

The Dentist

Generally the dentist is the team leader and often owns the dental practice. The role of the dentist is to diagnose and treat dental diseases, malformations, and injuries of the teeth and gums. He or she is the only dental team member who can legally make a diagnosis. Dentists repair teeth with fillings, crowns, and other restorations and extract teeth that are beyond repair or are nonfunctioning, such as wisdom teeth (Figure 2-1). Because teeth are dependent on healthy gums and bone to support them, dentists also focus on prevention and treatment of gum disease.

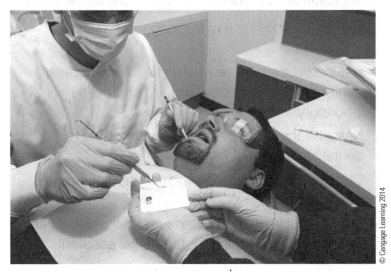

© Cengage Learning 2014

FIGURE 2-1 One of the duties a dentist performs is the repair of a damaged tooth by placing a crown.

Education and Licensure

To qualify to practice dentistry, the dentist must have graduated from a dental school accredited by the Commission on Dental Accreditation of the American Dental Association and be licensed in each state where the dentist works. Before being admitted to dental school, he or she must first earn an undergraduate degree that includes the required dental school prerequisites. Most dental school candidates obtain a degree in the biomedical sciences.

The prospective dentist then must attend dental school for an additional 4 years. During that time the focus of study is on dentistry. Clinical skills are practiced in a dental clinic operated by the school. Admission into a dental school is competitive and grades during undergraduate studies and the Dental Admission Test (DAT) are both used for selection along with other criteria. The DAT was created to measure general academic ability, comprehension of scientific information, and perceptual ability. All dental schools require applicants to participate in the Dental Admission Testing Program but test results are only one of many factors considered in evaluating the candidate for admission into a dental program.

After graduation from dental school, the dentist is addressed as doctor. The dentist earns either a DDS or DMD degree depending on the school attended. DDS stands for Doctor of Dental Surgery (this does not mean that the graduate is an oral surgeon); DMD stands for Doctor of Medical Dentistry (which does not mean that the graduate is a physician). According to the American Dental Association (ADA), 80 percent of all dental school graduates practice as family dentists and see a wide variety of dental patients and problems. The remaining 20 percent become dental specialists and focus on a specific aspect of dentistry.

Graduation from dental school does not guarantee that the dentist can treat patients. The new graduate must first apply for licensure in the state where he or she plans to practice. To become licensed the dentist is required to take a written exam, demonstrate clinical proficiency, provide character references, and pay a fee. The dentist must follow all rules, regulations, and statutes set forth by the State Dental Practice Act. To maintain the license, a periodic fee must be paid and most states require the dentist to engage in continuing education. The exact number of continuing education hours, timing of obtaining the hours, and subjects that qualify vary between states.

Recognized Dental Specialties

After graduation from an accredited dental school, the dentist may elect to pursue additional credentials in one the following nine recognized dental specialties. Each specialty has its own educational requirements and specific testing to earn Board Certification. Once a dentist becomes a specialist, he or she can limit the practice and scope of their dental treatment exclusively to that specialty. The nine dental specialties are the following:

- Prosthodontics
- Periodontics
- Oral and maxillofacial surgery
- Endodontics
- Pediatric dentistry
- Dental public health

- Oral and maxillofacial pathology
- Oral and maxillofacial radiology
- Orthodontics and dentofacial orthopedics

Prosthodontics Prosthodontics involves the restoration and replacement of teeth damaged by disease or injury. This dental specialist constructs crowns, bridges, fixed, and removable appliances with a variety of materials to restore a functional bite for the patient. Becoming a prosthodontist requires 36 months of postgraduate specialty training after obtaining a DDS or DMD. Training consists of rigorous preparation in basic sciences, head and neck anatomy, esthetics, biomedical sciences, function of the occlusion (bite), temporomandibular joint (TMJ), and treatment planning. Prosthodontists are called on to treat complex cases and full mouth restoration. Until the ADA recognizes the specialty of cosmetic dentistry, prosthodontics is the specialty under which esthetic dentistry falls.

Periodontics Periodontics is the corrective surgery of soft tissue (gums) and supporting structures (bone) to treat disease. Periodontists receive extensive training in these areas, including three additional years of education beyond dental school and are familiar with the latest techniques for diagnosing and treating periodontal disease. They are also trained in performing cosmetic periodontal procedures. A periodontist can contour and graft tissue and add bone to defects, changing the appearance of the soft tissue surrounding the teeth. This specialty is also very involved in the prevention and eliminating recurrence of periodontal disease.

Oral and Maxillofacial Surgery Oral and maxillofacial surgery is a specialty dealing with diagnosis and treatment of injuries, diseases, and defects of the face and jaws. Oral and maxillofacial surgeons care for patients with problem wisdom teeth, facial pain, and work with orthodontists to correct misaligned jaws. They treat accident victims suffering facial injuries; place dental implants; care for patients with oral cancer, tumors, and cysts of the jaws; and perform facial cosmetic surgery. Oral and maxillofacial surgeons have advanced training in anesthesia, which allows them to provide quality care with maximum patient comfort and safety in the office setting. Their four- to six-year residencies after earning a DDS or DMD degree incorporate extensive training in anesthesia administration, including local anesthesia, nitrous oxide, intravenous sedation, and general anesthesia, all of which the surgeon may safely administer in the oral and maxillofacial surgery office.

Oral and Maxillofacial Pathology Oral and maxillofacial pathology is the research and study of the causes and effects of the oral manifestations of diseases. Early diagnosis, treatment, and prevention of oral disease improve outcomes and provide the best in oral health care. Oral and maxillofacial pathologists also establish connections between oral disease and systemic disease. To become an oral pathologist requires three calendar years of study beyond dental school.

Orthodontics and Dentofacial Orthopedics Orthodontics and dentofacial orthopedics is the specialty that involves the repositioning of teeth to create a functional bite that will improve the appearance of the smile and make the teeth last longer by reducing abnormal biting stresses. Orthodontists are the uniquely educated experts in dentistry to straighten teeth and align jaws by studying two to three years beyond their DDS or DMD degree to specialize in orthodontics. Orthodontists not only straighten teeth with braces but can work together with an oral maxillofacial surgeon to change the position of the jaws.

Endodontics Endodontics is the diagnosis and treatment of injuries that are specific to the nerves and pulp that are found inside the tooth. After obtaining a DDS or DMD specializing in endodontics takes an additional two years or more of advanced study. People identify this specialist with root canals and during the lengthy specialty education the endodontist receives, he or she learns to perform all aspects of root canal therapy including routine as well as complex root canals and endodontic surgery.

Pediatric Dentistry Pediatric dentistry is the dental specialty that involves treating children and their special needs (Figure 2-2). Most patients are ready to move into an adult office by their teens but many pediatric dentists continue to treat adults with special needs throughout their lives. The two-year pediatric dentistry residency program is started after graduation from dental school with a DDS or DMD. It includes clinical and non-clinical experience. The student learns advanced diagnostic and surgical procedures, along with child psychology and clinical management, oral pathology, child-related pharmacology, radiology, child development, management of oral/facial trauma, care for patients with special needs, conscious sedation, and general anesthesia. A pediatric dentist will work not only in an office but also sees some patients in the hospital.

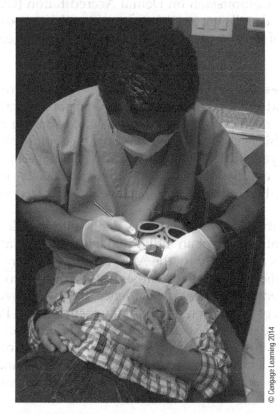

© Cengage Learning 2014

FIGURE 2-2 The pediatric dentist specializes in working with children.

Dental Public Health Dental public health develops policies and programs, such as health care reform, that affects the community at large. Public health dentists promote oral health by assessing the oral health needs of the community, developing and implementing oral health policy, and providing programs and services that address oral health issues. Dental public health specialists must have knowledge and skills in public health administration, research methodology, the prevention and control of oral diseases, and the delivery and financing of oral health care. This specialized field of dentistry takes one to two years beyond the DDS or DMD.

Oral and Maxillofacial Radiology Oral and maxillofacial radiology is the specialty dealing with the exposure and interpretation of traditional and digital radiographs to evaluate the oral-facial structures and determine health or disease. The residency program to receive a specialty credential in oral and maxillofacial radiology consists of a two-year program where diagnostic skills are augmented through clinical experience.

Future Specialties

For an area of dentistry to become a specialty it must be recognized that advanced knowledge and skill are essential to maintain or restore a patient's oral health. To begin the process an application of recognition is made to the ADA by a sponsoring organization. This organization must demonstrate that it has the ability to establish a certifying board, that the proposed specialty has direct benefit to some aspect of dental care, and that it requires knowledge and skills that are different from any other specialty or combination of specialties. Each specialty must have a minimum of two years of study in a curriculum approved by the Commission on Dental Accreditation (CODA) to provide the knowledge and skills required for practice of the proposed specialty. The following areas of dentistry are potential candidates for dental specialties in the future.

Dental Anesthesiology Dental anesthesiology recognizes the need for deep sedation and general anesthetic to manage pain and anxiety in patients for whom local anesthetic and lighter levels of sedation are ineffective or inappropriate. This is especially relevant for uncooperative children, developmentally delayed, autistic, and physically challenged patients as well as the elderly with cognitive defects. The American Society of Dental Anesthesiologists has applied to the ADA to become a recognized specialty.

Forensic Dentistry Forensic dentistry deals with the identification of bite marks or the identification of an individual by use of dental records. It is not yet recognized as a specialty by the ADA but does require specific training beyond dental school. A forensic dentist deals with the proper handling and examination of dental evidence. The evidence may be derived from teeth or in the identification of the person to whom the teeth belong. Paul Revere was a silversmith and a dentist; he was known for the identification of fallen revolutionary soldiers through dental evidence becoming one of the first forensic dentists. Forensic dentists identify found human remains and victims of mass fatalities, evaluate and assess bite mark injuries, help in cases of child abuse, and estimate age.

Cosmetic Dentistry Cosmetic dentistry is gaining in popularity as more and more people are seeking improvement in their looks through enhancements to their teeth and smile. Cosmetic dentistry includes teeth whitening as well as the improvement and repair of defects in teeth and oral structures. It is currently not recognized as a dental specialty but an increasing number of dentists are limiting their practices to esthetic or cosmetic dentistry. With the increasing number of patients seeking cosmetic dentistry and the volume of additional education available for dentists, this facet of dentistry may become a recognized specialty in the future.

The Dental Hygienist

The dental hygienist is a member of the dental team whose duties include the prevention of oral diseases and the preservation of the natural teeth. The dental hygienist cleans the patient's teeth, which is also known as oral prophylaxis (Figure 2-3). This cleaning is done to remove stains, dental plaque, and calculus. Preventive care also includes applying fluoride to strengthen the tooth surface or pit and fissure sealants to prevent decay in areas the toothbrush bristles can't reach. The hygienist exposes oral radiographs (x-rays) and provides preventive nutritional and oral hygiene instruction and counseling to patients.

The dental hygienist is not able to legally diagnose dental disease so most hygienists work under the supervision of a dentist (see Chapter 3, Legal and Ethical Regulations in Dental Office Management).

Education and Licensure

Requirements for becoming a dental hygienist include a high school degree or equivalent and a minimum of an associates' degree from a program accredited by the Commission on Dental Accreditation of the American Dental Association. Many hygienists go on to earn a bachelor's degree. Most hygiene programs require some prerequisite college level science courses before application. Admission into hygiene programs is competitive. During the two years of hygiene education, the hygienist practices his or her clinical skills

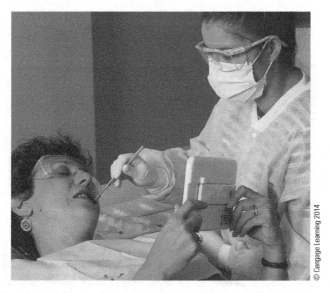

FIGURE 2-3 The dental hygienist cleans and polishes teeth.

in a dental clinic operated by the school and spends time in the community educating people about oral hygiene along with the importance of keeping their teeth healthy.

After graduation the dental hygienist must pass both written and clinical examinations to be licensed to practice in the state of employment. If the hygienist chooses to move to another state, a new license must be applied for before seeking employment at the new location. Upon satisfactory completion of the testing and licensing requirements, the hygienist becomes a **Registered Dental Hygienist** with **RDH** following his or her name. The hygienist must follow all rules, regulations, and statutes set forth by the State Dental Practice Act. To maintain the license, a periodic fee must be paid, and most states require continuing education. The exact number of continuing education hours, timing of obtaining the hours, and subject matter eligible vary between states.

Depending on the individual State Dental Practice Act, the dental hygienist may also be eligible to obtain certification for expanded duties. For example, after satisfactory completion of additional courses, the hygienist could administer local anesthetic.

The Clinical Dental Assistant

A clinical dental assistant, also called a **chairside dental assistant**, works directly with the dentist and patients in the treatment room. The clinical assistant sets up the treatment room, gets all the instruments and supplies that will be needed for the appointment, makes sure the patient is comfortable and helps the dentist during the appointment, and then disinfects the room after the appointment (Figure 2-4). While working with the dentist the assistant mixes and prepares dental restorative and impression materials and also evacuates debris and extraneous materials from the oral cavity. In most offices the clinical assistant exposes x-rays; however, states may have specific requirements that the assistant must meet. The clinical assistant may sterilize dental instruments and is most often the person responsible for infection control and sterilization requirements as set forth in government regulations and guidelines. If the office works with a dental laboratory, the clinical assistant will help prepare cases to be sent to the lab.

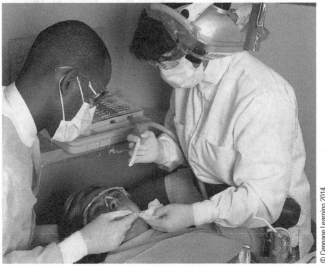

© Cengage Learning 2014

FIGURE 2-4 The dental assistant assists the dentist during procedures.

The clinical dental assistant works under the general or direct supervision of the dentist as described in Chapter 3 and is legally allowed to perform only those duties outlined by the State Dental Practice Act in the state of employment.

Education and Certification

The clinical assistant may be trained on the job or may have received formal training. Credentials that can be earned by the clinical assistant are certification, which is obtained through the Dental Assisting National Board (DANB), and registration, which is a state-specific designation. With additional training, the clinical assistant may also be credentialed in expanded functions, as permitted within the state of employment.

Certification may be earned in one of several areas: Certified Dental Assistant (CDA), Certified Orthodontic Assistant (COA), and Certified Preventive Functions Dental Assistant (CPFDA). Individuals desiring certification must meet one of the eligibility pathways and must pass the examination(s) related to the area of certification desired. Each pathway requires proof of cardiopulmonary resuscitation (CPR) certification from a provider approved by DANB.

Certified Dental Assistant (CDA)[1] The CDA exam consists of three components: General Chairside exam (GC), Radiation Health and Safety (RHS) exam, and Infection Control Exam (ICE). There are no prerequisites to take the radiation health and safety exam or infection control exam. The general chairside exam can only be taken by individuals who have graduated from an accredited dental assisting or dental hygiene program, have two years (3,500 hours) of assisting experience, or have previously held a CDA certification with a lapsed status of three months or more. These exams offered by the DANB are multiple choice and do not involve a clinical component.

Certified Preventive Functions Dental Assistant (CPFDA)[2] DANB establishes no prerequisites to take the Coronal Polishing (CP), Sealant Exam (SE), Topical Anesthetic (TA), and Topical Fluoride (TF) component exams. However, to earn CPFDA certification, candidates must meet certain requirements, such as holding current CPR certification, holding DANB CDA certification, graduating from a CODA–accredited dental assisting program, or holding an RDH license. Candidates may also need to submit proof of work experience, dentist verification of competency in the four functions, or complete coursework in a dental assisting program from a state that allows dental assistants to perform all four functions. Candidates must pass all four component exams within a three-year window to apply for CPFDA certification. Although the exams are multiple choice and non-clinical, candidates must provide proof of competency in the form of verification by a dentist.

---

[1] For more detailed information regarding any of the certification exams or qualification for certification, visit the Dental Assisting National Board (DANB) Website at www.danb.org.

[2] For more detailed information regarding any of the certification exams or qualification for certification, visit the Dental Assisting National Board (DANB) Website at www.danb.org.

Certified Orthodontic Assistant (COA)[3] The Orthodontic Assisting (OA) exam joins Infection Control (ICE) as one of two components of the Certified Orthodontic Assistant (COA) credential. The OA exam is multiple choice and is not an evaluation of clinical skills. Application for the COA requires specific documentation supporting eligibility. Candidates who successfully complete the OA exam may within five years of passing this exam apply their scores toward a DANB COA certification, as long as they have also passed the ICE within this same time period.

Registration

Registration is a state-specific credential and assistants who meet those requirements may use Registered Dental Assistant (RDA) after their name. Each state determines if they will require registration of dental assistants and if so what the qualification will be for that registration. An increasing number of states are adding this credential for dental assistants to ensure quality care for patients. The State Dental Practice Act for each state contains the criteria for registration, which may involve education and testing regarding radiology and/or infection control.

Assistants that have earned their Certified Dental Assisting credential will also have to apply for registration in states that require it. Those assistants may choose to use Certified Registered Dental Assistant (CRDA) following their name.

The Dental Laboratory Technician

The dental laboratory technician is a member of the dental team who works closely with the dentist to create corrective devices and replacements for natural teeth (Figure 2-5). The technician may work in a dental practice or with an independent laboratory that provides laboratory services for several dental practices.

There are two types of dental lab work that require the skill of a dental laboratory technician. *Restorative* laboratory procedures are performed when a patient loses a natural tooth through an accident or dental disease and needs a replacement to maintain normal function and appearance. *Orthodontic* laboratory procedures are provided when teeth must be moved or stabilized to optimize function or to prevent painful dysfunction.

The job of the laboratory technician is both an art and a science. It is an art because each tooth is unique and must simulate the function of the patient's natural tooth. The restoration should look completely natural. It is a science because the laboratory technician must have a keen understanding of the mechanics of the mouth and the dental devices that are fabricated.

The dental laboratory technician does not have to work under the direct supervision of the dentist and many technicians own their own business. However, they must adhere to any regulations set forth in the State Dental Practice Act. Dental lab technicians can join the American Dental Laboratory Technician Association (ADLTA), a professional organization.

---

[3] For more detailed information regarding any of the certification exams or qualification for certification, visit the Dental Assisting National Board (DANB) Website at www.danb.org.

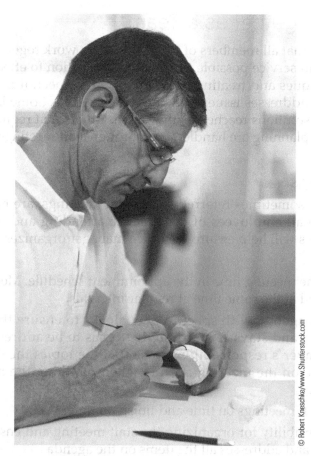

FIGURE 2-5 The dental laboratory technician specializes in the construction of corrective devices or replacements for natural teeth.

Education and Certification

The dental laboratory technician may be trained on the job or formally trained at one of 35 schools accredited by the Commission on Dental Accreditation of the American Dental Association. A successful dental laboratory technician has excellent hand–eye coordination, good color coordination, dexterity with small instruments, and enjoys detailed work.

Lab technicians who would like credentials can pass an examination to become a Certified Dental Technician (CDT) offered by the National Board for Certification in Dental Laboratory Technology. To be eligible to take the CDT exam, it is necessary to graduate from a formal lab technician program or have experience as a lab technician, have a working knowledge of the English language, and not have been found guilty of practicing dentistry illegally.

The CDT exam consists of three parts: a written comprehensive portion, a specialty practical exam for demonstration of skills, and a written specialty exam. Certification requires completion of all three parts of the exam within four years but they can be taken in any order. Graduates of recognized schools can waive the comprehensive part of the exam. The five specialty exam options are: complete dentures, partial dentures, crown and bridge, ceramics, and orthodontics.

Working Together as a Team

It is imperative that all members of the dental team work together to provide the best care and service possible to patients. In addition to effective communication techniques and treating each other with respect, it is vital that the team routinely addresses issues that affect the practice. Some issues may be addressed and solutions reached as they arise. Others that require additional discussion and planning are handled best through staff meetings.

Staff Meetings

Staff meetings, sometimes referred to as team meetings, are held on a routine basis with all employees of the practice attending and participating. These guidelines will help ensure the office manager organizes effective staff meetings:

- Block out the meeting time in the appointment schedule. Meetings should be scheduled at the same time at regular intervals.
- Prepare an agenda with specific time blocks to ensure the team stays on schedule and stays focused on the topics to be addressed. It is the office manager's responsibility to see that the topics the dentist wants covered are on the meeting agenda when planning the meeting with the dentist.
- Start the staff meetings on time and finish on time.
- Take responsibility for organizing the staff meeting and ensuring it stays productive and addresses all the items on the agenda.
- Assign a staff member to take notes and provide a written action plan resulting from the meeting.
- Provide a large newsprint pad, flip chart, or writing board to record brainstorming sessions and action ideas.

Although staff members assist in running the meeting, the dentist has the following responsibilities:

- To cast a deciding or final vote when the team is divided on an issue or where significant financial considerations apply.
- To aid the office manager in keeping the meeting on time and focused as necessary.
- To introduce significant changes in the practice.
- To review progress of action items with each staff member, if necessary, and then lead the team with follow-up and recognition.

Morning Meetings

The morning meeting is a brief gathering at the beginning of the day to set the tone, strategize procedures, and discuss patients' specific needs. It is the office manager's job to provide information to the dentist for the morning meeting to enhance communication and cooperation between business and clinical staff, to provide improved patient service, and to increase the overall productivity of the practice. The dentist should be provided a copy of the schedule ahead of the meeting so there is time to review it. The morning meeting may include the following:

- *Specific concerns from the previous day:* How could the schedule have run more smoothly?
- *Highlight today's schedule:* Who are the new patients? Are there any emergencies on the schedule and details of the problem?
- *Emergency and catch-up time:* Are there any flexible times where additional treatment could be accomplished? How much time is available?
- *Available production time:* When are the next available pre-blocked production times?
- *Financial concerns:* Do any of the patients need new financial arrangements made? Are any accounts overdue?
- *Marketing opportunities:* Who are the new patients on the schedule? What was the source of the new patient? How is the practice thanking those who refer new patients?

Office Goals

One of the important elements of staff meetings are setting and evaluating the office goals. During the time set aside for a staff or morning meeting there is time available for goals to be set and broken down into measurable results, such as quality and promptness of service, number of surfaces restored, percentage of recall patients scheduled, number of new patients, number of cancellations or failures, and amount of unscheduled time/downtime. The practice's productivity, and ultimately the staff's rewards, comes partly as a result of meeting practice goals, including production goals.

Quality Assurance

Establishing standards for the highest quality dental care is another essential that arises from staff meetings and goal setting. Quality to the dentist is equated with outstanding technical skill; to the patient it is a perception that includes outstanding communication, satisfaction, and being treated with courtesy and respect by the dentist and staff. In reality, *quality is a judgment that includes both technical skills and the management of communication exchanges between the patient and the practice.*

Continuous quality improvement and total quality management emphasize continuous improvement through understanding and knowledge about the procedures and techniques used to improve care, the health results achieved, and an emphasis on the patients' perceived needs and demands. This customer service philosophy reflects patients' involvement in their care and obtaining the necessary information they need to make informed decisions about their dental health (Figure 2-6).

Patient Perceptions That Determine Quality of Care

- How dental conditions affect daily function and well-being. If I have an abscessed tooth and fever, how will that affect my work performance today?

- Treatment needs. If my treatment plan includes a root canal, what will happen during the procedure? What will happen after it is done?

- Satisfaction with the care. How satisfied am I with elements of service, for example, when I called the office was the phone answered promptly by an actual person? Was I offered an appointment quickly? Was I greeted by the staff and dentist with courtesy and compassion? Were all my questions answered thoroughly?

- Treatment effectiveness. Did the root canal treatment relieve the discomfort? Did the prescribed medications control any symptoms? Did the final result meet or exceed my expectations?

- Follow-up. Did the dentist and staff take the time to contact me to make sure the treatment was effective?

© Cengage Learning 2014

FIGURE 2-6 Patient priorities that determine quality of care.

 Exploring the Web

Academy of Prosthodontics
www.academyofprosthodontics.org

American Academy of Periodontology
www.perio.org

American Association of Oral and Maxillofacial Surgeons
www.aaoms.org

American Academy of Oral and Maxillofacial Pathology
www.aaomp.org

American Association of Orthodontists
www.braces.org

American Association of Endodontists
www.aae.org

American Academy of Pediatric Dentistry
www.aapd.org

American Board of Forensic Odontology
www.abfo.org

American Academy of Cosmetic Dentistry
www.aacd.com

American Society of Dental Anesthesiologists
www.asdahq.org

American Dental Association
www.ada.org

American Dental Hygienists Association
www.adha.org

American Dental Assistants Association
www.dentalassistant.org

Dental Assisting National Board
www.danb.org

Skill Building

1. Working in a group, do a role-play of an office meeting. Discuss three problems that a practice might have to deal with, such as attracting new patients, a misunderstanding between staff members, and overscheduling resulting in the staff always working late. Work together to solve those problems.

2. Describe how a dental practice could improve the perception of quality to its patients.

3. Your office has interviewed three excellent potential employees. Describe what characteristics you would be looking for when considering adding an employee.

Challenge Your Understanding

1. A periodontist:
   a. Provides gingival (gum) treatment
   b. Does root canals
   c. Constructs fixed prosthetics
   d. None of the above

2. A dental specialist may become certified in one or more recognized specialties; currently how many recognized specialties are there in dentistry?
   a. 12
   b. 8
   c. 9
   d. 6

3. To work in private practice a dentist must be:
   a. A graduate of a dental school approved by the Commission on Dental Accreditation of the American Dental Association
   b. Licensed in all 50 states
   c. A member of the State Board of Dental Examiners
   d. All of the above

4. A certified dental assistant (CDA):
   a. Has met all requirements to practice in any state
   b. Has successfully completed all requirements of the Dental Assisting National Board
   c. Is qualified to diagnose dental disease
   d. Can perform expanded duties in any state

5. An oral surgeon is a dental specialist who:
   a. Extracts teeth
   b. Exposes impacted teeth
   c. Wires fractured jaws
   d. All of the above

6. The dental hygienist:
   a. Performs dental cleaning known as prophylaxis for patients
   b. Diagnoses dental disease
   c. Performs extractions
   d. All of the above

7. The dental hygienist must always work:
   a. In accordance with the State Dental Practice Act
   b. With a hygiene assistant
   c. Under direct supervision of a dentist
   d. All of the above

8. The clinical dental assistant:
   a. Performs deep scaling and curettage procedures
   b. Prepares instrument trays and anesthesia setups as required by the dentist
   c. Uses the initials RDH after his or her name
   d. Is required to be licensed in every state

9. The dental laboratory technician:
   a. Fabricates dental prostheses
   b. Must be licensed in the state in which he or she works
   c. Is required to work under the direct supervision of the dentist
   d. None of the above

10. The dental office manager can organize effective staff meetings by:
    a. Blocking out the meeting time in the appointment schedule
    b. Preparing an agenda to ensure the team stays on schedule and stays focused
    c. Assigning a staff member to take notes and provide a written action plan resulting from the meeting
    d. All of the above

CHAPTER 3

Legal and Ethical Regulations in Dental Office Management

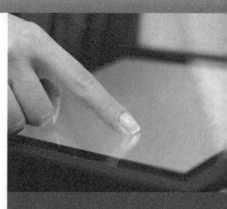

CHAPTER OUTLINES

- **Dental Jurisprudence**
- **Dental Ethics**
  Code of Ethics
- **State Dental Practice Act**
  State Board of Dental Examiners
- **Laws and Regulations Related to Office Management**
  Supervision of Staff
  Record Keeping
  Fair Hiring Practices
  Quality of the Work Environment
- **Americans with Disabilities Act**
  Protected Categories
  Effects of Americans with Disabilities Act on the Dental Office
- **Risk Management Strategies to Prevent Malpractice**
  Negligence
  Standard of Care
  Abandonment
  Burden of Proof
  Elements of Malpractice
  Causes of Malpractice Suits
  Steps to Prevent Malpractice
  Handling Accidents or Complaints
  Patient Discontinuation of Treatment

KEY TERMS

abandonment
abuse
Americans with Disabilities Act (AwDA)
benefits
burden of proof
compensation
direct supervision
disability
Equal Employment Opportunity Commission (EEOC)
ethics
general supervision
Health Insurance Portability and Accountability Act (HIPAA)
informed consent
job description
jurisprudence
liable
licensee
malpractice
negligence
noncompliance
overtime pay
paid leave
performance review
provisional employment
risk management
severance pay
standard of care

■ **Health Insurance Portability and Accountability Act**
HIPAA in the Dental Office
■ **Reporting Suspected Abuse**
Signs and Symptoms of Abuse and Neglect
Reporting and Documenting Procedures

LEARNING OBJECTIVES

Upon completion of this chapter, the reader should be able to:

1. Define and describe the terms ethics and jurisprudence.
2. List the duties of the State Board of Dental Examiners.
3. Be familiar with the content and implications of the *American Dental Assistants Association Principles of Ethics and Professional Conduct*.
4. Define and describe the difference between general and direct supervision.
5 Describe legal and financial aspects and hiring practices associated with the dental office.
6. Describe the provisions and implications of the *Americans with Disabilities Act* (AwDA) as it pertains to the dental office.
7. Describe the importance of risk management in preventing dental malpractice.
8. Describe the legal requirements of dental offices to report suspected cases of abuse.
9. Describe the Health Insurance Portability and Accountability Act and its statutes.

Dental Jurisprudence

Dental jurisprudence is the application of legal statutes and other regulations that pertain to the State Dental Practice Act. Jurisprudence is a philosophy of law or a set of legal regulations set forth by each state's legislature. By law, dental professionals must understand the obligations and privileges granted by their license or registration; they must follow these rules and be aware of dental duties legally allowable in the state where they practice. For example, a state has a law requiring a state-approved course for an individual to expose dental radiographs also known as x-rays. Dental professionals must be aware of this requirement and must not expose radiographs until they have completed the approved course. For example, Susan, who has been a clinical dental assistant for 10 years and has been taking x-rays during that time, moves to a neighboring state. This state requires dental assistants who take dental x-rays to prove knowledge of safety procedures, infection control, and correct film placement. It is Susan's responsibility to know the law and to comply with it.

Dental Ethics

Ethics is a moral obligation that encompasses professional conduct and judgment imposed by the members of a particular profession. The ethical standards are developed by the professional organizations; those who participate in the profession are morally obligated to act within an ethical or moral manner. Ethics is considered a higher standard (moral) than jurisprudence (legal) requirements. Unlike the law, ethics are constantly changing and evolving just as personal values and morals change. For example: Is it ethical to enter into a personal relationship with a patient? Is the dental professional obligated to tell the patient everything regarding treatment?

Code of Ethics

A professional code of ethics is that which stands above the legal requirement of the dental profession. The American Dental Assistants Association has developed and published the *Principles of Dental Ethics and Code of Professional Conduct*, to which all practicing assistants are morally obligated to adhere (Figures 3-1 and 3-2).

American Dental Assistants Association Principles of Ethics

Each individual involved in the practice of dentistry assumes the obligation of maintaining and enriching the profession. Each member may choose to meet this obligation according to the dictates of personal conscience based on the needs of the human beings the profession of dentistry is committed to serve.

The spirit of the Golden Rule is the basic guiding principle of this concept. The member must strive to at all times maintain confidentiality, and exhibit respect for the dentist/employer. The member shall refrain from performing any professional service which is prohibited by state law and has the obligation to prove competence prior to providing services to any patient. The member shall constantly strive to upgrade and expand technical skills for the benefit of the employer and the consumer public. The member should additionally seek to sustain and improve the Local Organization, State Association, and the American Dental Assistants Association by active participation and personal commitment.

Reprinted with permission of the ADAA

FIGURE 3-1 American Dental Assistants Association Principles of Ethics.

American Dental Assistants Association Code of Professional Conduct

As a member of the American Dental Assistants Association, I pledge to:

- Abide by the Bylaws of the Association;
- Maintain loyalty to the Association;
- Pursue the objectives of the Association;
- Hold in confidence the information entrusted to me by the Association;
- Serve all members of the Association in an impartial manner;
- Recognize and follow all laws and regulations relating to activities of the Association;
- Maintain respect for the members and the employees of the Association;
- Exercise and insist on sound business principles in the conduct of the affairs of the Association;
- Use legal and ethical means to influence legislation or regulation affecting members of the Association;
- Issue no false or misleading statements to fellow members or to the public;
- Refrain from disseminating malicious information concerning the Association or any member or employee of the American Dental Assistants Association;
- To not imply Association endorsement of personal opinions or positions;
- Maintain high standards of personal conduct and integrity;
- Cooperate in a reasonable and proper manner with staff and members;
- Accept no personal compensation from fellow members, except as approved by the Association;
- Promote and maintain the highest standards or performance in service to the Association;
- Assure public confidence in the integrity and service of the Association.

ADAA House of Delegates, (1980)

FIGURE 3-2 "American Dental Assistants Association Code of Professional Conduct" (Reprinted with permission of the ADAA).

State Dental Practice Act

The dental practice act is a group of regulations that govern the practice of dentistry in each state. It is changed and updated by the Board of Dental Examiners regularly to reflect changes in the dental field. Although some regulations are similar among different states, each practice act is unique. The State Dental Practice Act for each state is available on the state's board of dentistry Website. To locate the board of dentistry, use your search engine with the name of the state and board of dentistry.

State Board of Dental Examiners

Each state has a separate State Board of Dental Examiners, empowered by the legislature to enforce the State Dental Practice Act to protect the health, safety, and welfare of the people residing in the particular state. The state board also regulates the standards for dental licensees within the state and issues and renews licenses and registrations for dental personnel practicing within the state. It monitors licensees and enforces discipline for noncompliance.

A licensee is a person who has met the requirements set forth in the State Dental Practice Act to provide patient services as regulated by the state. When the applicant applies for a license he or she agrees to treat patients according to state laws. Failure to follow the laws and regulations is called noncompliance and can result in the loss of the individual license to practice in the state.

Each State Board of Dental Examiners regulates and enforces the limit and scope of allowable duties for dental assistants and hygienists within its Dental Practice Act. Working beyond the scope of the Dental Practice Act may be considered practicing dentistry without a license and is a serious offense.

Laws and Regulations Related to Office Management

It is the responsibility of the dental staff to stay up to date on the laws and regulations that govern dentistry. The office manager needs to be familiar with state laws when hiring new staff or scheduling existing staff.

Supervision of Staff

By law, the dentist is responsible for all acts committed within the practice. This includes delegation of duties to properly trained personnel. Most dentists have insurance that covers them if an employee does something wrong *in good faith*. For example: the hygienist is asked to do a sealant for a patient and undetected decay is deep in the groove, causing it to become larger under the protection of the sealant. In this case the hygienist was following the dentist's exact instruction and doing something he or she has been trained to do and is legally allowed to do under state law. The dentist is responsible because the act was committed in the practice. On the other hand, if the hygienist decided to seal a tooth before it was examined, he or she might be determined to have practiced outside of the law. While the dentist is still responsible because the hygienist is a staff member, the insurance company or state may see it as practicing outside of legal limits because the hygienist could not legally diagnose that the tooth was safe for the sealant.

Your dental office manual and specific job descriptions can be important for all staff to understand their duties in the practice.

General Supervision

General supervision, in most states, means the dentist is responsible for all acts delegated to and performed by staff (within the law) but that the act itself may be done while the dentist is not physically present in the office. Examples of a dental assistant's duties under general supervision might be sterilizing instruments or ordering supplies. For hygienists duties under general supervision could include prophylaxis and exposing radiographs for a patient of record or a patient whom the doctor has seen in the past, and not for a new patient.

Direct Supervision

Direct supervision includes overseeing of specific delegated duties, as stipulated in the State Dental Practice Act as allowable for trained staff to perform. The dentist must be present in the facility while these procedures are being performed. Examples of this, for an assistant, might be exposing radiographs for patients or performing coronal polish procedures. For hygienists, administering local anesthetic might be legal only under direct supervision.

Record Keeping

Record keeping means creating a history of everyone and everything in the office. The general rule is "if it isn't written down, it didn't happen"; obviously with the increase in paperless charting that statement includes electronic records that aren't literally written. Dental records are legal documents for both patient and employee.

Employee Records

Accurate and thorough record keeping is the lifeline of the practice. Not only does this include the patients' clinical and accounting records, but also employee records. These records are confidential and include payroll, tax, disability, worker compensation, unemployment, and other information required by Occupational Safety and Health Administration (OSHA), including management of accidental injuries and work site accidents.

Dental offices are required to retain employee records for the duration of employment plus an amount of time determined by federal and state laws. In the event of the death of the doctor or sale of the practice, the records become the property of the new owner.

Importance of an Office Manual

An office manual is a reflection of the management style of the practice that outlines the practice philosophy, policies, procedures, and employee behavior. Having a single source of written office policies and procedures is essential for preventing misunderstanding. It also provides a standard of fairness and consistency for all employees, especially in larger clinics or group practices. The office manual may be the "final word" when office policies are questioned. It is important that the office manager makes sure the manual is updated or adapted to reflect changes in employment laws or other government regulations.

All new dental employees should be provided with a copy of the office manual when hired. Current dental staff should review the manual annually. Many offices ask that employees sign a document stating that they have read and understood the office manual.

It is important to note that the office manual also provides protection for the employee in the event of exposure to a potentially hazardous substance or an accidental injury. An office may have several different manuals because of the volume of information and wide variety of procedures. For example, an office might have separate manuals for personnel issues, hazard communications, and Material Safety Data Sheets (MSDS). (The latter two are also addressed in Chapter 4.)

Personnel Policies For optimal communication and to prevent misunderstandings, most offices have written guidelines in the form of a personnel policy manual. In many states the courts have ruled personnel policies, procedures manuals, and employee handbooks may be legally binding contracts.

Employee Behavior The office manual should outline specific expectations of employee behavior, including keeping office hours, policies on tardiness, and personal use of office equipment including computers and the Internet. The office manual should address the use of personal cell phones and other electronic devices in the office.

Written Job Descriptions To avoid misunderstandings and to clearly communicate the expectations of the employer, it is essential that a written job description be made available to the job candidate. A copy of each staff member's job description should be included in the office manual and a copy should be provided to the candidate at the employment interview (Figures 3-3 through 3-5).

As job responsibilities change, the job description should also be updated. A printed copy along with the date on which it was updated should be provided

RECEPTIONIST/OFFICE MANAGER DUTIES

Name_____

Date_____

Routinely Perform	Occasionally Perform	Never Perform		Trainee	Assistant	Senior Receptionist	Principal Receptionist
			1. Schedules new patients for appointments to see.	Procedure Training	Procedure Competency	Procedure Competency	Procedure Competency
			2. Schedules patients (both new and recall) to see the Dental Hygienist.				
			3. Maintains patient records.				
			4. Develops and maintains an effective recall system for patients who have completed treatment.				
			5. Develops and maintains effective inventory control of recyclable, consumable and expendable supplies.				
			6. Orders all supplies for clinical and business office use.				
			7. Discusses financial arrangements with patients.	Training	Procedure Competency	Procedure Competency	
			8. Arranges payment schedule for patients receiving treatment.				
			9. Submits statements monthly to all patients with account balances.				
			10. Maintains patient accounts to minimize delinquent accounts.				
			11. Collects fees from patients.				
			12. Maintains business records of the practice.	Training			
			13. Submits payment for office expenses.				
			14. Reconciles check book with bank statement monthly.				
			15. Cooperates with other professional and auxiliary staff.				

Minimal Desirable Qualifications
1. High school graduation.
2. Ability to work in a semi-autonomous manner.
3. Good secretarial skills.
4. Bookkeeping skills.

Work Schedule
The normal work schedule for this individual will be eight hours per day five days each week for a total of 40 hours per week.
It is expected that this individual will work 50 weeks per year, with two weeks paid vacation after the first full year of employment. There will be five to eight paid holidays per year.

Salary
1. Annual Salary of_____.
2. _____% of all office gross above_____.

Courtesy of Drs. Thomas M. Cooper and John A. DiBaggio from Applied Practice Management

FIGURE 3-3 Sample job description: dental receptionist/office manager.

DENTAL ASSISTANT DUTIES

Name_____

Date_____

Routinely Perform	Occasionally Perform	Never Perform	Duties	Trainee Assistant	Senior Assistant	Principal Assistant
			1. Perform basic administrative office procedures.	Procedure Training	Procedure Competency	Procedure Competency
			2. Assist the dentist in four-handed dentistry.			
			3. Prepare tray setups for commonly performed procedures.			
			4. Record oral examinations as directed by the dentist.			
			5. Prepare and clean instruments.			
			6. Prepare and sterilize instruments.			
			7. Pour and trim diagnostic models.			
			8. Construct custom acrylic trays.			
			9. Assist in administration of local anesthetics.			
			10. Prepare dental materials as indicated for treatment.			
			11. Assist with placement and removal of rubber dam.			
			12. Assist with placement of bases and liners.			
			13. Assist in insertion and finishing of temporary restorations.			
			14. Assist in insertion and finishing of composite restorations.			
			15. Assist in placement and removal of matrices.			
			16. Assist in insertion and carving of amalgam restorations.			
			17. Assist with first aid and emergency procedures.	Training	Procedure Competency	
			18. Aid in the presentation of post-operative instructions.			
			19. Expose, process and mount radiographs.			
			20. Assist with advanced dental procedures.			
			21. Instruct other auxiliaries in dental assisting.		Training	
			22. Conduct demonstrations in assisting.			
			23. Evaluate new personnel for the purpose of grading.			
			24. Conduct ongoing in-service training for auxiliaries.			

Minimal Desirable Qualifications
1. High school graduation
2. Three years experience as dental assistant.

Work Schedule
The normal work schedule for this individual will be eight hours per day five days per week for a total of 40 hours per week.
It is expected that this individual will work 50 weeks per year, with two weeks paid vacation after the first full year of employment. There will be five to eight paid holidays per year.

Salary
1. Annual Salary of_____.
2. _____% of gross above_____.

Courtesy of Drs. Thomas M. Cooper and John A. DiBaggio from Applied Practice Management

FIGURE 3-4 Sample job description: dental assistant.

to the employee. At the time of the annual performance review, both the dentist-employer and the staff member should review the written job description. The office manager may conduct the annual review on behalf of the employer. It is the job of the dentist and office manager to make sure the job descriptions reflect the State Dental Practice Act and all employees are practicing within the law.

Fair Hiring Practices

A well-run office is one in which all staff and the dentist work together as a team to serve patients. One key to keeping the workflow productive is sound communication skills that build positive relationships within the office. This should be emphasized during the interview process and reinforced at staff meetings.

DENTAL HYGIENIST DUTIES

Name_____

Date_____

Routinely Perform	Occasionally Perform	Never Perform		Assistant Dental Hyg.	Senior Hygienist	Principal Hygienist
			1. Promotes the maintenance of dental health among patients.			
			2. Scales and polishes teeth.			
			3. Scales and planes root surfaces.			
			4. Topically applies caries preventive agents.			
			5. Desensitizes hypersensitive teeth and oral mucosa.			
			6. Maintains relative asepsis.			
			7. Removes overhanging margins.			
			8. Removes and recements space maintainers.			
			9. Initiates or assists in administering emergency care for patients, and removes sutures and surgical packs from oral cavity.			
			10. Coordinates the office Preventive Dentistry Program.			
			11. Designs and maintains an effective recall program.			
			12. Trains members of the dental team in preventive procedures.			

(Column labels: Pro. Competency / Training / Procedure Competency / Procedure Competency / Training)

Minimal Desirable Qualifications
1. Graduation from a two-year accredited certificate program.
2. Must be licensed in this state.
3. Two years clinical experience.

Work Schedule
The normal work schedule for this individual will be eight hours per day five days each week for a total of 40 hours per week.
It is expected that this individual will work 50 weeks per year, with two weeks paid vacation after the first full year of employment. There will be five to eight paid holidays per year.

Salary
1. Annual Salary of_____.
2. _____% of all office gross above_____.

Courtesy of Drs. Thomas M. Cooper and John A. DiBaggio from Applied Practice Management

FIGURE 3-5 Sample job description: dental hygienist.

When hiring a new employee, consensus of the team is essential to ensure a successful training period and introduction to the practice's procedures and philosophy.

Employer and prospective staff members must be aware of specific topics that may or may not be discussed during an interview for employment. These standards are set by the Federal Government through the Equal Employment Opportunity Commission (EEOC) under Title VII of the Civil Rights Act of 1964. The EEOC is responsible for ensuring all individuals have the right to compete for employment opportunities, as well as to reduce the potential for hiring discrimination based upon a variety of factors. These include, but may not be limited to, questions regarding race, color, religion, sex, national origin, age, or disability. It is also illegal to discriminate against a person because the person complained about discrimination, filed a charge of discrimination, or participated in an employment discrimination investigation or lawsuit.

The dentist as employer, by law, has the right to select whomever she or he believes is the best-qualified candidate to perform the responsibilities and duties of a specific job. Under current employment laws the employer is not required to select the *most qualified candidate*; he or she is only required to select a candidate who meets the *minimum requirements* of the job. The EEOC covers offices with 15 or more employees (20 in the case of age discrimination) so many small dental offices are not bound by their authority.

Provisional Employment

After completing a successful interview, which could include not only a traditional interview but also a working interview, the dental practice may elect to hire a new staff member but with agreement that employment is conditional on the employee being able perform tasks required by the practice. This conditional employment is referred to as provisional employment, and is defined by written notice on letterhead, outlines the starting date, the rate of compensation, the work hours, and any other benefits included along with the position. The benefit of entering into provisional employment is that either the dental practice or the staff member may, at any time during the provisional period (customarily 90 days), elect to discontinue the employment arrangement without prior notice and without cause (reason). Under provisional employment agreements, no unemployment benefits are awarded. During the provisional employment period, the staff member may not be offered benefits that will be a part of the compensation later; for example, health care benefits, uniform allowance, or reimbursement for continuing education.

Temporary Employment Services

Many dental practices work with outside agencies to provide temporary employees to cover staff vacation time, maternity leave, or extended leaves of absence. Dental staff members who are employed by these agencies apply directly with them and are paid by them. The dental practice pays a fee directly to the staffing agency. These agencies may also provide long-term employees on a contract basis by taking care of the employee screening, administration of payroll, sick days, vacation, and benefits. This type of arrangement gives the dentist more time to devote to the practice of dentistry. Agencies may also offer permanent placement services helping to match employees and dental practices. Fees paid to an agency for temporary or contract staffing can be significant.

Performance Reviews

Performance reviews, most often conducted annually, are essential to sustaining positive dentist–staff relationships. Performance reviews are based upon the objectives of performance expectation outlined in the individual staff member's written job description (Figure 3-6). Often a rating scale is used to evaluate how well an employee has performed. Performance reviews can be extremely helpful for an employee to understand his or her strengths and weaknesses. Problems in performance should not be saved for the annual review; they should be addressed as needed. Regardless of the setting, formal or informal, record of a review should be retained in the employment file. Often, the office manager assists the dentist with performance reviews.

The performance review can be done separately from a salary review; neither an annual performance review nor a salary increase is mandated by law.

Termination

The terms of employment and termination should be outlined clearly in the office manual and should be explained to all new hires. Termination is the act of

PERFORMANCE REVIEW

NAME: DATE OF EMPLOYMENT:
STARTING SALARY: EXPERIENCE:

REVIEW DATE: EVALUATION AND COMMENTS:
SALARY CHANGE:

REVIEW DATE: EVALUATION AND COMMENTS:
SALARY CHANGE:

REVIEW DATE: EVALUATION AND COMMENTS:
SALARY CHANGE:

REVIEW DATE: EVALUATION AND COMMENTS:
SALARY CHANGE:

REVIEW DATE: EVALUATION AND COMMENTS:
SALARY CHANGE:

REVIEW DATE: EVALUATION AND COMMENTS:
SALARY CHANGE:

Courtesy of Drs. Thomas M. Cooper and John A. DiBaggio from Applied Practice Management

FIGURE 3-6 Sample performance review form

leaving a job whether it is the choice of the employer or employee. Sometimes the word "termination" is thought of as being "fired" but it simply means the end of employment. Understanding what happens when employment ends not only prevents misunderstandings, but it also reduces stress levels, eliminates anxiety, and creates a common understanding between employer and employee.

When leaving a position, often, the employee will provide a two-week notice. This has been a standard of business practice for many years; it is a formal courtesy and not governed by law. Thus, a staff member desiring to terminate her or his employment may give a two-week written notice. However, the employer-dentist is not legally or ethically bound to continue the employment during this period.

Likewise, in the event the employer-dentist elects to terminate an employee, service may be terminated with little or no notice. Many employers, however, may choose to award **severance pay**, an allowance based upon the length of service, or award unused vacation pay at termination. These terms should be outlined in the office manual and may differ depending on the circumstances of the termination.

Wrongful Dismissal

Wrongful dismissal stems from an employee alleging he or she was wrongly terminated from employment. Grounds may include age discrimination, failure to comply with office policies, disputes arising from uncompensated overtime or vacation pay, or attitude. Whether pursued through the court system or through state employment commission grievance procedures, the burden is on the employee to prove beyond a reasonable doubt that the employer was guilty of wrongful discharge. This is often very difficult to prove.

Quality of the Work Environment

The dentist as employer must ensure that all state laws regarding quality of the work environment are upheld for the health, welfare, protection, and safety of all employees. Failure to uphold these codes may result in fines, penalties, or restriction of practice. For example, the employer must ensure that hazards such as poor ventilation, protection from radiation, and potential for accidents and injuries are minimized.

Harassment

The law contains specific wording on the nature and definition of harassment in the workplace. Simply defined, harassment consists of any unwanted or unwelcome advances by an employer or supervisor toward a subordinate employee or between employees, especially where continued employment, advancement, or favors are implicit or explicit based upon compliance. Many office manuals contain a copy of guidelines regarding harassment.

Employee Salary and Benefits

Compensation to the employee is often paid on an hourly rate but it could also be as a salary or even as a daily pay rate. Overtime pay may be awarded to full-time hourly wage employees for working beyond the standard work week as defined in the office manual. The rate of overtime pay can vary according to state regulations or office policy and should be clearly outlined in the office manual or in the offer of employment letter.

In addition to hourly or weekly pay, benefits, usually provided only to full-time employees, represent a significant form of nontaxable compensation provided by the employer. Benefits may include paid vacation, sick days, and compensation for reaching production goals, health insurance, or pension plan contributions.

Many employers provide quantitative information with the pay stub or annual wage and benefit statement that outlines the total value of the job, including employee benefits (Figure 3-7).

Paid Leave

Paid leave includes time away from the office taken for earned vacation, federal holidays, or sick time. Vacation pay or annual leave is customarily one or two weeks earned after one full year of employment. With additional years of service, many employers provide an additional week's paid leave.

The six recognized paid federal holidays include, but may not be limited to, New Year's Day, Memorial Day, Independence Day, Labor Day, Thanksgiving, and Christmas. Some employers may also recognize additional holidays such as Martin Luther King Jr. Day, President's Day, Columbus Day, and Veteran's Day.

Employee Name:			
Annual Employee Total Compensation/Cost			
A. Direct Compensation	_ _ _ _ (estimate)	_ _ _ _ (actual)	_ _ _ _ (actual)
Gross Base Salary (Includes Vacation/Sick pay)			
Overtime (Pre-Tax Amount)			
Bonuses (Pre-Tax Amount)			
Employee Tax (Estimate 10% of Gross Salary)			
or FICA			
State Unemployment/FUTA			
Worker's Compensation Insurance			
*Retirement Plan Contribution (if 100% vested)			
Retirement Plan Administration Allocation			
B. Employee Fringe Benefits			
*Cafeteria Plan Reimbursement			
*Medical Insurance and Reimbursements			
*Group Life Insurance			
*Uniforms			
*Child Care ($5,000 Max)			
Tangible Awards Program (every 5 years)			
Annual Gift ($25 Max)			
Dental Care			
C. Career Benefits			
Dental Continuing Education			
Tuition and Travel Reimbursement			
Lodging and Meals			
Inoculations and OSHA Safety			
*Professional Dues & Subscriptions			
TOTAL COMPENSATION/COST			
D. Hidden Compensation			
Tax Savings (example for Illinois: FICA .07 + FED .28 + State .03 = 38% x all *)			
True per Hr. Wage (Total Compensation/Hrs.)			

Courtesy of Dental Economics

FIGURE 3-7 Employee compensation.

Paid sick time or personal days are awarded at the discretion of the employer.

Office policies regarding recognized holidays and sick time should be outlined by the employer in the office manual.

Unpaid Leave

Some employers provide unpaid leave, that is, time away from the office for which the employee is not compensated. Unpaid leave may include maternity leave (after any vacation and sick days are used), personal leave for family emergencies, and bereavement leave for the death of an immediate family member, or jury duty. The specific terms must be outlined by the employer in the office manual.

Additional Benefits

By law, the cost of required hepatitis B vaccine and personal protective equipment required by OSHA safety regulations must be provided by the employer to employees at risk of contact with bloodborne pathogens.

Other benefits not directly included in the paycheck but provided by the employer may include health and life insurance, retirement (pension plan), and uniform allowances. Many practices make these additional benefits available, some on a copayment basis where the employer and the employee share in the cost or contribution toward the benefit. Some employers, especially those who require standard uniforms of matching clinic attire, provide an annual uniform allowance toward the cost of these items.

Bonus or incentive programs may be offered to staff for exceptional performance on the job. Bonuses may be based upon goals set within the practice such as new patients, production, recall program retention, or collection of overdue accounts.

The cost of child or elder care may be an additional benefit shared by the employer and employee. Many employers also provide or share the cost of continuing education with the employee. Examples include attendance at dental seminars, dental meetings, lodging and meals, paid subscriptions to dental periodicals, and certification, registration, or licensure renewal fees. Dental offices provide cardiopulmonary resuscitation (CPR) instruction and certification because it is a requirement for both administrative and clinical staff members. The dentist must provide a safe environment for patients, and every staff member needs to be ready to assist a patient who is not breathing or whose heart has stopped beating. CPR certification is a benefit for the employee and is also valuable for the dentist and patients.

Employees may receive dental treatment at reduced fees for themselves and their immediate family members as an additional benefit. Some practices may even offer free dental care to employees and immediate family members. Employees may need to pay for lab work or other costs.

Any additional benefits provided to employees should be outlined in the office manual.

Americans with Disabilities Act

The **Americans with Disabilities Act (AwDA)** became law in 1990 and prohibits discrimination in access to services and employment against persons who are disabled (Figure 3-8). Provisions enacted in 1992 specifically apply to dental offices requiring facilities are accessible to physically or mentally compromised patients.

Protected Categories

To be protected by the AwDA, one must have a disability or have a relationship or association with an individual with a disability. An individual with a disability is defined by the AwDA as a person who has a physical or mental impairment that substantially limits one or more major life activities, a person who has a history or record of such impairment, or a person who is perceived

What Is the Americans with Disabilities Act?

The *Americans with Disabilities Act* is a federal legal provision designed to prevent discrimination of handicapped persons. It provides a national mandate for the elimination of discrimination against individuals with disabilities and provides clear, strong, enforceable standards addressing discrimination against disabled people. The *AwDA* is broken down into five titles; *Titles I* and *III* have the greatest relevance to dental practices.

- *Title I* – eliminates discriminating employment policies.
- *Title II* – prohibits discrimination against the disabled in the use of public transportation.
- *Title III* – requires that public accommodations operated by private entities not discriminate against individuals with disabilities.
- *Title IV* – prohibits discrimination against the disabled in the area of communication, especially the hearing and speech impaired.
- *Title V* – contains miscellaneous provisions regarding the continued viability of other state or federal laws providing disabled persons with equal or greater rights than the *Act*. This section also prohibits state or local governments from discriminating against individuals with disabilities.

© Cengage Learning 2014

FIGURE 3-8 Five provisions of the *Americans with Disabilities Act*.

by others as having such impairment. The AwDA does not specifically name all of the impairments.

Effects of Americans with Disabilities Act on the Dental Office

The principles of the nondiscrimination requirements of the AwDA include the following:

- Equal opportunity for the disabled person to participate as a patient in the practice and receive dental treatment,
- Equal opportunity for the disabled person to benefit from dental treatment, and
- The opportunity for the disabled person to receive treatment in the most integrated setting possible.

Violations of the AwDA include civil monetary penalties: up to $50,000 may be assessed for the first violation and up to $100,000 for subsequent violations. In addition, a violator (dentist) may be ordered to provide services that are found to have been wrongfully denied. A dentist who employs 15 or more people for a minimum of 20 weeks annually must comply with the AwDA Title 1 requirements regarding discriminating employment policies.

The AwDA does not require the dental practice to remove all barriers to accessibility, providing a plan of priorities is established. The Department of Justice recommends barriers be removed based upon the following priorities:

- *Access to premises:* Providing access from public sidewalks, parking, and public transportation. This can be done by providing wider entrances, ramps, and accessible parking spaces, including designated handicapped spaces.

Equipping the Office for Improved Accessibility

The Department of Justice recommends the following modifications to barriers that may be readily achievable under the *Americans with Disabilities Act:*

- Installing ramps
- Installing curb cuts (areas where the sidewalk dips down to accommodate wheelchairs or vehicles)
- Designating handicapped parking spaces
- Installing raised letters and Braille on elevator controls
- Providing visual alarms
- Widening doors and doorways
- Installing grab bars
- Installing raised toilet seats and large stalls
- Repositioning paper towel dispensers in restrooms
- Installing paper cup dispensers at existing water fountains
- Eliminating high-pile, low-density carpeting

© Cengage Learning 2014

FIGURE 3-9 Department of Justice recommendations.

- *Access to service areas:* Creating physical access, as well as eliminating barriers for the visually and hearing impaired.
- *Access to restrooms:* Widening doorways, installing ramps, adding appropriate signage, widening toilet stalls, and installing grab bars in restrooms.
- *Access to other areas of the practice:* Providing equal services to the disabled.
- Additional modifications are outlined in Figure 3-9.

All attempts should be made by the dental team to integrate disabled patients into the practice. No service can be denied, nor can an individual patient be excluded, segregated, or otherwise treated differently than other patients, simply because the patient has a disability.

Risk Management Strategies to Prevent Malpractice

Dental legal and ethical concerns continue to grow as the number of dental malpractice suits rises. The dental office manager must keep in mind that while lawsuits cannot be eliminated or prevented, the risk for potential must be kept to a minimum. Thus, the term **risk management** is used as a preventive strategy to reduce this potential. Although the dentist is the primary person listed in a malpractice suit or complaint, all members of the dental team may be held **liable** (responsible).

The wise office manager is alert to strategies for risk management and ways to reduce the potential for malpractice suits against the practice. The following concepts are important to the office manager in preventing malpractice suits.

Negligence

In most states, negligence is defined as a dentist who "does an act within his or her profession that a responsible dentist would not do, or fails to do an act that a reasonable dentist would do." If a lawsuit is filed against the dentist, it must be shown that the dentist acted negligently and that this negligence was the cause of the patient's injury for an award to be made. While the dentist, as primary care practitioner and/or owner of the practice, is most often the one against whom a suit is filed, any member of the dental staff may also be held accountable for negligence or harm done to a patient.

In most states, if the dentist is found negligent, this is an adverse action, reported to the National Practitioner Data Bank (NPDB). The adverse action is also automatically reported to the respective dentist's State Board of Dental Examiners. The NPDB functions as a national reporting entity to track and monitor complaints against licensed health care professionals. The Health Care Quality Improvement Act of 1986, brought about the creation of the NPDB as a central repository for information on paid malpractice claims and adverse reports of health care licensees.

Standard of Care

An unsatisfactory treatment outcome does not confirm negligence on the part of the dentist. It must be proven that the dentist provided treatment that deviated from an applicable standard of care, and that this departure resulted in the injury sustained by the patient.

In health care, there are no "absolute" standards of care; rather, treatment guidelines that a dentist with the same knowledge, skill, and care in the same community would provide. Thus, the standard of care may be interpreted to mean "Did the dentist act reasonably at the time and under the circumstances?"

Abandonment

Abandonment is defined by the ADA in its Principles of Ethics and Code of Professional Conduct as once a dentist has started a course of treatment, the dentist should not discontinue that treatment without giving the patient adequate notice and the opportunity to obtain the services of another dentist. Care must be taken not to jeopardize the patient's oral health. Abandonment of patients is considered unprofessional conduct in most State Dental Practice Acts and may also constitute malpractice. Under this provision, the dentist may not withdraw treatment of a patient unless both reasonable notice of the withdrawal and replacement dentist(s) are offered to the patient. Failure to treat a patient whose needs are apparent and for which the opportunity to treat the patient exists may be considered negligence. Record keeping is extremely important because the burden of proof is on the dentist.

Burden of Proof

In a malpractice case, the burden of proof requires that the patient seeking to impose liability against the dentist must supply the more convincing evidence that the dentist's action caused resulting harm or injury. The dentist's records can be subpoenaed and used as a legal document.

Let's look at an example: A patient comes into the office in a great deal of discomfort with an abscessed tooth. The patient begins root canal therapy but does not return. After the initial treatment he is comfortable so sees little reason to keep his subsequent appointments. The dental office contacts him numerous times to try and schedule his next visit. Once he even schedules and doesn't show up. Within a few months the tooth breaks and must be extracted; now he needs an expensive implant.

If the dental office doesn't have a record of phone calls and missed appointments, he might have a case for abandonment, however, if they do, the burden of proof that the root canal was defective and was the dentist's fault is on the patient.

Elements of Malpractice

All dental staff are legally obligated to adhere to the standard of care set forth in the State Dental Practice Act. As an example, many states require all dental staff to have CPR certification with periodic renewals. In addition to familiarity with the terms set forth in the State Dental Practice Act, the dentist and staff must possess an awareness of treatment procedures and protocols that fall within the standard of care. Malpractice is the incorrect or negligent treatment given to a patient by a doctor, dentist, or health care provider. Failure to perform any of the following may be considered cause for malpractice (Figure 3-10).

- The first element is a *duty to act*. A health care practitioner has a legal and ethical duty to respond when treatment is required.

- The second element is an act of *omission* or an act of *commission*. Omission means failing to carry out something that should be done to prevent harm or injury; commission means committing an act that contributes to or directly causes harm or injury.

  Failure to provide CPR to a patient in cardiopulmonary arrest would be an act of omission. Breaking and leaving a root canal instrument in the tooth without informing the patient would be an act of commission.

- The third element is proof of injury or harm caused to the patient by the dentist. This most commonly refers to physical injury, but may include emotional or psychological harm. To claim malpractice, there has to be some definable harm. Did incorrect diagnosis or substandard treatment cause something bad to happen? Did failure to review the patient's health history result in physical harm or illness?

Elements of Malpractice

Four elements must be proven to establish malpractice:

1. Duty to act or render care
2. Acts of omission or commission
3. Injury to the patient
4. Failure to act was the proximate cause of the patient's injury

---

FIGURE 3-10 Elements of malpractice.

- The fourth element is failure to act as a reasonable, prudent person was the proximate cause of the patient's injuries. An example would be spilling acid etch material on a patient's skin resulting in burning.

Causes of Malpractice Suits

More than two-thirds of the claims made in health care malpractice suits are directly relevant to *unexpected outcomes* or *unrealistic expectations* perceived by the patient. The following sequence of events is often what leads up to a patient filing a malpractice suit:

1. A dental problem occurs that may be unexpected but not unusual under the circumstances.
2. The patient is unhappy with the situation or result.
3. The patient contacts the dentist for clarification or solutions.
4. The patient is dissatisfied with attempts or explanations made by the dentist about the perceived problem or result associated with treatment.
5. The patient files a malpractice suit.

Another very common reason patients' file malpractice is *poor communication* on the part of the dentist or staff. The patient feels that the treatment was not as described or more commonly costs more that he or she thought. Patients under stress often misunderstand treatment and the dental team that provides treatment everyday forgets that the patient doesn't know everything that they do.

Failure to diagnose or inform the patient of a specific clinical finding is another common reason for filing a malpractice suit. This problem is a great example: a patient has lost a tooth and the dentist recommends a bridge. A bridge is expensive, somewhat time consuming, and relies on the teeth adjacent to the space to support it. However, the support of the adjacent teeth is compromised by bone loss and the bridge is destined to fail; adding to the problem, the additional stress on the adjacent teeth causes them to be lost as well. So, the dentist's failure to diagnose the problem with the adjacent teeth or tell the patient the risk has resulted in the loss of the bridge and two additional teeth. This could result in a malpractice claim.

Failure to diagnose and treat or refer for treatment to a specialist is common cause for malpractice. Sometimes problems are not apparent on the surface and the dentist underestimates it. Referring a patient to a specialist is sometimes the most conservative approach to treatment.

Failure to explain treatment options and the expected, realistic outcome, and/or consequences of no treatment is another cause of malpractice suits. Explaining treatment is difficult, time consuming, and it is sometimes hard to know what the patient understands. It is important to have treatment options for the patient if they exist. The ability to choose a course of treatment makes them responsible for the outcome.

Steps to Prevent Malpractice

The following risk management steps are important to reduce the possibility of a lawsuit against the dentist. The dental office manager must ensure that these steps are followed and that all team members are familiar with them.

1. Always obtain **informed consent**, written, signed, and dated, prior to proceeding with treatment. If the patient is a minor or is mentally incompetent, the office manager must obtain informed consent from a parent or guardian on behalf of the patient.

   > **Note:** *Implied consent, which simply interpreted means the patient sits in the dental chair and implies that she or he consents to whatever dental treatment is needed, is no longer sufficient.* Informed consent is more than obtaining permission to examine or treat a patient. It includes the ailment, disease, or problem; the recommended treatment and the risks involved; alternative treatments and the risks; inadequate or non-treatment risks; and fees.

2. Always obtain a thorough medical and dental history, signed and updated; again, if the patient is a minor or is mentally incompetent, request this information from a parent or guardian. It is the office managers responsibility to ensure that updates to this information are made at each recall visit or at a minimum annually.

3. Make sure all records are complete and accurate. These include up-to-date radiographs, a written treatment plan, diagnosis, and dated treatment progress notes. Also document that the reasons for recommended treatment were explained to the patient, including possible complications of delayed treatment or noncompliance with recommended treatment. Document that all treatment options and their corresponding prognosis were explained to the patient. If the patient elects not to accept or proceed with recommended treatment, request that she or he sign a detailed, dated wavier rejecting treatment and stating that he or she understands the consequences.

4. Document all patient complaints, comments, and reasons for seeking treatment.

5. Always enter chart notations in blue or black ink when using paper charts. Never erase, cover up, white out, or attempt to amend records. If an error is made, draw a single line through the error, initial and date the error, and make the correction immediately next to the original chart entry (Figure 3-11). All staff members, including the dentist, must initial chart entries. When using paperless charting, patient records can be edited until the system is backed up daily. Errors caught after the backup should be handled by noting the error and making a correct entry.

6. If an additional treatment note is required, enter it on a new line in the chart with the date it was added.

7. Never discard inactive patient records without consent of the dentist. Store them in a separate *secured* area and retain them according to the laws of the state where the practice is located. Always keep treatment, financial, and personal patient documentation and records on separate forms. When legally ready to destroy patient records make sure it is done in accordance with Health Insurance Portability and Accountability Act (HIPAA) and as recommended by the ADA.

8. Follow a uniform chart entry system to ensure conformity and lessen the likelihood of omission of relevant information.

9. If records are requested or subpoenaed, forward high quality duplicates—never the originals!

10. Never berate another dentist's treatment. Clinical records and related discussion and documentation should include only the patient's condition as

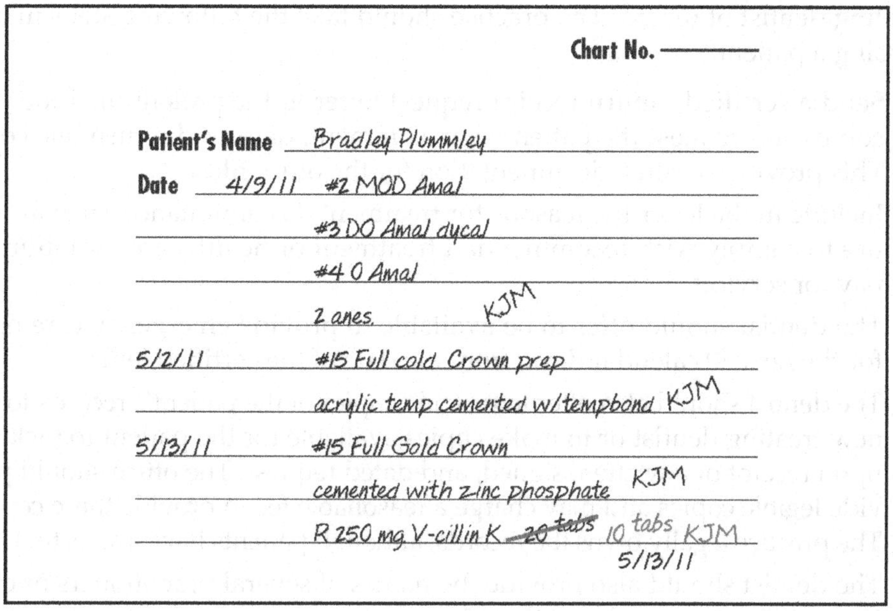

Chart No. ————

Patient's Name _____Bradley Plummley_____

Date _____4/9/11_____ #2 MOD Amal

#3 DO Amal dycal

#4 O Amal

2 anes.   KJM

5/2/11   #15 Full cold Crown prep

acrylic temp cemented w/tempbond KJM

5/13/11   #15 Full Gold Crown

cemented with zinc phosphate KJM

R 250 mg V-cillin K ~~20 tabs~~ 10 tabs KJM
                                5/13/11

© Cengage Learning 2014

FIGURE 3-11 Proper way to correct a medical record.

diagnosed, objective observations, patient's comments relating to the situation, and the recommended necessary treatment plan.

11. Document in the record, all telephone conversations with patients, referring specialists, and other authorized people.

12. Make sure all medications (prescription as well as over the counter) are entered into the patient's chart.

13. Document all cancellations, late arrivals, and failed appointments in the patient record.

14. Enter the date of all radiographs or diagnostic casts in the record.

15. Enter specific postoperative instructions or note that standard postoperative instructions were given to the patient.

16. Note the type of (generic or brand name) of materials used for all dental procedures.

17. Never make treatment guarantees. Instead, educate patients that their active participation and cooperation have a substantial effect on the success of their treatment outcomes.

Handling Accidents or Complaints

If an accident occurs, especially resulting in undue injury or harm to a patient, or if there is a complaint by a patient, the office manager should collect the information and say nothing to the patient. Instead, she or he should alert the doctor to the nature of the patient's injury or complaint and let the doctor handle it appropriately.

Patient Discontinuation of Treatment

In the event that a patient chooses to discontinue planned treatment that the doctor feels is in the patient's best interest to seek dental treatment elsewhere, or the practice has been sold, great caution must be taken in releasing the patient from the doctor's care. This is to reduce the likelihood of the patient claiming abandonment and also to ensure that the patient finds another treating dentist of record. The practice should take the following steps in dismissing a patient:

1. Send a certified, return receipt request letter to the patient. Include two copies and request the patient sign, comment, date, and return one copy. This provides written documentation for the office files.

2. Include in the letter the reasons for treatment discontinuance, such as failure to comply with recommended treatment or health care, or failure to pay for services.

3. The dentist should offer to be available to provide emergency care only, for the next 30 calendar days, from the date of the certified letter.

4. The dentist should also offer to provide copies of the patient's records to the new treating dentist or to make copies available for the patient to pick up, upon receipt of a written, signed, and dated request. The office should provide legible copies and may charge a reasonable fee to provide these copies. The practice legally owns the records, although patients have access to them.

5. The dentist should also provide the names of several practitioners or clinics available to provide continued care.

Health Insurance Portability and Accountability Act

The **Health Insurance Portability and Accountability Act (HIPAA)** of 1996 is a federal law that consists of two parts or titles.

- *Title 1* went into effect in 1997 and guarantees that a person covered by health insurance from one employer can obtain health insurance through a second employer if they change jobs.

- *Title 2* is the administration simplification and protection and security of Personal Health Information (PHI). It was published in 2003 and beginning in 2005 health professionals including dentists had to comply with this law. This is commonly known as the privacy rule and protects personal information as described under administrative simplification.

There are five parts of HIPAA administrative simplification:

- *Transaction and code set standards*. This sets national standards for electronic health-care transactions and code sets, unique health identifiers, and security. This requires the use of ADA coding for all dental procedures thus simplifying filing insurance claims.

- *Identifier standards*. These were set when it was recognized that advances in electronic technology could erode privacy. Provisions were created that mandated the adoption of federal privacy protections for individually identifiable health information. This included unique subscriber numbers instead of using a social security number.

- *Privacy rule*. This sets up national standards for protection of individually identifiable health information into three types of covered entities; health plans, health care clearing houses, and health care providers. Although protecting a patient's privacy has always been an important part of the doctor patient relationship, this sets specific guidelines regarding any release of patient information to third parties. This rule restricts communication regarding treatments to those people specifically authorized, provides rules regarding patient access to medical records, restricts patient information used for marketing purposes, and sets a procedure for complaints.

- *Security rule.* This sets national standards for protecting the confidentiality, integrity, and availability of electronic protected health information. With the growth in the use of electronic transmission of information, this rule mandates certain security measures be put into place to safeguard information.

- *Enforcement rule.* In 2006, the final enforcement rule for HIPAA was released. This enforcement rule specifies the procedure for complaints of HIPAA violations and provides for civil monetary penalties that can be assessed for violations of HIPAA. The U.S. Department of Health and Human Services, in conjunction with other state and/or federal departments, are responsible for the enforcement of HIPAA.

HIPAA in the Dental Office

Every dental office must have a HIPAA privacy officer to oversee compliance with all HIPAA regulations (Figure 3-12). The dental office manager either assumes this role or delegates it to a trusted staff member. The job of the compliance officer is to develop and post HIPAA regulations in the office, make decisions regarding HIPAA, and maintain records. The dental office must obtain an acknowledgement from patients that they have read and understood the Notice of Privacy Practices.

The office compliance officer also coordinates the training of employees regarding Personal Health Information (PHI) and privacy along with documenting that training. The dental office must also designate a contact person for patients that have a complaint or wish to obtain additional information.

Basic *Notice of Privacy Practices and Acknowledgement of Receipt* only apply to provision of medical/dental treatment and the use of information in obtaining payment for treatment; for example, dealing with an insurance company. These do *not* apply to anything that involves the use of PHI for any marketing, for which a higher level of authorization is required. Authorization is also

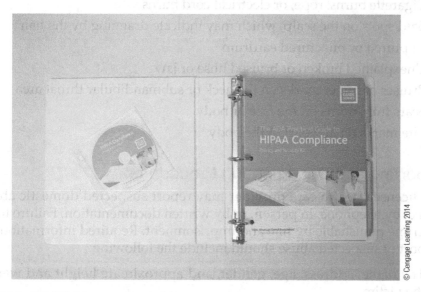

FIGURE 3-12 HIPAA compliance kit.

generally needed for release of PHI to schools, employers, and other non-health entities. Note that reminders for periodic or ongoing care are generally not considered marketing.

Reporting Suspected Abuse

All 50 states have laws requiring licensed and in some cases unlicensed health care professionals, including dentists and dental hygienists, to report cases of suspected domestic abuse, including violent or active abuse and neglect or passive abuse. In some states the dental assistant may also be legally required to report suspected abuse. Under these laws, the licensed dental professional is immune from prosecution for reporting abuse, even when no legal foundation confirms the suspected or alleged abuse.

Domestic abuse most often involves child abuse but also encompasses spousal abuse committed against a marital partner or significant other living in the same household, or elder abuse against a geriatric relative or dependent.

Signs and Symptoms of Abuse and Neglect

Abuse is defined as maltreatment or negligent treatment by a spouse or partner, guardian, other caretaker, or relative. Abuse is an act of commission; neglect is an act of omission. Abuse may be characterized by broken bones, cigarette burns, human bite marks, starvation, or sexual molestation.

Abuse may be suspected with any of the following unexplained signs:

- Injuries around the head and neck
- Black eyes or blood clots in the nostrils
- Bruises or severe lacerations of the oral mucosa
- Oral radiographs that exhibit healed or recent fractures
- A child with suspected sexually transmitted diseases that would indicate sexual abuse
- A fractured nose or broken or of false teeth
- Cigarette burns, rope, or electrical cord burns
- Bald spots on the scalp, which may indicate dragging by the hair
- Ruptured or punctured eardrum
- Unexplained broken or bruised nose or jaw
- Bruises or finger marks on the neck or submandibular throat area
- Scars from burns on the face or body
- Bite marks on any part of the body

Reporting and Documenting Procedures

Any licensed health care provider may report suspected domestic abuse or neglect by telephone, in person, or by written documentation. Failure to do so is a crime punishable by fine and imprisonment. Required information to file a report of suspected abuse should include the following:

- The name, address, age, gender, and approximate height and weight of the victim
- The name and address of the responsible custodial adult or partner

- A description of the physical emotional abuse and/or neglect of the patient
- The supporting clinical evidence of previous neglect or injuries
- Supportive information that may help establish the cause or source of the injuries
- The nature of the patient's condition or injuries
- Photographs, radiographs, or sketches showing the nature and location of the injuries

Some state protective agencies permit the health care provider to photograph injuries without a patient or guardian's consent (in cases of abuse of a minor). Other states allow only designated authorities to photograph injuries arising from abuse.

It is also important to carefully document in the patient's record any findings of suspected neglect or abuse, including the following:

- The time and date that the injury was observed and noted
- The location and number of injuries
- The color and size of each lesion, bruise, or injury
- The caretaker's verbal response to the cause of the injuries

It is also essential to have another individual witness the examination and initial or cosign the documentation to corroborate any suspected domestic abuse or neglect.

Exploring the Web

Federal Fair Hiring Practices
www.eeoc.gov/employers/index.cfm

Americans with Disabilities Act, *U.S. Department of Justice*
www.ada.gov

HIPAA, *U.S. Department of Health and Human Services*
www.hhs.gov/ocr/privacy/hipaa/understanding/index.html

National Practitioner Data Bank (NPDB)
www.npdb-hipdb.hrsa.gov/

Dental Practice Act, *unique to each state*
Search: State+Dental Practice Act

Skill Building

1. Discuss and describe the difference between ethics and jurisprudence. Give an example of each.

2. List and describe the duties of the State Board of Dental Examiners and give at least three reasons why its role is important.

3. On your own or in a group prepare a list of reasons why dental assistants and office managers should maintain high ethical standards. Imagine an incident in which a dental assistant or office manager may be asked to make an ethical decision and provide possible solutions.

4. Prepare a list of three scenarios of legal and/or financial aspects of hiring practices. Determine if each was legal or illegal.

5. Discuss the following scenario: You are hired in an office where the dentist permits staff to perform functions that are outside the scope of the State Dental Practice Act. You become aware of this. What should you do?

6. A patient of record calls to make an appointment for a disabled family member. What information should the office manager obtain prior to making the appointment? What, if anything, should you do before scheduling the appointment? Is it illegal for the office to refuse to treat a disabled patient?

7. List 10 things the staff can do to lower the practice's potential for a malpractice suit.

8. An eight-year-old child is seated for his first appointment. He appears to have signs of neglect or abuse. What measures should the office manager or dental assistant take? Should she report her suspicions directly to the authorities? Why?

9. What does the abbreviation HIPAA stand for? How does it affect the dental practice? What are its four parts?

 Challenge Your Understanding

1. In a dental malpractice suit, which of the following people may be held liable?
   a. The dentist
   b. The dental hygienist
   c. The dental office manager
   d. Any/All of the above

2. The dental office manager must keep in mind:
   a. Proper record keeping can eliminate malpractice
   b. Lawsuits cannot be eliminated
   c. The potential risk must be kept to a maximum
   d. The patient is always right

3. Dental jurisprudence:
   a. Requires understanding of regulations that pertain to the State Dental Practice Act
   b. Is a philosophy of law or a set of legal regulations enacted by the legislature
   c. Contains rules and legally allowable duties that may be performed by qualified dental personnel
   d. All of the above

4. Ethical requirements are:
   a. Considered a lower standard than jurisprudence requirements
   b. Considered a higher standard than jurisprudence requirements
   c. Constant and never changing
   d. Part of HIPAA

5. The State Board of Dental Examiners:
   a. Protects the health, safety, and welfare of the public
   b. Regulates the criteria for dental licensees within the state
   c. Monitors licensees and enforces discipline for noncompliance
   d. All of the above

6. Under supervision rules stipulated in the State Dental Practice Act, the dentist:
   a. Is responsible for all acts delegated to and performed by staff
   b. Must be physically present in the office when staff perform direct supervision procedures
   c. Must be physically present in the office when staff performed general provision procedures
   d. a and b only

7. The office manual:
   a. Provides a single source of written office policies and procedures
   b. Provides a standard of fairness for all employees
   c. Is considered legally binding
   d. All of the above

8. Under current employment laws:
   a. The dentist as employer is required to select the most qualified candidate for the position
   b. The dentist does not need to comply with EEOC rules if the practice has fewer than 15 employees
   c. The dentist needs to select a candidate that meets minimum job requirements
   d. All of the above

9. All of the following fall under current law regarding employee records except:
   a. All records are confidential
   b. The records may not be released to the employee upon the death of the dentist or sale of the practice
   c. The records become property of the employee when she leaves the practice
   d. All of the above fall under current law

10. The Americans with Disabilities Act covers patients with:
    a. Advanced age
    b. Obesity
    c. Any physiological disorder or condition
    d. A history of domestic abuse

11. When dismissing a patient from the practice the dentist should:
    a. Be available to provide emergency dental care for the next 90 days
    b. Inform the patient in person
    c. Inform the patient in writing by certified mail upon return receipt requested
    d. Hold the clinical records until the patient's balance has been paid

12. Child abuse may be suspected when the patient exhibits signs of which of the following?
    a. Cigarette burns, rope or electrical cord burns
    b. Black eyes or blood clots in the nostrils
    c. Venereal warts or HIV-associated lesions, such as oral candidiasis indicating sexual abuse
    d. Any/all of the above

13. When filing a report of suspected domestic abuse, the dentist should include:
    a. The nature of the patient's condition or injuries
    b. The name and address of the responsible custodial adult or partner
    c. Supporting clinical evidence of previous negligence or injuries
    d. All of the above information should be included

14. If an accident occurs or a complaint is made by a patient, the office manager should:
    a. Say nothing until contacted by an attorney
    b. Alert the dentist the nature of the patient's injury or complaint
    c. Attempt to calm the patient down and offer a refund for the treatment rendered
    d. a and b only

15. The dental professional may be found negligent:
    a. When he or she commits an act any responsible dentist would not do
    b. When he or she fails to do an act that a responsible dentist would do
    c. If the patient injury was caused by the dentist
    d. All of the above

16. Which of the following does not fall within the scope and authority of the National Practitioner Data Bank (NPDB)?
    a. It is a national reporting entity that tracks and monitors complaints against licensed healthcare professionals.
    b. It is a central repository for information on paid malpractice claims and adverse reports on health care licensees.
    c. It has the power to revoke dental licenses.
    d. All are within the in NPDB's scope of authority.

17. Under a provisional employment agreement:
    a. The employee earns unemployment benefits
    b. Is guaranteed permanent employment after the probationary period
    c. Is given the guidelines of provisional employment in writing
    d. Is only allowed to observe

18. As total compensation, the dental office manager's package may include:
    a. An hourly or weekly salary and paid vacation and holidays
    b. A uniform allowance
    c. Reimbursement for attending continuing education courses
    d. Any/all of the above

19. Health Insurance Portability and Accountability Act:
    a. Is abbreviated HIPAA
    b. Must be followed by all dental offices
    c. Is only mandated in offices of over eight employees
    d. a and b only

20. HIPAA rules include:
    a. Provisions for disabled patients
    b. Security rules dealing with PHI
    c. Mandates for regulating malpractice suits
    d. Reporting protocol for abuse cases

CHAPTER 4

Hazard Communication and Regulatory Agency Mandates

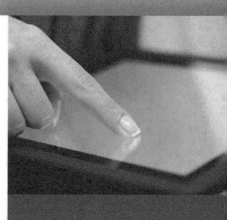

CHAPTER OUTLINES

- **The Role of Government Agencies in the Dental Office**
  Occupational Safety and Health Administration (OSHA)
  The Centers for Disease Control and Prevention (CDC)
  The Environmental Protection Agency (EPA)
  The Food and Drug Administration (FDA)
  The Organization for Safety and Asepsis Procedures (OSAP)

- **Hazard Communication Standard**
  Product Warning Labels and Stickers
  National Fire Protection Association Color
    and Number Codes
  Material Safety Data Sheets (MSDSs)
  Staff Training
  Training Recordkeeping
  Reducing Hazards in the Dental Office
  Handling Hazardous Materials

- **Bloodborne Pathogens Standard**
  OSHA Engineering and Work Practice Controls
  Standard (Universal) Precautions
  Handling and Laundry of Reusable PPE
  Decontamination of Surfaces
  Waste Management
  Hepatitis B Vaccination
  Exposure Incidents
  Recordkeeping

- **Waterline Biofilms**

- **Fire and Emergency Evacuation Procedures**
  Signage Requirements

- **The Safety Coordinator's Duties**
  Practice Compliance Check List

KEY TERMS

bioburden
biofilms
bloodborne pathogens
biohazard warning label
Bloodborne Pathogens
  Standard
Centers for Disease
  Control and Prevention
  (CDC)
engineering controls
Environmental Protection
  Agency (EPA)
exposure incident
exposure-control plan
Food and Drug
  Administration (FDA)
hazard communication
  standard
hepatitis B vaccination
material safety data
  sheets (MSDS)
medical waste
occupational exposure
Occupational Safety and
  Health Administration
  (OSHA)
Organization for
  Safety and Asepsis
  Procedures (OSAP)
personal protective
  equipment (PPE)

Other Potentially
  Infectious Material
  (OPIM)
Standard Precautions
work practice
  controls

LEARNING OBJECTIVES

Upon completion of this chapter, the reader should be able to:

1. Describe the role of government regulatory agencies and how they affect the dental office.
2. Describe the importance of maintaining a hazard communication program and the necessary components.
3. List ways to reduce hazards inherent in the dental office.
4. Describe the necessary procedures for handling hazardous materials in the dental office.
5. List and describe the components of *OSHA's Bloodborne Pathogens Standard* and the responsibilities of the dental team to implement them.
6. Describe the necessary recordkeeping required by the government with regard to staff training.
7. Describe the inherent dangers of biofilms in the dental unit waterlines and methods to reduce the risk of cross-contamination associated with them.
8. List fire and other required emergency evacuation procedures.
9. List the duties of the office safety coordinator.

The Role of Government Agencies in the Dental Office

A variety of government agencies have responded to the demands of patients for protection from diseases and other potential hazards associated with dental care. New regulations, as well as stringent enforcement of older regulations, require dental practices to follow guidelines and recommendations set forth by government regulatory agencies. There are many government regulatory agencies that affect the way dental practices protect their employees and patients from potential hazards associated with dental treatment.

Occupational Safety and Health Administration (OSHA)

The **Occupational Safety and Health Administration (OSHA)** requires employers, including those in the health care profession, to establish and carry out a wide range of procedures designed to protect employees, implement and maintain employee exposure-incident records for the duration of employment plus 30 years, and provide specific personal protective equipment (PPE) to protect staff from infectious diseases and other potential hazards.

OSHA's Bloodborne Pathogens Final Standard covers all dental employees who could reasonably anticipate coming into contact with blood and other potentially infectious material (OPIM) during the course of employment. It is designed to help minimize occupational exposure to bloodborne illnesses and thus protect employees from possible resulting illness.

Dental office employees are placed into one of three risk categories depending on their possibility of exposure:

- Category 1 includes employees whose daily job responsibility involves exposure to blood, salvia, or tissue. This group would include the dentist, hygienist, and clinical dental assistant.

- Category 2 includes employees whose job does not involve regular contact with blood, saliva, or tissue but might unintentionally come into contact with them. Office managers and administrative assistants would fall into this category.

- Category 3 would include employees who would never be subject to exposure such as an office accountant or management consultant.

The Centers for Disease Control and Prevention (CDC)

The goal of Centers for Disease Control and Prevention (CDC) is providing necessary information to communities and individuals to protect their health. The organization educates people regarding new health threats as well as provides necessary information to prevent existing diseases, possible injury, or disability. The CDC has set forth specific guidelines for infection control and disease containment. Although the CDC does not have enforcement power over dental practices, OSHA is charged with investigation and enforcement of the CDC's guidelines.

The Environmental Protection Agency (EPA)

The Environmental Protection Agency (EPA) regulates and registers certain products used in dental practices, including surface disinfectants. The EPA requires products to undergo and pass specific testing requirements prior to approval for registration.

The Food and Drug Administration (FDA)

The Food and Drug Administration (FDA) regulates marketing of medical devices that include equipment and disposable items. The FDA reviews product labels for false or misleading information and sufficient directions for use. As such, the FDA regulates many chemical germicides used as antiseptics, disinfectants, drugs, and sterilizers.

The Organization for Safety and Asepsis Procedures (OSAP)

The Organization for Safety and Asepsis Procedures (OSAP) is a national organization of teachers, practitioners, dental health care workers, and manufacturers and distributors of dental equipment and products. It is specifically concerned with the safe and infection-free delivery of oral health care. The OSAP communicates standards and information on aseptic technique to dental practices and educational institutions and assists them with infection control programs. The role of OSAP is to act as a source of information and training to its members, and it does not make or enforce laws or regulations.

Hazard Communication Standard

The focus of OSHA's Hazard Communication Standard is the employee's right to know law, which addresses the right of every employee to know the possible dangers associated with hazardous chemicals and other related hazards in the workplace. This law also requires employers to provide methods for corrective action.

To comply with the Hazard Communication Standard, the dentist must develop and implement a written compliance program. This must include an exposure-control plan (including the Bloodborne Pathogens Standard), a written hazard communication program, waste and sharps handling management, and injury and illness prevention.

The dentist must also ensure that hazardous chemicals used in the office are properly labeled and hazardous substances have corresponding Material Safety Data Sheets (MSDS) available for staff training and review.

The dentist must designate a program coordinator to provide staff training to new employees and once annually thereafter. The dentist must develop ways to reduce hazards in the office, and provide a safe means for handling of hazardous materials.

Product Warning Labels and Stickers

Warning labels must be attached to containers, products, or other hazardous materials used in the dental office. The most common of these include mercury (used in silver filling material to create amalgam), nitrous oxide sedation gases (used for conscious sedation), and disinfectants used on surfaces and chemicals used in processing dental radiographs (developer and fixer).

The label or sticker must contain appropriate warnings by hazard class, including routes of entry into the body and target organs of the body that may be affected. Product labels must contain the identity of the chemical, the appropriate hazard warnings, and the name and address of the manufacturer (Figures 4-1 through 4-3).

A container properly labeled when received from the manufacturer or supplier does not require an additional label. The exception for labeling is single-use or single-dispensing items or products.

All members of the dental team should familiarize themselves with the labels of hazardous substances and be aware of how to clean up spills or handle other emergencies that may arise when handling these products. The most basic elements required for a hazardous spill kit include absorbents to soak up any liquids, a scooping device to pick up materials using a "no-touch" method, and a hazardous waste bag with a biohazard warning label (Figure 4-4). Hazardous products moved from one container to another must have an appropriate warning label or sticker affixed to the new container.

RED: FIRE HAZARD	YELLOW: REACTIVITY
4 = Danger: Flammable gas or extremely flammable liquid	4 = Danger: Explosive at room temperature
3 = Warning: Flammable liquid	3 = Danger: May be explosive if spark occurs or if heated under confinement
2 = Caution: Combustible liquid	2 = Warning: Unstable or may react if mixed with water
1 = Caution: Combustible if heated	1 = Caution: May react if heated or mixed with water
0 = Noncombustible	0 = Stable: Nonreactive when mixed with water

BLUE: HEALTH HAZARD	WHITE: PPE	
4 = Danger: May be fatal	A	Goggles
3 = Warning: Corrosive or toxic	B	Goggles, gloves
2 = Warning: Harmful if inhaled	C	Goggles, gloves, apron
1 = Caution: May cause irritation	D	Face shields, gloves, apron
0 = No unusual hazard	E	Goggles, gloves, mask
	F	Goggles, gloves, apron, mask
	X	Gloves

Courtesy of POL Consultants

FIGURE 4-1 National Fire Protection Association's color and number method.

Chemical Warning Label Determination

The Hazard Communication Act contains specific labeling requirements. Labels must be on all hazardous chemicals that are shipped to and used in the workplace. Labels must not be removed. Material safety data sheets for all chemicals will be available to employees.

Manufacturer Requirements: Chemical manufacturers are required to evaluate chemicals, determine status as hazards, provide material safety data sheets (MSDSs), and label all shipped chemicals properly. Manufacturer labels must never be removed. The best way to determine the hazards of the chemical is to read the MSDS, obtain an OSHA designated list or State Hazardous Substance list. For most mixed chemicals, it is necessary to contact the manufacturer for MSDS.

Office Chemicals: Search through your office and write down all chemicals you have in the office. Most pharmaceuticals and common household products do not come under this standard. Ingredients can then be compared to a list of regulated substances or MSDSs will provide necessary information.

Employer's Responsibility: Any hazardous chemical used in the workplace that is not in its original container **must** be labeled with the identity of the chemical and hazards. "Target Organ" chemical labels may be used. The label must include the chemical and common name, warnings about physical and health hazards, and the name and address of the manufacturer. The employer is to compile a chemical inventory list that is to be updated as needed. MSDS information should be located in a place where it is accessible to all employees. Label and MSDS information should be provided during the safety training program.

Identity: The term *identity* can refer to any chemical or common name designation for the individual chemical or mixture, as long as the term used is also used on the list of hazardous chemicals and the MSDS.

Note: If a chemical is poured into another container for immediate use, it does not need to be labeled.

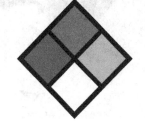

Chemical name

Common name

Manufacturer

Courtesy of POL Consultants

FIGURE 4-2 A chemical warning label.

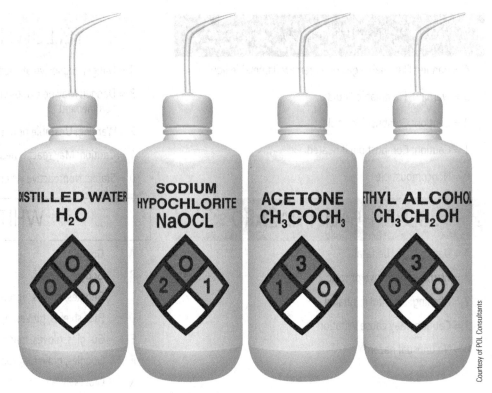

FIGURE 4-3 Containers with chemical warning labels.

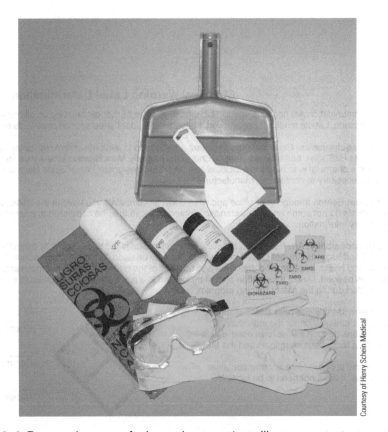

FIGURE 4-4 Proper clean up of a hazardous waste spill.

National Fire Protection Association
Color and Number Codes

The National Fire Protection uses a four-color and number coded system to easily identify hazardous ingredients. These labels not only inform staff of harmful contents but also fire fighters should a fire occur.

Red: Fire Hazard

Red items are coded 4-0, with 4 being dangerous materials such as flammable gas or extremely flammable fluid to 0 for noncombustible material.

Yellow: Reactivity

Yellow items are coded 4-0, with 4 being dangerous material explosive at room temperature to 0 for stable nonreactive materials when mixed with water.

Blue: Health Hazard

Blue items are coded 4-0, with 4 being dangerous potentially fatal items and 0 being items with no unusual hazard.

White: PPE

The white codes indicate what PPE will be needed when dealing with the red, blue, or yellow item. Codes are A–F and X. A is for goggles; B for gloves and goggles; C for goggles, gloves, and apron; D for face shield, gloves, and apron; E for goggles, gloves, and mask; F for goggles, gloves, apron, and mask; and X for gloves only.

Mercury

Concerns about the effects of mercury on the environment have increased over the years. Although mercury is a naturally occurring metal, human activity accounts for about half of the mercury released into the environment. According to the American Dental Association (ADA), less than 1 percent of the environmental mercury is a contribution from dentistry but even that small amount can be reduced if mercury is disposed of properly.

Mercury is one component of amalgam dental restorations but is considered stable in the form of dental amalgam. However, it should not be disposed of in the garbage, infectious waste "red bag," or sharps container. Amalgam must not be rinsed down the drain. These cautions are important because some communities incinerate waste products that might contain dental amalgam if the amalgam has not been disposed of properly.

Safety recommendations during preparation and placement of amalgam are as follows:

1. Use only precapsulated amalgam alloys. The ADA recommends against the use of bulk alloy and bulk elemental mercury, also referred to as liquid or raw mercury, in the dental office. If you still have bulk elemental mercury in the office, it should be recycled according to guidelines.
2. Use an amalgamator with a completely enclosed arm.
3. If possible, recap single-use capsules after use, store them in a closed container, and recycle them.

4. Use care when handling amalgam. Avoid skin contact with mercury or freshly mixed amalgam.

5. Use high-volume evacuation systems (fitted with traps or filters) when finishing or removing amalgam.

ADA recommendation for recycling dental amalgam waste is as follows:

1. Stock a variety of sizes when ordering amalgam to minimize the amount of product waste generated.

2. Use gloves, mask, and protective eyewear when handling amalgam waste.

3. Contact an amalgam waste recycler about special requirements that may exist in your area for collecting, storing, and transporting amalgam waste.

4. Store amalgam waste in a covered plastic container labeled "amalgam for recycling" or as directed by your recycler.

5. Look for a recycler who complies with the ADA-ANSI standard. This standard is meant to encourage recycling.

Any free mercury in the office that was used prior to encapsulated amalgam should be disposed of according to the amalgam recycling procedure or as suggested by your recycling company.

Material Safety Data Sheets (MSDSs)

Material Safety Data Sheets (MSDSs) provide written information about the content of any chemicals used in the office and are on file in the office. By law, MSDSs must be provided by manufacturers or suppliers of products. It is the responsibility of the dental practice, however, to ensure that these sheets are obtained and kept up to date.

MSDSs must always be available, accessible and up to date for all employees to review. It is common for an office to use large three ring binders to organize the information, making it easy to divide available information into categories such as disinfectants or restorative materials. The categories chosen will be unique to the practice. Everyone in the office should know where the MSDSs binders or files are stored.

OSHA requires each MSDSs contain (Figure 4-5):

- Identification (chemical and common names)
- Hazardous ingredients
- Physical and chemical characteristics (boiling point, vapor pressure, etc.)
- Fire and explosion data
- Health hazard data
- Reactivity data
- Spill and disposal procedures
- Protection information
- Handling and storage precautions, including waste disposal
- Emergency and first aid procedures
- Date of preparation of the MSDSs
- Name and address of the manufacturer

Material Safety Data Sheet

I—Product Identification

Company Name: We Wash Inc.

	Tel. No.:	(314) 621-1818
	Nights:	(314) 621-1399
Address: 5035 Manchester Avenue	CHEMTREC:	(800) 424-9343
Freedom, TX 79430		

Product Name: Spotfree   Product No.: 2190
Synonyms: Warewashing Detergent

II—Hazardous Ingredients of Mixtures

Material:	(CAS#)	% by Wt.	TLV	PEL
According to the OSHA Hazard Communication Standard, 29 CFR 1910.1200, this product contains no hazardous ingredients.		N/A	N/A	N/A

III—Physical Data

Vapor pressure, mm Hg: N/A   Vapor density (air=1) 60–90F: N/A
Evaporation rate (ether=1): N/A   % Volatile by wt.: N/A
Solubility in H_2O: Complete   pH @ 1%   Solution 9.3–9.8
Freezing point F: N/A   pH as distributed: N/A
Boiling point F: N/A   Appearance: Off-white granular powder
Specific gravity H_2O=1 @25C: N/A   Odor: Mild chemical odor

IV—Fire and Explosion

Flash point F: N/AV   Flammable limits: N/A

Extinguishing media: The product is not flammable or combustible. Use media appropriate for the primary source of fire.

Special firefighting procedures: Use caution when fighting any fire involving chemicals. A self-contained breathing apparatus is essential.
Unusual fire and explosion hazards: None known.

V—Reactivity Data

Stability: Conditions to avoid: None known.

Incompatibility: Contact of carbonates or bicarbonates with acids can release large quantities of carbon dioxide and heat.

Hazardous decomposition products: In fire situations, heat decomposition may result in the release of sulfur oxides.
Conditions contributing to hazardous polymerization: N/A

Spotfree
VI—Health Hazard Data

Effects of overexposure (medical conditions aggravated/target organ effects)
A. Acute (primary route of exposure)   Eyes: Product granules may cause mechanical irritation to eyes.
   Skin (primary route of exposure): Prolonged, repeated contact with skin may result in drying of skin.
   Ingestion: Not expected to be toxic if swallowed; however, gastrointestinal discomfort may occur.
B. Subchronic, chronic, other: None known.

(continues)

(continued)

VII—Emergency and First Aid Procedures

Eyes: In case of contact, flush thoroughly with water for 15 minutes. Get medical attention if irritation persists.
Skin: Flush and dry Spotfree from skin with flowing water. Always wash hands after use.
Ingestion: If swallowed, drink large quantities of water and call a physician.

VIII—Spill or Leak Procedures

Spill management: Sweep up material and repackage, if possible.
Spill residue may be flushed to the sewer with water.
Waste disposal methods: Dispose of in accordance with federal, state, and local regulations.

IX—Protection Information/Control Measures

Respiratory: None needed.   Eye: Safety glasses. Glove: Not required.

Other clothing and equipment: None required.

Ventilation: Normal.

X—Special Precautions

Precautions to be taken in handling and storing: Avoid contact with eyes. Avoid prolonged or repeated contact with skin. Wash thoroughly after handling. Keep container closed when not in use.
Additional information: Store away from acids.

Prepared by: D. Martinez   Revision date: 04/11/__

Seller makes no warranty, expressed or implied, concerning the use of this product other than indicated on the label. Buyer assumes all risk of use and/or handling of this material when such use and/or handling is contrary to label instructions.

While Seller believes that the information contained herein is accurate, such information is offered solely for its customers' consideration and verification under their specific use conditions. This information is not to be deemed a warranty or representation of any kind for which Seller assumes legal responsibility.

FIGURE 4-5 Sample MSDS.

Staff Training

By law, the dentist must provide staff training regarding potential hazardous chemicals. The training must be provided to new employees at the beginning of their employment, whenever a new hazardous material is introduced into the office, and at least annually thereafter.

The dentist is legally responsible to provide this training; however, she or he may delegate training responsibilities to the office manager, safety coordinator, or other team member.

OSHA also requires that hazard communication training include methods and observations that may be employed to detect the presence or release of a hazardous substance in the work areas, for example, continuous radiation, nitrous oxide monitoring devices, or particular odors associated with chemicals.

OSHA hazard communication training must include:

- A copy of the Bloodborne Pathogens Standard and specific information regarding the meaning of the standard
- Information about bloodborne pathogens, both the epidemiology and symptoms of the diseases

- Information about the cross-contamination pathways of bloodborne pathogens
- A written copy or means for employees to obtain the employer's/office's written exposure-control plan
- Information on the tasks, category placement of classifications, and how each is identified in relation to bloodborne pathogens and OPIM
- Information regarding the hepatitis B vaccine
- Information about exposure reduction, including PPE: work practices; standard precautions, including universal precautions; and engineering practices
- Information about selection, placement, use, removal, disinfection, sterilization, and disposal of PPE
- Information about what to do and whom to contact if an emergency involving blood or OPIM arises
- Information about the procedure to follow if an incident blood exposure occurs, how to report the incident, and what type of medical follow-up is available at no cost to the employee
- Information about the post-exposure and follow-up the employer provides
- A copy of the OSHA Hazard Communication Standard
- MSDSs and information about labeling and hazardous waste
- An opportunity for employees to ask questions of the individual giving the information

Physical and health hazards of these chemicals used in the work area must be addressed, for example, avoidance of handling mercury with ungloved hands or the potential for acid etch to burn skin or clothing.

Training must also include measures employees can take to protect themselves from hazardous materials, such as by using PPE, including protective gloves, eyewear, and face masks, which must be supplied by the employer, in appropriate sizes for all clinical staff members.

The employer or staff representative is also responsible for explaining the details of the hazard communication program, including the labeling system, the use and nature of MSDSs, and ways employees can obtain and use appropriate hazard information for their safety.

Employee training may be conducted at staff meetings, using audiovisuals, lectures, or at continuing education courses offered through accredited providers. It is essential that the training be conducted in such a way that employees understand the information presented and that their questions are answered. Training must be conducted at no cost to employees, during standard working hours.

Training Recordkeeping

Verification of training must also be documented, indicating when and where the training took place and those present for training (Figure 4-6). Training records should be maintained for a minimum of three years. Training records must be available to employees upon request for review and copying.

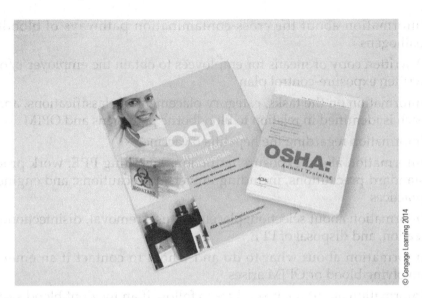

FIGURE 4-6 OSHA staff training manual.

A training summary should contain a description of the content and nature of the training, the names of those in attendance, and qualifications of the safety training coordinator.

In the event the practice is sold or transferred, employee records must be transferred to the new owner. If the practice is permanently closed because of death or retirement of the dentist, these records should be offered in writing to the National Institute for Occupational Safety and Health (NIOSH) 90 days prior to the anticipated close of the office.

Reducing Hazards in the Dental Office

It is the responsibility of all members of the dental team to reduce hazards and the potential hazards. This can be accomplished by:

- Keeping the number of hazardous materials to a minimum
- Reading all product labels and following directions for use
- Storing hazardous chemicals in their original containers
- Keeping containers tightly closed or covered when not in use
- Avoiding the combination of two or more known hazardous chemicals; for example, mixing household chloride bleach with ammonia may cause an explosion; inhaling the fumes may be fatal
- Wearing appropriate PPE when using hazardous chemicals or when there is potential for accidental exposure on contact with body fluids
- Washing and thoroughly drying hands before and after wearing gloves
- Keeping the office well ventilated and avoiding skin contact with known hazardous substances
- Keeping a functional fire extinguisher in the office
- Knowing proper cleanup procedures in the event of a chemical spill
- Disposing of all hazardous chemicals and other substances in accordance with MSDSs instructions or the product labels

Handling Hazardous Materials

Because contact with hazardous materials is inevitable when working in the dental office, there are measures the dentist and staff can take to protect themselves. The most significant measure is using PPE, part of the standard precautions mandated by OSHA.

As part of the hazard communication program, the office must have a written procedure for handling and disposing of used or outdated materials that cannot be poured down the sanitary sewer or treated as routine or medical waste. These items include, but are limited to, outdated radiography solutions, vapor sterilization fluid, lead foil from dental x-ray packets, scrap amalgam, and glutaraldehyde or other disinfection solutions.

Dental team members must be instructed on how to handle spills and cleanup of hazardous substances and chemicals. In the event of an accidental spill, staff should follow the manufacturer's instructions found on the label or on the MSDSs and wear PPE.

Bloodborne Pathogens Standard

The Bloodborne Pathogens Standard is the most significant OSHA regulation affecting health care practices. To understand the standard, it is first necessary to understand the term bloodborne pathogen; bloodborne pathogens are infectious microorganisms present in blood that can cause disease in humans. These pathogens include but are not limited to, hepatitis B (HBV), hepatitis C (HCV), and human immunodeficiency virus (HIV), the virus that causes AIDS. The standard protects workers who can reasonably be anticipated to come into contact with bloodborne pathogens, placing them at risk for serious or life-threatening illnesses.

The standard requires employers to do the following:

- Establish an exposure-control plan. This is a written plan to eliminate or minimize occupational exposures.

- *Employers must update the plan annually* to reflect changes in tasks, procedures, and positions that affect occupational exposure, and also technological changes that eliminate or reduce occupational exposure. Employers must also document that they have solicited input from frontline workers in identifying, evaluating, and selecting effective engineering and work practice controls.

- Implement the use of standard precautions. Treat all human blood as if known to be infectious for bloodborne pathogens.

- Identify and use engineering controls. Engineering controls are devices that isolate or remove the bloodborne pathogen hazard from the workplace, for example, sharps disposable containers, self-sheathing needles, and safer medical devices like needleless systems and sharps with sharps injury protection.

- Identify and ensure the use of work practice controls.

- Provide PPE such as gloves, gowns, eye protection, and masks.

- Make available hepatitis B vaccinations to all workers with occupational exposure.

- Make available post-exposure evaluation and follow-up to any occupationally exposed worker who experiences an exposure incident.

- Use labels and signs to communicate hazards.
- Provide information and training to workers.
- Maintain worker medical and training records.

OSHA Engineering and Work Practice Controls

The office must use proper engineering controls, which means the use of specific equipment or devices that facilitate prevention of accidental exposure, such as capping needles, for example. Work practice controls means changing the way procedures are currently performed to ensure a higher degree of safety or protection from accidental exposure.

OSHA requires engineering controls such as making appropriate hand-washing facilities available and accessible to all staff members. Contaminated sharps, especially needles, must be handled appropriately and disposed of to prevent accidental exposure. A minimum of one eyewash station must be immediately available to all personnel. Other engineering controls applicable to dentistry include high-volume evacuation and use of dental dam.

OSHA guidelines require that offices put into place work practice controls that prohibit eating, drinking, smoking, applying cosmetics or lip balm, and handling of contact lenses in areas of the office where there is a reasonable potential for occupational exposure. Work practice controls would be the office rules contained in the office manual. In addition, all food and beverages should be stored separately from areas where bloodborne pathogens and OPIMs are present. Work practice controls also include proper hand washing, handling of sharps, and containment of regulated waste.

Standard (Universal) Precautions

The term "universal precautions" was developed in the 1980s specifically to protect health care workers from bloodborne pathogens. Standard precautions is an expanded version of universal precautions that includes not just blood but more body fluids. Following standard precautions must be observed with *all* patients at *all* times regardless of their age, gender, diagnosis, or whether they are being treated for a specific disease. Standard precautions emphasize employing engineering and work practice controls to reduce the level of contamination that may be involved during an accidental exposure.

Personal Protective Equipment

Personal protective equipment (PPE) consists of a minimum of four items, which must be worn by chairside personnel, who have a reasonable potential to come into contact with infectious diseases. These items are gloves, protective eyewear, face masks, and gowns (Figure 4-7). In some instances, a face shield may be substituted for protective eyewear, but does not replace a facemask. If preferred, goggles may be used as protective eyewear over contacts or prescription eyeglasses. If eyeglasses are worn as PPE, they must have side shields to protect the wearer from spatter or contact with infectious microorganisms.

Lab jacket, gowns, or other PPE may be disposable or made of cotton polyester. If, during the course of a procedure, disposable items are torn or saturated, the procedure must be stopped and the torn or visibly saturated item must be replaced.

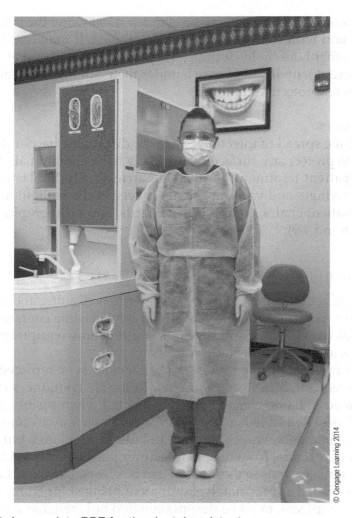

FIGURE 4-7 Appropriate PPE for the dental assistant.

When working away from chairside, such as in the dental lab or when preparing instruments for sterilization, all personnel must protect themselves by wearing PPE. In the sterilization area, reusable utility gloves that can be sterilized may be worn instead of disposable gloves.

The employer must provide, maintain, and ensure use and laundry of PPE, at no charge to staff. PPE must be worn when there is a potential for an employee to come into contact with blood or OPIMs.

In instances where a dental staff member is known to be sensitive to PPE — for example, an allergy to latex gloves — the employer must provide alternatives, such as vinyl gloves or cotton glove liners.

Handling and Laundry of Reusable PPE

Handling of reusable PPE, the items that are not single-use disposables, must be kept to a minimum. It is the dentist's responsibility to provide laundry or dry cleaning services for reusable lab jackets or scrubs worn during invasive procedures. Contaminated laundry in the office must be placed into containers that are red or labeled with the biohazard symbol.

Dental staff may not wear outer protective clothing worn for invasive procedures to and from the office; nor may they wear it when leaving the office during the day, such as during a lunch hour.

Outer protective clothing may be laundered following the manufacturer's directions and with standard laundry detergents. It may not, however, be done with other household clothing. They must be laundered at the office or at a commercial laundry. Staff may launder their clothing, at home, worn underneath outer protective clothing.

Barrier Devices

To prevent the spread of infectious diseases, disposable barrier devices must be placed to protect any surface that is likely to be contaminated during the course of patient treatment. Protective barriers include plastic sleeves on air/water syringes and vacuum tubing, covers on dental light handles, light switches, patient chairs, computer keyboards, and radiography tube heads (Figures 4-8 and 4-9).

Decontamination of Surfaces

The standard requires the office to have a written cleaning and maintenance schedule for surfaces and other areas that may become contaminated with blood or saliva. This description should outline how equipment and treatment rooms are decontaminated.

For example, all plastic covers and barriers must be replaced when contaminated as well as between patients. Reusable containers that become contaminated must be cleaned and disinfected when visibly soiled or on a routine basis. Reusable containers are a common way to contain the cost of materials in a dental office. Buying in bulk saves money but a container other than the original from the manufacturer must be adapted for the product. Make sure any reusable container can be cleaned with surface disinfectant and is labeled appropriately. Equipment being shipped for repair, such as dental handpieces, must be decontaminated or labeled as a biohazard.

Waste Management

Regulated **medical waste** is defined as liquid or semiliquid body fluid. This includes any items in the dental office contaminated with regulated waste (e.g., cotton rolls or gauze) that release **bioburden** (contaminated hazardous or infectious material) when compressed, items caked with dried

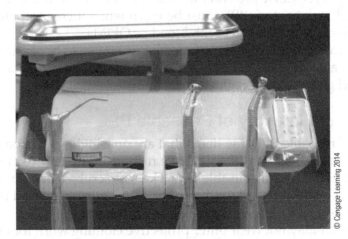

© Cengage Learning 2014

FIGURE 4-8 (a) Barrier covers for the dental handpieces, air-water syringe, saliva ejector, and high volume evacuator.

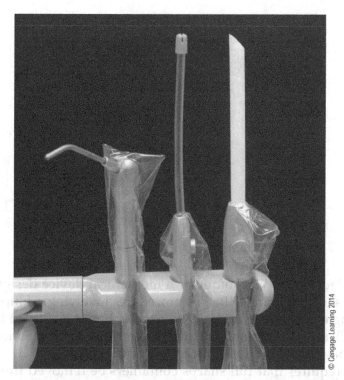

FIGURE 4-8 (b) Barrier covers for the dental handpieces, air-water syringe, saliva ejector, and high volume evacuator.

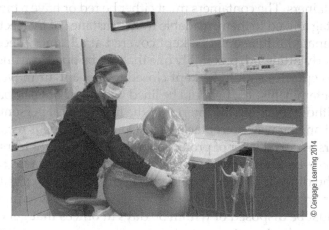

FIGURE 4-9 Barrier cover for the dental chair.

body fluid that have the potential to release bioburden during handling, contaminated sharps, and pathological and microbial wastes containing body fluid.

Any type of disposable sharps, that is, any item capable of puncturing the skin (needles, scalpels, burs, and orthodontic wires) must be disposed of in puncture-resistant, color-coded or labeled, red, closable, leakproof containers. Sharps containers must be located as close as possible to where sharps are used in the office. They must also be kept upright and must be closed during transport.

Needles must not be recapped by hand; nor may they be broken or sheared by hand prior to disposal. Instead, dental personnel should use either

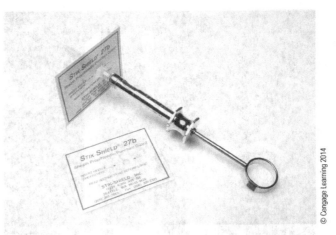

© Cengage Learning 2014

FIGURE 4-10 Needlestick protector.

a one-handed "scoop" technique or a mechanical device designed to hold the needle sheath (Figure 4-10). For procedures involving multiple injections using a single needle, the unsheathed needle should be placed in a location where it will not become contaminated or contribute to unintentional percutaneous (through the skin) needlesticks between injections.

OSHA requires that full sharps containers be removed from the office within seven days of reaching the "fill line" on the container.

Other regulated waste products, including those items saturated or visibly caked with blood or saliva, must be disposed of in closable, leak proof bags or covered containers. The containers must either be red or have a biohazard warning label or tag affixed to them, readable from a distance of five feet (Figure 4-11).

Contaminated refuse must be kept covered at all times. Receptacles must have a properly fitting lid, preferably one that can be opened using a foot pedal.

Waste receptacles should be kept closed to prevent air movement and the spread of contaminants. They should be lined with sturdy plastic bags that can be removed without touching the interior of the liner. Dental personnel must wear PPE when changing waste receptacle bags. Double-bagging is recommended because it offers a second layer of protection if the bag breaks or tears off.

Laws vary by state and region regarding proper waste transport and tracking. The office manager should check with the local regulatory agency in his or her area for additional regulations. As a general requirement, medical waste must be disposed of within 30 days in offices that generate less than 20 pounds of medical waste a year.

Hepatitis B Vaccination

OSHA requires that the hepatitis B vaccination be administered to all full-time employees who are at potential risk for exposure to bloodborne pathogens. The employer must make the vaccination available to all employees at no charge. In rare instances where employees refuse the vaccination, they should sign a waiver, acknowledging their refusal of the vaccine and that they do not hold the employer liable for the consequences.

Exposure Incidents

If a member of the dental team sustains an exposure incident, directly related to the nature of employment, the dentist is required to follow specific steps.

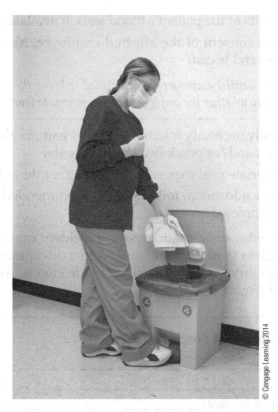

FIGURE 4-11 Contaminated medical waste needs to be placed in biohazard containers.

According to OSHA, an exposure incident consists of "specific eye, mouth or other mucous membranes, non-intact skin or parenteral contact with blood or OPIMS that directly results from the performance of an employee's duties." Most common examples of occupational exposures occur when dental staff accidentally cut themselves on a contaminated dental instrument or sustain a needlestick injury from a contaminated anesthesia syringe.

If an exposure incident occurs, the staff member should stop his or her immediately and report the incident to the office manager and to the dentist. If the exposure involves the hands, the employee should remove the gloves.

The injury should be treated with scrupulous first-aid measures, including the following steps:

1. If the affected area is bleeding, the staff member should squeeze it gently until a small amount of blood is released.

2. Wash the affected area thoroughly with antimicrobial soap and water that is comfortably warm to hot.

3. After drying the affected area, a small amount of antiseptic should be applied and the injury covered it with a bandage.

The employer must follow specific OSHA guidelines, including providing an independent medical evaluation of the exposure incident. The employers must do the following:

- Document the route or routes of exposure and how the incident occurred
- Attempt to identify the source individual (the patient who was treated using the specific instruments or needle) if possible

- Obtain the results of the patient's blood tests, if available
- With informed consent of the affected employee, have the employee's blood collected and tested.

> **Note:** *By law the dentist-employer is not entitled to know the results of the employee's blood test, only whether the employee is fit to return to work.*

- Obtain medically necessary injections, such as gamma globulin, hepatitis B vaccine booster, and/or possibly a tetanus booster
- Provide appropriate post-exposure counseling for the employee
- Ensure that any additional follow-up as recommended by the attending physician is completed

An employee who sustains an exposure incident may choose to decline the exposure incident follow-up, but must sign a disclaimer waiving the employer's responsibility for future results or side effects. All documentation must be recorded (Figure 4-12).

Exposure Incident Report Form

Employee: _____

Date: _____

Place and Time of Incident: _____

Those Present: _____

Route of Exposure: _____

Description of the Exposure Incident: _____

_____

_____

Engineering Controls in Place: _____

_____

Work Practice Controls Employed: _____

_____

List PPE used at time of Exposure Incident: _____

_____

Source Patient: _____

Was Source Patient Tested? ☐ Yes   ☐ No

HIV Status: ☐ Positive   ☐ Negative

Name of Lab: _____

Date of Testing: _____

Employee Tested? ☐ Yes   ☐ No

If Employee Refused, was Waiver signed: ☐ Yes   ☐ No

Explain: _____

Post-Exposure Prophylaxis: _____

Physician's Follow-Up: _____

Physician's Written Opinion on File? ☐ Yes   ☐ No

FIGURE 4-12 Sample exposure incident report form.

Recordkeeping

Medical records of staff must be kept confidential and must be retained by the dentist for the duration of employment plus 30 years. They should include the names and social security numbers of all employees, copies of all employees' hepatitis B vaccination records, and any other medical records pertinent to the employees' ability to receive the vaccination, circumstances surrounding any exposure incidents, and documentation of all follow-up procedures, including the treating physician's written opinion.

Waterline Biofilms

Biofilms can be found virtually anywhere moisture and a suitable solid surface exist. They are composed of millions of microorganisms that accumulate on surfaces inside moist environments. These film-forming microbes excrete a glue-like substance that anchors them to metals, plastic, tissue, and soil particles. Biofilms attach themselves to the inner surfaces of the plastic tubing used to keep handpieces cool and supply air-water syringes, where they create an ideal environment for growth.

This results in a nearly stagnant condition of the tubing's inner wall surface, even when water actively flows through the tubing. A vast number of bacteria, fungi, and viruses living inside dental units become highly concentrated, significantly increasing a patient's susceptibility to transmissible diseases.

To avoid the buildup of dental unit waterline biofilms, the CDC, the ADA, and OSAP recommend dental personnel flush their dental unit waterlines at the start of the day and between patients.

To help reduce bacterial counts, the ADA suggests dental professionals follow these guidelines to improve the quality of water in their lines and minimize disease transmission:

- At the start of each day, run and discharge water from the dental unit waterlines for several minutes.
- Run high-speed handpieces to release air and water for 20–30 seconds after each patient.
- Always follow the manufacturer's instructions for proper maintenance of handpieces and waterlines.
- Consider other options to improve water quality such as special filters, chemical therapeutics, and separate water reservoirs.

Fire and Emergency Evacuation Procedures

OSHA requires the employer to have a written fire safety policy, consisting of training in the use and maintenance of fire extinguishers. A diagram must be provided that clearly marks the exit routes in the event of a fire. Posting of emergency telephone numbers for police, fire, and rescue is also required.

Written evacuation and safety procedures should be provided in areas susceptible to severe weather conditions, including hurricanes, tornadoes, floods, and earthquakes.

Signage Requirements

In addition to signage required by the Americans with Disabilities Act, signs should be posted to include office exits and potential exposure hazards, such as radiography machines, ultrasonic machines, and microwaves. Exit signs must be illuminated and be a minimum of five inches high. Doors to other rooms should also be appropriately marked with such signs as "storage," "private," "not an exit," etc.

The Safety Coordinator's Duties

The office manager or clinical assistant may be delegated the responsibilities of office safety coordinator by the dentist. The safety coordinator may be responsible for any or all of the following to ensure compliance with government regulations:

- Constantly review infection control, hazardous materials, and other office safety procedures and protocols
- Prepare, review, and constantly upgrade the office exposure-control plan and all manuals, including MSDSs, hazardous materials log, employee exposures, and so on
- Develop procedures that provide written, step-by-step instructions for office safety
- Provide training updates regularly
- Monitor compliance with office safety procedures and regulations in compliance with the government
- Ensure that all employees have received the hepatitis B vaccine at no charge to them
- Initiate procedures for management of accidental exposure of staff
- Review the circumstances surrounding accidental exposure and steps taken to reduce or prevent their recurrence
- Maintain required items to protect staff as required by the government (e.g., gloves, masks, eyewear) and other necessary equipment
- Ensure that spore-testing of office sterilizers is done routinely and that proper biological monitoring of records is maintained
- Document and follow medical waste disposal requirements
- Ensure that warning labels and MSDSs, and the hazardous materials log, are maintained and updated as necessary
- Maintain clearly marked exit signs and evacuation routes in the event of fire or other emergency
- Maintain radiography equipment certification
- Prepare and maintain all necessary records and forms

Practice Compliance Check List

This checklist may be helpful to the office manager in organizing the practice's compliance list:

- Appropriate licenses, registrations, certificates, and OSHA posters posted in plain view
- Licenses and registration of staff if required by the State Dental Practice Act
- A record of hepatitis B vaccination and any other appropriate vaccines administered
- Infection control manual, hazard communication manuals, hazardous materials log, and MSDSs accessible and available for review
- Appropriate handwashing procedures
- Appropriate use of PPE, available in sizes to fit respective clinical staff members
- Appropriate use of barrier wraps and disposable coverings for treatment room and laboratory
- Appropriate use, management, and disposal of single-use items
- Appropriate surface disinfection of all splash areas
- Appropriate aseptic technique followed by all personnel
- Appropriate sterilization/disinfection of contaminated, reusable instruments
- Appropriate biological monitoring as recommended
- Appropriate instrument sterilization/instrument recycling area
- Nitrile gloves for presoaking, cleaning, and processing of instruments prior to sterilization
- Appropriate disposal and tracking of regulated waste and OPIMs, including sharps
- Eyewash stations in each operatory
- Appropriate infection-control precautions for radiographic procedures
- Appropriate cross-contamination prevention in the dental laboratory area
- Appropriate safety checks and inspections for fire extinguishers, smoke detectors, radiation, and nitrous oxide monitors

WWW Exploring the Web

OSHA — U.S. Department of Labor — Quick Reference Guide to the Bloodborne Pathogens Standard
www.osha.gov/SLTC/bloodbornepathogens/bloodborne_quickref.html

FDA — U.S. Food and Drug Administration
www.fda.gov

OSAP — Organization for Safety and Asepsis Procedures
www.osap.org

CDC — Centers for Disease Control and Prevention
www.cdc.gov

EPA — Environmental Protection Agency
www.epa.gov

Skill Building

1. List reasons why the federal government requires the dentist to maintain a hazard communication program and the necessary components.

2. List five ways to reduce hazards inherent in the dental office.

3. Describe the necessary procedures for handling hazardous materials in the dental office.

4. Develop a chart listing the necessary recordkeeping required by the government for staff training.

5. Pretend you have been assigned the role of office safety coordinator. Develop a list of duties you might be expected to perform.

6. Work in a group to discuss the steps you would take if a clinical assistant in your office had sustained a needlestick. She comes to you with a droplet of blood oozing out of her glove. Complete a sample exposure incident report.

7. With your group describe the steps you would take if a patient vomited at the front desk following a tooth extraction.

Challenge Your Understanding

1. OSHA requires employers, including those in the health care profession to:
   a. Establish and carry out procedures to protect employees
   b. Implement and maintain employee exposure-incident records for the duration of employment plus 30 years
   c. Provide personal protective equipment (PPE) to protect staff from infectious diseases and other potential hazards
   d. All of the above

2. Hazard communication training must be provided for:
   a. New employees at the beginning of employment
   b. Any time a new hazardous material is introduced into the office
   c. At least annually
   d. All of the above

3. OSHA's Bloodborne Pathogens Standard is designed to:
   a. Limit occupational exposure to blood and OPIMs
   b. Mandate topics covered in regular training sessions
   c. Assist dental offices in setting up an exposure-control plan
   d. All of the above

4. OSHA's Bloodborne Pathogens Standard covers:
   a. All dental employees
   b. Those employees in category 1
   c. Those employees in category 3
   d. Dental patients

5. The Environmental Protection Agency:
   a. Regulates and registers certain products used in dental practices
   b. Requires products to undergo and pass specific testing requirements prior to approval for registration
   c. Reviews product labels for false or misleading information and sufficient directions for use
   d. All of the above

6. Warning labels or stickers must contain appropriate warnings according to:
   a. Hazard class, including routes of entry and target organs that may be affected
   b. The identity of the chemical and the appropriate hazard warnings
   c. The name and address of the manufacturer
   d. All of the above

7. Hazardous products moved from one container to another:
   a. Must have a warning label or sticker affixed to them
   b. Do not need a label because the product is labeled somewhere in the office
   c. No label as long as an MSDSs sheet is in the office binder
   d. All products must remain in their original packaging

8. Which element is not a requirement of a basic hazardous spill kit?
   a. Absorbent material
   b. A scooping device
   c. An EPA registration label
   d. A hazardous waste bag with a biohazard label

9. The office must maintain Material Safety Data Sheets on every product that has a potential hazard. MSDSs must:
   a. Provide written information about the content and potential hazard of a specific product
   b. Be provided by the manufacturer or supplier
   c. Always be available and accessible to all employees for review and be kept updated
   d. All of the above

10. Dental sharps must be disposed of in containers that is/are:
    a. Puncture- resistant
    b. Color-coded or labeled
    c. Closable and leakproof
    d. All of the above

11. When recapping needles, dental personnel should:
    a. Use a one handed "scoop" technique or a mechanical recapping device
    b. Use both hands making sure the device is secure when recapping
    c. Not recap as it is not necessary when the needle is disposed of in a sharps container
    d. Wear gloves and capture the needle within the glove as it is removed and immediately dispose of it in the hazardous waste.

12. Sharps containers should be:
    a. Located as close as possible to where sharps are used in the office
    b. Be filled as full as possible to avoid shifting during transport
    c. Shipped in an upright position
    d. Both a and c

13. Personal protective equipment includes:
    a. Scrubs
    b. Shoe covers
    c. Protective eyewear
    d. Both b and c

14. Following standard precautions means:
    a. Treating each and every patient as though potentially carrying an infectious disease
    b. Using the same standards of personal protection when treating all patients
    c. Employing engineering and work practice controls to reduce the level of contamination that may be involved during an accidental exposure
    d. Both a and b

15. Hepatitis B vaccination must be:
    a. Provided by the employer to all full-time employees who may be exposed during the course of their jobs
    b. Provided at no cost to employees
    c. Documented in the employee medical history records
    d. All of the above

16. The Hazardous Materials Log must:
    a. List the hazardous material
    b. Clearly state where the material is located in the office
    c. Give the quantity on hand
    d. All of the above

17. Whether conducted by the dentist, the office safety coordinator, or the office manager, staff training must include:
    a. Hazards of chemicals and their proper handling
    b. The availability of MSDSs
    c. An explanation of the labeling of hazardous chemicals and an explanation of OSHA regulations
    d. All of the above

18. Members of the dental team may reduce hazards and their potential by:
    a. Reading all product labels and following directions for use
    b. Avoiding the combination of two or more known hazardous chemicals
    c. Wearing appropriate personal protective equipment (PPE) when using hazardous chemicals or when there is potential for accidental exposure or contact with body fluids
    d. All of the above

19. Which is not a requirement of the hazard communication program?
    a. Having a written procedure for handling and disposing of used or outdated materials that cannot be poured down the sanitary sewer or treated as routine or medical waste
    b. Instructing dental team members on how to handle spills and cleaning up of hazardous substances and chemicals
    c. Joining OSAP
    d. Maintaining a hazardous materials log

20. To prevent the spread of infectious diseases, disposable barriers must be placed to protect splash surfaces likely to be contaminated during the course of patient treatment. Protective barriers include:
    a. Plastic covering around the base of the dental chair
    b. Plastic covering over patients' shoes
    c. Plastic covering on radiography tube head
    d. Plastic covering over computer monitors

SECTION II

Practice Communications

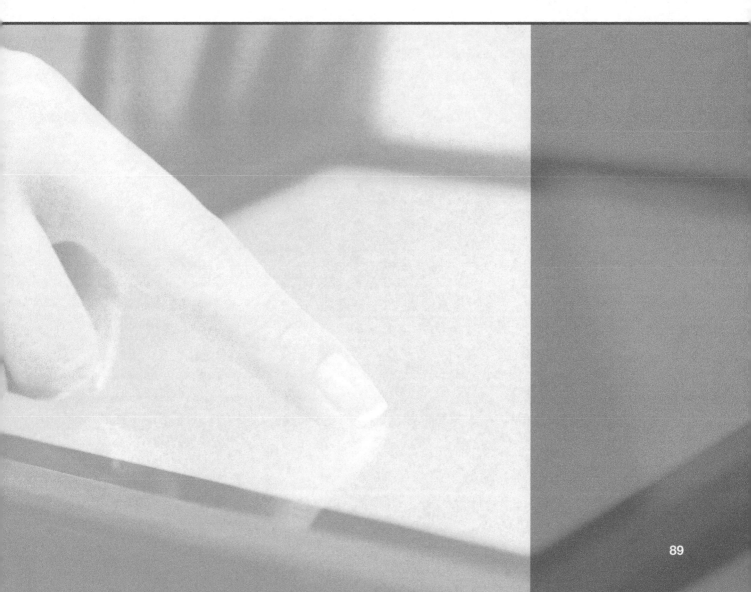

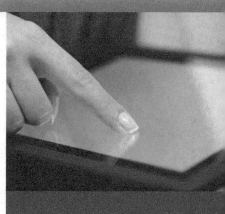

CHAPTER 5

The Dental Office Manager as a Patient Relations Specialist

CHAPTER OUTLINES

KEY TERMS

amenities
anxiety
etiquette
impression
patient flow
phobia
protocol
reception area

LEARNING OBJECTIVES

Upon completion of this chapter, the reader should be able to:

1. List the three goals of a patient relations policy with regard to greeting patients.
2. Describe at least seven amenities of a modern dental office reception area.
3. Describe the role of the office manager in assisting new patients to complete necessary forms.
4. Describe the importance of understanding and communicating patients' rights.
5. Discuss five steps to defuse a patient's anger.
6. Discuss the differences between the anxious patient and the phobic patient.
7. Describe the protocol involved in introducing the patient to the other members of the dental team.
8. List and describe aspects of nonverbal communication and how they convey positive patient relations and perceptions.
9. Be familiar with rules of common courtesy and office etiquette.
10. Describe two important factors in making follow-up calls to patients.
11. Describe the role of the office manager in providing referrals and extended services.

Welcoming Patients as Guests

Although every member of the dental team is a patient relations representative, the office manager is most often the first and last contact most patients have with the office. It is the role of the office manager as patient relations specialist to acknowledge and greet patients when they enter. Every office should have a patient relations policy for greeting and handling patients throughout the duration of their dental visits. The goals of the patient relations policy are to:

- Focus on the patient and the patient's chief concerns rather than on the procedure
- Manage patient flow so that there is a smooth process of events between the patient's arrival and departure
- Control the environment as much as possible to facilitate optimum dental care

THINK Green

Communications is a great place to think about making the practice more eco-friendly. Throughout this section ideas for a greener practice will be presented.

Prior to the New Patient's First Appointment

The expression, "you never get a second chance to make a first **impression**," is very appropriate in dentistry as a service profession. Prior to the new patient's first appointment, many offices send out a variety of get-acquainted materials to make the patient feel welcome and facilitate the first visit. These materials may include a new patient packet, a map or printed instructions about the office location and parking, a copy of the practice newsletter, acquaintance forms, office policies, and information about the doctor's professional training and background.

Greeting the Patient

A patient visiting for the first time may feel anxious about the choice of a new dentist, finding the building and a place to park, locating the office if it is part of a larger complex, and interacting with people whom he or she has never met.

The office manager can alleviate much of the patient's anxiety by acknowledging him or her by name within the first 30 seconds of entry into the **reception area** (Figure 5-1). If the patient is visiting for the first appointment, the office manager or receptionist should anticipate the new patient's arrival and be ready to introduce her or himself, "Good morning. You must be Mr. Wilson. My name is Mary/John. We're delighted to welcome you to our practice." If the office is in a large complex of professional offices, he or she may further inquire, "Did you have any problems finding the office?" This helps ease any awkwardness or shyness the new patient might feel in an unfamiliar environment. It establishes

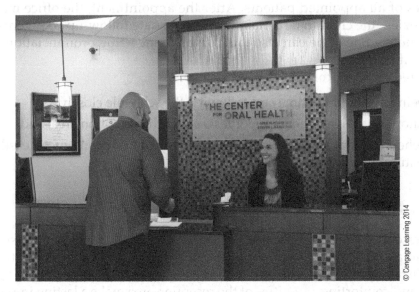

© Cengage Learning 2014

FIGURE 5-1 The office manager's greeting of the patient can set the tone for the office visit.

the office manager as the appropriate professional to whom the patient can address questions or concerns. It "breaks the ice" by

- beginning the conversation;
- supplying a name for ease of asking questions or requesting assistance;
- initiating the new patient's orientation; and
- guiding the patient, new or existing, to the next step of the visit.

Patients should always be guided as to "what happens next?" If the patient needs to complete or update paperwork, invite the patient to complete the forms in a comfortable place and return the forms to you when finished. When the forms are complete, inform the patient of the next step, such as "Please have a seat and Debbie, Dr. Crawford's assistant will be here in a moment." If you know it will be more than a few minutes, let the patient know such as by saying, "Thank you Mrs. Smith for being so prompt today; Dr. Crawford is just completing treatment for a patient. It will be about 10 minutes. Can I get you something to drink or a magazine?" By keeping the patient informed, she or he can relax.

Patients of record must be greeted as a welcome guest. Again, immediate acknowledgment within 30 seconds of arrival is necessary to reassure the patient, reestablish the relationship, and keep scheduled procedures on time. Even though the patient is familiar with the office routine he or she still needs to know "what's next"; this allows the patient to take a moment to unwind and relax.

An effective office manager notes on an attachment to the patient record events in a patient's life that should be recalled at the next visit, such as a vacation or a graduation or wedding in the family. These notes are reviewed before the patient arrives and may even be shared at the morning meeting. When the patient arrives the event can become part of the conversation. These notes are not a part of the patient's formal legal treatment record and should not be made in the clinical record.

The office manager should review the schedule frequently to learn the names of all appointed patients. After the appointment, the office manager can review the chart to be certain that appropriate follow-up comments have been noted. She or he can also indicate phonetic name pronunciation in the notes, if necessary.

Greeting protocol can be mastered by

- being aware of the time and following the schedule closely;
- knowing which patients and guests are in the reception area; and
- rehearsing names when necessary so they can be pronounced easily and naturally as patients enter the office.

The Reception Area

The reception area is a reflection of the practice's philosophy and personality. It also assures the new patient of the doctor's values, such as treating the whole family and welcoming friends as prospective new patients. The appearance and comforting amenities of the reception area make a lasting impression upon patients and communicate that the dentist and staff find their comfort important. The reception area should never be referred to as the waiting room.

It is important for the reception area to be clean because it reflects the cleanliness of the entire practice. In clinical areas, cleaning solutions are mandated for their ability to disinfect and sterilize. Consider using more environmentally friendly products in the reception areas. They can effectively clean the area and smell better too.

Creating a Comfortable Atmosphere

By furnishing the reception area with hospitality in mind, the office manager can impact a patient's sense of relaxation and add an element of enjoyment to the time spent waiting for family members or awaiting his or her treatment. Many practices today have removed the frosted privacy glass and the reception window, opening the area to make a receiving counter where patients feel comfortable approaching personnel. Designating a small consultation area away from the front desk allows private discussions to remain private.

The traditional hardback chairs have been replaced by living room-like furnishings that make patients and their families feel at home (Figure 5-2).

Organizers and Signs

A coat rack, boot tray, umbrella stand, and mirror help patients feel that the office has anticipated their needs. These conveniences seem minor but they help put a patient at ease. Signs that direct patients to information are also helpful and may help the patient relax in the new environment.

Reading Materials

The reception area is the ideal place to provide educational and recreational reading materials. Most dental offices provide racks and specialized brochures

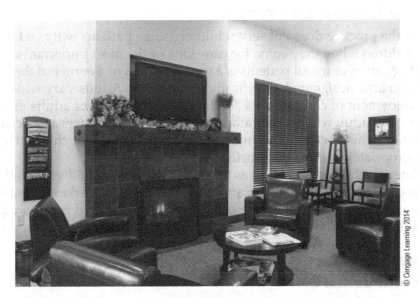

FIGURE 5-2 Many offices now design the reception area to have a very relaxed "homey" feeling to put patients at ease.

THINK Green

- Check your lighting to make sure it is as effective as possible. You can save the office money on electricity while you are greening your practice.
- Your mother was right! Turn off lights in rooms when not in use.
- Use energy-efficient light bulbs.

that focus on a variety of oral health topics. Many also provide a DVD player that features dental health subjects.

The creative office manager experiments with reading materials to find an appealing mix of literature. Attractively bound "coffee table" books can be displayed if space permits. A book of cosmetic dental procedures with actual patient "before and after" photos is also popular. Magazines, cookbooks, or other books must be kept up to date and in good condition. If you provide age-appropriate children's books, they must be checked frequently for damage and cleanliness.

Lighting, Ventilation, and Aroma Therapy

Optimal lighting should be provided in the reading areas throughout the reception area. An excellent way to determine if lighting is sufficient is for the office manager to seat herself or himself in the reception area from time to time with a book or magazine to see where inadequate light creates a problem.

Proper ventilation helps reduce the dental office odors associated with traditional practices. Minimizing "dental odors" is important because for patients smells may increase anxiety. Many offices use automatic aroma therapy dispensing systems that release small doses of odor-neutralizing vapor into the air. Light fragrances are popular. Be careful not to overwhelm one bad smell with one that is even worse.

Special Touches for Children

Even if the practice does not serve children, some patients will need to bring their children when they come for care. One of the most important comforts the office can offer for all patients is a reception area or a corner of the general reception area designated specifically for children. Adults vary widely with their enjoyment of children so a "children's corner" serves adults as well as children. An adult who would rather not deal with youngsters appreciates the separation. Those who enjoy children are happy to see that children's needs are appropriately met by the practice.

Materials that lend themselves to quiet activities for children include individual coloring sheets, crayons, and washable colored markers. Jigsaw puzzles keep many children happily occupied. Toys separated into storage bins and activity boxes labeled for age appropriateness are also a welcome amenity.

THINK Green

Toys must be cleaned often with nontoxic cleaners.

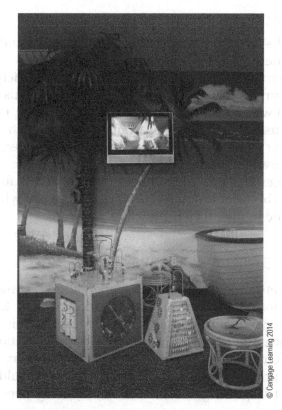

FIGURE 5-3 A pediatric practice may design the reception area around a kid-friendly theme such as this aquatic themed office.

Practices that treat a large number of children, often, have a reception area reserved exclusively for kids that may offer more lively diversion such as video games or popular movies on DVD (Figure 5-3).

As in all decisions regarding the practice, the philosophy and image should prevail. As practice relations specialist, the office manager is attuned to the task of supporting and promoting the practice philosophy in all the details of its management.

Refreshments

It has become increasingly common for dental practices to provide light refreshments in the reception area as a sign of hospitality. Complimentary coffee, tea, juices, hot chocolate, and bottled water promote relaxation and make any wait seem shorter.

THINK Green

If the practice is providing water to patients in plastic water bottles consider using the most environmentally efficient products possible and consider smaller bottles. An alternative is a water cooler with a large refillable bottle and small paper cups. Depending on the individual office and usage, it might be a nice touch to use coffee cups with the office logo that can be put into the dishwasher. Remember even though they are reusable, to wash them requires water, electricity, and detergent. Think carefully and choose wisely.

Sound System and Internet Access

A quality sound system is another effective way to provide a comforting, pleasant atmosphere that helps patients relax.

Just as pleasurable aromas mask smells that induce anxiety, relaxing music can also cover sounds that might trigger fear or subconscious anxiety. Another bonus associated with background music is added privacy. Patients feel more comfortable discussing their financial arrangements or treatment options with the office manager when they sense that the music in the reception area helps to make these conversations inaudible to the other patients.

Many practices also provide wireless Internet access for patients in the reception area. This enables guests or parents to work while in the office, making their time in the office productive.

Assisting Patients with Necessary Forms

The best way to ensure that all office documentation is correct and complete is to oversee it carefully. It is the role of the office manager to offer assistance to patients when completing forms. More importantly, this assistance offers a valuable opportunity to establish a personal, caring relationship with each patient and reinforces this communication of concern at every visit. If the forms were completed prior to arriving at the office, patients should be asked if they have any questions regarding the forms when they bring them to the front desk.

Patient's Rights

As in any other service organization, in the dental office patients are the customers and have specific rights regarding information about their diagnosis and treatment. A Dental Patient's Rights (Figure 5-4) has been adapted from the medical/hospital system to define patients' rights. Some practices develop their own version and display a framed copy in the reception or business office areas for patients to see, whereas others include it with the new patient introductory forms.

Introducing the New Patient to the Dental Team

When the patient has satisfactorily completed the necessary forms, the clinical staff should be informed that the patient is ready. The patient should be introduced to staff members who will be responsible for the next step in the patient's visit. The staff members name must be pronounced clearly, even if an earlier introduction has been made, so the patient can comfortably ask questions or initiate a conversation about the proposed treatment.

Many dental offices consider staff nametags an essential part of the team uniform and require all employees to wear them.

Office Tours

Some practices make it a matter of policy to give each new patient a tour of the office, introducing the patient to all team members. The benefits to the patient include increased familiarity, a sense of being treated as a partner in the health care decision-making process, increased understanding of the routine procedures of the office, and an opportunity to ask questions about sterilization procedures.

A Dental Patient's Rights

Patients enrolled in our practice are entitled to be treated fairly and with dignity. We hold our patients in high regard and strive to treat them with the finest quality of care and service. Our patients are guaranteed to:

1. Be treated with respect and consideration for their dental needs.
2. Be informed **of** all aspects regarding dental treatment, including type of treatment and necessity for referral, when indicated.
3. Be informed of appointment times and fees for service.
4. A review of all personal financial and clinical records.
5. Obtain a thorough evaluation of oral needs.
6. Be treated as a partner in his or her care and decision making related to treatment planning and delivery, as well as, an estimate of fees prior to rendering service.
7. Receive information and feel assured of quality treatment and materials.
8. Expect confidentially of all records pertaining to dental care.
9. Receive information of the dentist's participation in various third-party payment plans.
10. Obtain appropriate referrals for consultation, specialty care, and /or second opinions.
11. Receive instruction in maintaining good oral home care.
12. Receive treatment to prevent, reduce, or eliminate future dental or related oral disease.
13. Expect continuity of treatment and to be informed of the necessity of change in a treatment plan, should the need arise.
14. Be charged a fair and equitable fee for services.
15. Have appointment times maintained and respected.
16. Be treated by all members of the dental team with courtesy and respect.

© Cengage Learning 2014

FIGURE 5-4 A Dental patient's rights.

Office managers who conduct introductory tours find that patients enjoy learning more about the office staff members, infection control methods, types of radiography and imaging, as well as state-of-the-art equipment used for dental care. Touring the inner workings of the dental office they seldom see gives patients the sense of feeling welcomed as a friend in addition to the expected professional relationship and treatment outcome.

Patients concerned about disease transmission via dental equipment can see firsthand and ask questions about the practices compliance with government-mandated guidelines for infection control management.

Patients who suffer from a fear of dental care find walking through the office helps to demystify the experience and reassures them when they see other patients who are comfortable and that the staff is friendly and professional. Remember all patients have a right to privacy under Health Insurance Probability and Accountability Act (HIPAA); before offering a tour, you must make sure you have the consent of any patient being treated.

Parents of young children especially appreciate the tour because it provides their family members with an interesting and positive introduction to dental care. Children may be invited to take a ride in the dental chair as a preliminary introduction to the treatment room prior to their first visit.

An important part of the introductory tour is a prize for each child and a professional handout or information packet for the patient or prospective patient's parent. Sometimes the prize is a toothbrush that the patient is allowed to select or many offices have a reward box where patients choose a trinket. Many children have a positive opinion of their dental experience because of a sparkly ring or bracelet.

Using Communication to Create Patient Comfort

The key to understanding patient relations is managing anxiety. Often dental patients feel anxious about anticipated pain, temporary loss of control in the situation, financial concerns, and/or the amount of time required for maintaining their oral health. The office manager and members of the dental team can help alleviate these concerns through professional education and effective communication. By fostering ongoing professional relationships with patients of record, as well as prospective patients, the office manager can successfully anticipate problems that prevent patients from seeking dental care. At the same time he or she can generate referrals of new patients from satisfied patients of the practice.

The Anxious Patient

Many patients feel some degree of anxiety (a normal but enhanced feeling of concern) about dental appointments. An attentive office manager displays awareness and a willingness to accommodate patients to help alleviate their anxiety.

The office manager can emphasize that the anxiety is normal and many patients experience those same feelings. Reassure the patient that the practice considers calming fears and resolving concerns an important part of patient care.

There is a difference, however, between the anxious patient and the true dental phobic patient.

The Phobic Dental Patient

A phobia refers to a type of anxiety disorder that interferes with normal pursuits. A true dental phobic is so traumatized by the environment of the dental office that it is clinically impossible to treat him or her until the phobia is controlled.

Some dentists premedicate phobic patients. Others prefer the use of behavior modification techniques, such as visualization, hypnosis, or biofeedback. Often the dentist contacts the patient's therapist prior to the first dental visit to discuss various methods of handling appointments with the phobic patient. Some phobic patients may bring along the therapist for the first visit or for the first several visits, as required.

Some practices offer scheduling considerations for extremely anxious or phobic patients, such as times when there are no other patients in the office or short visits that permit the patient to adapt gradually to the fearful situation.

Patients with dental phobias are encouraged to bring a friend, spouse, counselor, or other support person. Some also bring along an item that may be clutched for comfort; maybe a pillow, blanket, stuffed animal, or anything that helps put them at ease. This permits the patient to bring a part of his or her comfortable environment into a frightening one and helps the phobic patient maintain a sense of control.

Some practices schedule a reception area only visit for the phobic patient during normal office hours. At this visit, the doctor, hygienist, or assistant may come out and greet the patient but there is no treatment scheduled and the patient goes no further than the reception area.

At the next scheduled visit, the phobic patient enters the treatment room but does not sit in the chair. At a subsequent visit, the patient enters the treatment room and sits in the chair but does not recline. Eventually the patient will go into the treatment room, sit, and recline in the chair for 10 minutes and practice deep breathing exercises.

When the patient is ready, an oral examination is scheduled. By using small, successive steps, many phobic patients gain a sense of self-mastery over anxious situations such as dental visits. In extreme cases of dental phobia, the dentist may admit the patient to the hospital for treatment under general anesthesia or if the dentist has appropriate training, use sedation in the dental office.

The Angry or Agitated Patient

On a rare occasion, a patient may feel angry or briefly agitated about a specific event in the practice. Most often the office manager as patient relations specialist is the person responsible for addressing the patient's anger or agitation. There are strategies the office manager can use to respectfully help diffuse the situation and calm the patient down (Figure 5-5).

Five Steps to Diffuse a Patient's Anger

1. **Let the patient release the anger**—Allow him or her to vent these feelings without being interrupted. Attempts to initially intervene or resolve the situation tend to fuel further anger.

2. **Don't try to lead or second guess where the patient is going with the conversation**—instead, listen! Trying to anticipate his or her comments can further frustrate the patient. What most patients want is to feel understood and to be taken seriously.

3. **Respond only after the patient has fully vented his or her feelings**—Speak in a low, calm voice, breathing slowly to reduce your rate of speech. This reduces the tendency toward defensiveness. Use neutral comments that communicate to the patient that you care about resolving the situation. For example, "How can I help?" or "I can see this is upsetting to you and I'd like to help." Express concern and clarify the problem by asking questions.

4. **Use the three Fs: feel, felt, and found**—A way to remember this is: "I know how you feel; I've felt that way myself sometimes, and I've found this may help."

5. **Avoid the urge to argue**—Clarify the facts, be empathetic but use caution about agreeing with the patient.

© Cengage Learning 2014

FIGURE 5-5 Five steps to diffuse a patient's anger.

Nonverbal Communication

Much of the professionalism and trustworthiness the office manager hopes to express to each patient is portrayed nonverbally. Up to 80 percent of all communication is nonverbal. So our facial expressions and body posture are the most important part of the messages we send to our patients. The professional appearance of the team, the attitude and etiquette of each staff member, and the appearance of the office instill confidence and promote relaxation in patients.

Personal Appearance

The office manager must project herself or himself as an authoritative but approachable person. Personal appearance emphasizes the professional role of the staff members. Hairstyle should be low maintenance and not require significant care during the course of the professional day. Long hair should be pulled away from the face and collar.

Many offices have rules regarding tattoos and piercings. These rules will often be found in the office policies. Employers may require that visible tattoos are covered or a piercing is removed as a condition of employment.

Because hair spray, colognes, aftershave, or cosmetics trigger allergic reaction in some patients, these items should be used sparingly or not at all. The best smell for the closed environment of the dental office is personal cleanliness.

During working hours the office manager must present a conservative, polished, professional image (Figure 5-6). Particular attention must be directed to hands and nails, which must be cared for and clean. Nails should be short, well-manicured, not calling attention to them. Artificial nails are discouraged for the administrative staff as they harbor microscopic pathogens, create undue noise on the computer keyboard, and promote fungal infections in susceptible individuals. Artificial nails are never acceptable for the clinical staff.

A reliable antiperspirant or deodorant is a must, and all staff members should follow professional courtesy of informing each other privately when

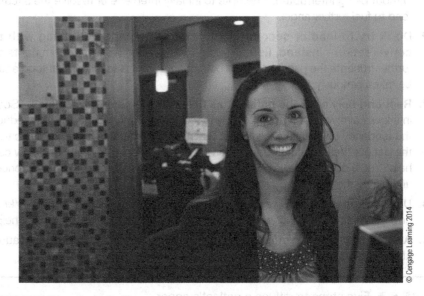

© Cengage Learning 2014

FIGURE 5-6 The dental office manager should have a professional and neat appearance.

there is an issue with personal hygiene or professional attire. The professional office manager needs to be prepared to take this responsibility if requested by the dentist or staff members.

Posture

One of the most important nonverbal communicators is posture. By standing poised to respond and looking a patient in the eye, an office manager can immediately take control of the conversation and identify herself or himself as a person in authority. Many office managers make it a practice to get down to the physical level of patients in wheelchairs by pulling their chairs together to speak in a friendlier manner. Similarly office managers and staff will sit or kneel when they need to speak to a young child rather than towering above him or her from intimidating height. These are examples of postures and body language that facilitate professional communication.

Slouching communicates boredom, or unwillingness to participate. Energetic, alert posture communicates helpfulness and interest. One of the most basic yet most powerful body language signs is when a person crosses his or her arms across the chest. This posture can indicate that the person is putting up an unconscious barrier between himself or herself and the person with whom they are speaking.

Other closed postures, such as hugging oneself or crossing ankles or knees, are usually perceived as compensatory or adaptive postures. They show insecurity, hostility, or withdrawal. The experienced office manager conducts herself or himself gracefully and with authority by keeping hands open and relaxed, poised for helpful gestures or necessary actions, keeping both legs straight with weight evenly distributed. The office manager sits naturally, with both feet on the floor and the ankles crossed.

Attire

Expectations of apparel for dental office managers have undergone fashion changes but the standard should always reflect the role and purpose of the professional combined with the individual practice image.

The current trend for office managers and administrative staff attire is consistent with a business professional. This will vary with different parts of the country being much less formal than others. As a guideline for what professional dress is in your area visit your local bank to see how employees there are dressed. They would be an example of acceptable business professional attire. Members of the clinical dental team wear matching or coordinating scrubs. This can vary depending on the practice, its location, and duties of staff members. Care must be taken that all team members comply with Occupational Safety and Health Administration (OSHA) requirements for attire and footwear. Regardless of the type of clothing it should always be neat, clean, and allow the employee to do the job comfortably. Clothing that is too small restricts movement and the employee runs the risk of overexposure. Excessive cleavage or an exposed midriff is not appropriate in the dental office.

Team Portraits

In addition to formal introductions, many office managers hang framed portraits of the staff members, including the doctor, in the reception area. These serve as a patient relations mechanism in several ways. A picture is the obvious way to become more familiar with the dental team members. The reception area gallery serves as an organizational chart, showing you at a glance the staff members' roles, their names, titles, and credentials.

Portraits convey a strong sense of importance to the dental team. They indicate that each member is a professional. Portraits with plaques showing the credentials of the personnel assure patients that they are in capable and trained hands.

The portraits help patients associate names with faces making further communication much more effective. Portraits also promote pride in the practice. Patients immediately feel a sense of community and a sense of belonging when they enter a practice with portraits in the reception area. The portraits should be taken in office attire to enhance this impact. As new team members join the practice, their portraits should be added as quickly as possible.

If the office has a high staff turnover rate another method of highlighting staff members may be considered. Patients notice and are concerned about potential underlying problems in an office where staff members leave quickly. Having a photo gallery can emphasize how quickly team members come and go. On the other hand, if the dental team has been together for a long time a photo wall can accentuate that also.

Courtesy Communicates Respect

Courtesy and other forms of verbal communication convey a wealth of information to perspective patients and dental team members. This includes a positive, confident attitude, as well as etiquette and courtesy.

Attitude

No discussion on communication is complete without exploring the impact of attitude. Attitude shows in posture, grooming, attire, and spoken communication, as well as unspoken messages. It is crucial to the success of the practice.

Positive attitudinal qualities a dental office manager should strive to maintain include self-confidence, the quality of being genuine, willingness to remain open to new or unfamiliar experiences, and intrinsic appreciation for the varying backgrounds or cultures of others, assertiveness, and integrity.

Etiquette

Etiquette is practicing good manners, knowing how to behave in a given situation, and knowing how to interact with people. Proper etiquette is appropriate everywhere but you may also see the terms professional and social etiquette to define what is appropriate in a business setting or among friends or acquaintances. Professional etiquette helps you make a great first impression for yourself and your practice. Professional etiquette includes nonverbal communication such as a handshake, posture, eye contact, facial expressions, and confidence. It also involves verbal communication including knowing the right thing to say, the right manner in which to phrase it, and the circumstances that require specific comments. Underlying these conventions are cooperation and consideration for the common benefit of all; communication is key. In a professional environment such as a dental practice, *"please"* and *"thank you"* are always required. The office manager says *"Follow me please"* when directing patients. This is more appropriate than *"Would you follow me?"* Each time the patient complies with the request the office manager should say *"Thank you."* During busy office times the dental staff may need to ask a caller if he or she would like to be placed on *"hold"* the term *"hang on"* should never be used in the dental office. An appropriate phrase is *"Would you please hold?"* Always wait for a response after asking the question; never assume you know the answer and always remember to thank the patient.

Professional office managers remember patient's names. When first introduced, the name is always repeated as part of the greeting. It is repeated again when the conversation ends and/or when the patient leaves the office. Terms of endearment are never substituted for names. It is never appropriate to call a patient *"honey"* for example. It is wise to ask the patient what variation of his or her name is preferred. Offices often include this question on an acquaintance form that the patient is asked to complete. Many people have a strong preference for their given names over a common nickname, whereas, others almost never use their given names. It is an important aspect of etiquette to honor the patient's preference consistently.

Patients who use wheelchairs or have some other form of physical disability should be addressed personally. It is not appropriate to speak to the escort as if the disabled person is not capable of conducting a conversation independently.

Simple common courtesy is required as a normal and expected part of office etiquette. Although every office is slightly different, Figure 5-7 provides common sense rules of etiquette when addressing patients or team members.

Follow-up Phone Calls after Treatment

In many practices the office manager or treatment coordinator contacts patients that have had treatment as a courtesy to ensure there are no complications or to answer questions regarding the treatment. In addition to expressing care and concern for the patient, this may prevent unnecessary emergency calls or reduce risks associated with unusual bleeding or swelling, dry sockets, lost temporaries, failure for sensation to return following local anesthetic, ensuring appropriate pain control, or avoiding unnecessary drug reactions. In the long run, this prevents misunderstandings and communicates their commitment to continuity of care for all patients. For the dental office manager this also provides valuable feedback regarding patient satisfaction.

Offering Extended Services

Many practices offer extended services as an expression of hospitality that demonstrate care and concern for their patients' total well-being. Extended services may include referrals to other dental and medical members of the community for tobacco cessation counseling, weight management, massage therapy, nutrition counseling, and hypertension management. Offices may also offer or sponsor cardiopulmonary resuscitation (CPR) classes, oral cancer screening, chewing tobacco education, and sports-related injury awareness and education.

The office manager plays a vital role in providing referral information to patients under the direction of the dentist.

Commonsense Etiquette and Good Manners

- Always use correct grammar; avoid the use of slang or extensive dental jargon when speaking to patients.
- Do not interrupt another person who is speaking.
- Never eat, drink, smoke, or chew gum in front of patients.
- Avoid creating unnecessarily loud noises, such as banging of a patient history clipboard on a countertop or slamming the telephone receiver or file drawer.
- Always hand a piece of paper or chart to another person; do not toss or fling it onto the countertop or desk for the other person to pick up.
- Never lick your fingers when handling paperwork or turning pages of the document. (Think how the next person handling the paper feels!)
- Always introduce unacquainted people. Repeat each person's name for the emphasis.
- If two people are engaged in conversation, avoid standing or sitting within voice range. If you must speak to one of them write a short note or speak to the person later. Only interrupt if it is an emergency.
- Always find a way to complement or praise another person.
- Respect another person's privacy.
- If the phone rings while you are in a conversation with a patient allow another team member to answer it or let it go to voice mail and return the call. Each patient deserves 100% of your attention.
- Avoid extensive or excessive conversations that do not involve the practice or patients.
- Avoid forming office clicks or engaging in office gossip. Remember a staff member that is willing to gossip with you is willing to gossip about you.
- Refrain from nervous mannerisms that distract others, such as fingernail drumming, humming, whistling, lip smacking, or excessive hand or foot movement.
- Always look the other person directly in the eye when engaging in conversation.
- Recognize that people are from different cultures, walks of life, and experiences, and thus have different values.

FIGURE 5-7 Commonsense etiquette and good manners.

 Exploring the Web

Green Dentistry
  www.dentistryiq.com/practice-management/green-dentistry.html
  www.ada.org/goinggreen.aspx

Phone Etiquette
  www.library.thinkquest.org /2993/phone.htm

Proper Etiquette
  www2.binghamton.edu/career-development-center/quick-reference-guides
  /etiquette.pdf

Skill Building

These optional activities and exercises are designed to help the student put into practice information learned in this chapter.

1. Think of at least three experiences you have had recently as a guest. These could be at the homes of friends or strangers, businesses, or professional offices. Divide a sheet of paper into two columns by drawing a vertical line down the center. Label the left column negative and label the right column positive. List the pleasant feelings or events under the second column and the frustrating and frightening, or awkward feelings or events under the first. Using this table as your inspiration, create a list of ideas for a comforting, pleasant, welcoming dental reception area. Use your imagination! Take turns sharing your list with the class and describe how those experiences felt.

2. Have volunteers from the class role play demonstrations of common courtesy, first using the wrong way, then correcting the same situation to the right way. Provide constructive feedback.

3. Imagine you have been put in charge of designing a dental office of the future where patients are treated like important clients or guests. Make a list of amenities and other personal touches you would provide. Share your list with the class.

4. Working in teams role-play handling a very angry patient. Provide constructive feedback.

Challenge Your Understanding

Select the response that best answers each of the following questions. Only one response is correct.

1. The goals of an office patient relations policy are to:
   a. Focus on the patient rather than the procedure
   b. Manage patient flow
   c. Control the environment as much as possible to facilitate optimum dental care
   d. All of the above

2. Get-acquainted-to-the-practice-materials may include any or all of the following except:
   a. A map or printed instructions about office location and parking
   b. Office policies and information about the doctor's professional training
   c. The patient's initial diagnosis
   d. A copy of the practice's newsletter

3. All patients should be greeted as a welcome guest within _____ seconds of their arrival.
   a. 10
   b. 30
   c. 45
   d. 60

4. Special touches for the children's area of the reception room may include all the following except:
   a. Coloring sheets and markers
   b. Jigsaw puzzles
   c. Coffee table books
   d. Video games

5. Proper ventilation and automatic aroma therapy may help reduce the dental office odor associated with traditional practices.
   a. True
   b. False

6. The benefits of taking the new patient on an office tour include:
   a. An increase familiarity
   b. A sense of partnership in health care decisions
   c. An opportunity to ask questions about sterilization procedures
   d. All of the above

7. A normal but enhanced feeling of concern when visiting the dentist is called:
   a. Dental phobia
   b. Dental terror
   c. Dental anxiety
   d. Dental paranoia

8. Which of the following common fears is not typically a problem in the dental office?
   a. Fear of getting lost or not being able to find the office
   b. Fear of heights
   c. Fear of losing control
   d. Fear that treatment will be too expensive

9. What is communicated nonverbally by slouching?
   a. Helpfulness
   b. Boredom
   c. Alertness
   d. Assertiveness

10. Greeting protocol can be mastered by:
    a. Keeping aware of the time and schedule
    b. Monitoring guests in the reception area closely
    c. Rehearsing names when necessary so they can be pronounced easily and naturally as patients enter the office
    d. All of the above

11. Why should the office manager wear business attire if he or she is not required to wear scrubs?
    a. He or she may be sued for impersonating a surgeon
    b. He or she should wear only flattering colors

   c. He or she is more effective at communicating if the attire suggests a business professional

   d. Scrubs are too warm for most dental office

12. Which of the following is not a desirable attitude for a dental office manager to cultivate?
   a. Self-confidence
   b. Self-absorption
   c. Appreciation for diverse backgrounds and cultures
   d. Assertiveness

13. Team portraits displayed in the office:
   a. Help patients familiarize themselves with names and faces
   b. Display team pride
   c. Introduce team members as professionals
   d. All of the above

14. Most patients prefer to be addressed as honey or another similar term of endearment
   a. True
   b. False

15. If two people are engaged in conversation, common courtesy dictates the office manager should:
   a. Avoid standing or sitting within voice range
   b. Leave a short note or speak to the person later
   c. Interrupt briefly to communicate the issue
   d. All of the above

16. Providing the follow-up care phone calls:
   a. Answers patients questions regarding treatment
   b. Communicates care and concern for the patient
   c. Addresses postoperative complications or drug reactions
   d. All of the above

17. When handling concerns of an angry patient, the office manager should interrupt periodically so the patient can take a moment to calm down.
   a. True
   b. False

18. When placing a patient on hold:
   a. Politely ask the patients permission
   b. Remember to do so quickly to save time
   c. *"Hang on"* is appropriate in some geographical areas
   d. *"Would you please hold"* implies consent

Marketing the Practice

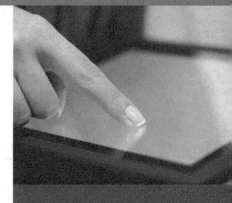

CHAPTER OUTLINES

KEY TERMS

advertising
direct marketing
  campaign
event marketing
external marketing
focus group
internal marketing
marketing
media
patient attributes
patient profiles
target audience
target mailings
social networking

LEARNING OBJECTIVES

Upon completion of this chapter, the reader should be able to:

1. Describe the need for marketing in dentistry.
2. Define and differentiate between marketing and advertising as they relate to dentistry.

3. Describe the necessity of a marketing budget and related terminology.

4. Describe the types of internal and external marketing programs as they relate to dentistry.

5. Discuss the importance and rationale of tracking results of marketing efforts in the dental practice.

6. Explain the rationale and importance of referral source management.

7. Discuss the importance of an office website and social network marketing.

The Necessity for Practice Marketing

During the past decade, the need for dental practices to market themselves has developed as a result of increasing competition for patients. Significant changes in dental practices have evolved owing to rising costs of dental care, declining birth rate, reduced dental insurance benefits, an increase in managed care programs, and rising dental school enrollments. Marketing concepts that have evolved from other professions, when applied ethically and professionally, can be used successfully to gain new patients, create an increased demand for dental services from the existing patient base, and generate additional referrals.

Although many people use the terms interchangeably, advertising and marketing are different. **Advertising** is the promotion of products or services provided by a business or organization through a variety of **media**, including telephone directories, newspapers, magazines, radio, television broadcast, and billboards.

By contrast, **marketing** is creating the demand, need, or awareness for a product or service the consumer (in this case the patient) may have desired but may have been unaware that it was available. Today, many practices effectively and ethically promote their individualized services using a variety of internal and external marketing strategies.

The American Dental Association (ADA) offers a variety of publications, reports, and booklets on ethical marketing for dental practices. Practices having questions about ethical marketing may contact the ADA for further information. Marketing a profession such as dentistry is unique because a skill or service is being sold rather than a product. Dentists have established guidelines concerning promoting their practices while still maintaining the dignity of the profession. The ADA through its membership directs the ethical marketing of a dental practice.

Some dental advertising may also be regulated under the State Dental Practice Act so the dental office manager should be aware of any laws pertaining to the advertising or marketing of a dental practice.

Key Elements of Dental Marketing

Four key elements of successful dental marketing campaigns that office managers should be familiar with include:

1. Create a need
2. Demonstrate expertise
3. Emphasize affordability
4. Offer convenience

Create a Need

Only about one half of the American population visits the dentist regularly, and fewer than that take advantage of specialized dental services. Many expanded dental services include not only the dental treatment itself, but offer a cosmetic benefit as well. Thus, a practice that wishes to increase the number of crowns and veneers, cosmetic bonding cases, or tooth bleaching procedures it does may promote cosmetic dentistry as a benefit or feature associated with service.

The patient's psychological association of elevated self-esteem, increased self-confidence, a youthful appearance, or preservation of his or her natural smile, are benefits often used to create a need for services in the mind of the patient. Terms such as "whiter teeth," "straighter teeth," "fresher breath," and "a more attractive smile" are often used as benefits of cosmetic dental procedures (Figure 6-1).

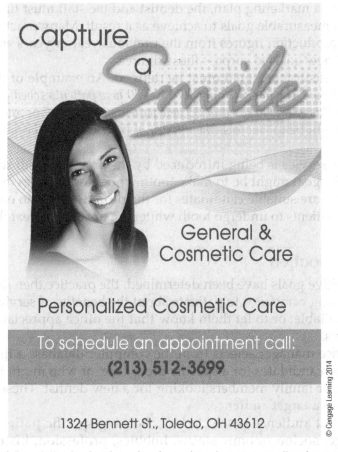

FIGURE 6-1 Advertizing in dentistry is often aimed at personalized care and enhancement of patient appearance.

Demonstrate Expertise

After the need has been created, the marketing-minded practice must demonstrate its expertise in solving patients' perceived problems to produce desired results. Many practices stress the dentist's specialized education and continuing education training to meet the identified need. Patients as consumers often perceive that special training offers a higher level of service or aesthetic result.

Emphasize Affordability

Practices who promote themselves through marketing programs must also provide ways to make it easy for the patient to afford their services. Types of payment plans to meet patient needs are addressed in Chapter 13 (Managing Accounts Receivable).

Offer Convenience

Patients as consumers expect convenience as a primary factor in making purchasing decisions. Dental practices that offer expanded treatment days, extended hours, or multiple locations, emphasize these conveniences to patients and prospective patients in their marketing campaigns.

Goal Setting

To formulate a marketing plan, the dentist and the staff must first brainstorm to establish measurable goals to achieve as a result. Many practices began by reviewing production figures from the previous year or years and then strategize to set new goals to surpass those figures.

To be measurable a goal must be defined. An example of the definable goal would be: *"The practice currently has 30 new patients scheduled per month. Our goal for this year is to schedule 35 new patients per month"* or another measurable goal might be to *"increase the number of veneers during the next quarter from 45 to 50."*

If a new service is being introduced by the practice, tooth whitening, for example, the goal might be to make tooth whitening services available to all patients who are suitable candidates for the procedure and to enroll a certain number of patients to undergo tooth whitening during the next three months.

Patient Selection

Once definitive goals have been determined, the practice then develops a direct marketing campaign to patients about the benefits of services, new procedures available, or to let them know that the office appreciates referral of new patients.

The office manager selects from the computer database a list of patients who may be candidates for a specific procedure, or who might have friends, coworkers, or family members looking for a new dentist. These patients are referred to as a target audience.

The target audience is selected by choosing specific patient attributes, such as age, socioeconomic status, hobbies, profession, history with the practice, ability to tolerate an elective procedure, and oral health suitable

THINK Green

Even though the computer itself uses additional electricity, using it to print materials only to a target audience can minimize printing materials you don't need. Marketing to patients by email can be a highly effective green practice because the message is received almost immediately and no paper or ink needs to be used.

to undergo the service. Working with the dentist, the office manager determines these specific attributes and prints out a list of suitable candidates to whom to market.

Use of the Computer in Marketing the Practice

For many office managers, the practice's computer is an invaluable tool for implementing, driving, analyzing, and tracking marketing programs directed toward patients. The office manager uses the practice's computer to create patient profiles containing specific attributes or items for each patient.

These patient attributes may be used for specific target mailings identified by patient profiles. The office manager uses the computer to print out lists of specific patients targeted to receive mailings on the topic or dental technique of interest in any category of the computer software's selection criteria.

The office manager also uses the computer to print out mailing address labels or to address postcards or envelopes directly to patients who comprise the target audience.

The Marketing Budget

A marketing budget must be established prior to devising a marketing plan. On average, most dental offices spend 5 percent of their total overhead (expenses) on their marketing programs. If, for example, the practice has a yearly gross (total amount of dentistry produced and collected) of $600,000 and the overhead (expenses required to run a practice) is 65 percent, or $390,000, 5 percent of the overhead equals $19,500 as a total yearly marketing budget for the practice.

Internal Marketing

Internal marketing includes any promotional efforts directed toward patients and their families currently enrolled in the practice. An internal marketing campaign may encompass one or more types of promotions. One common internal marketing promotion is giving a prize or free service such as whitening for the referral of friends or family. Another example of internal marketing might be encouraging patients to have dentistry before the end of the year to receive a tax deduction or to maximize their insurance benefits.

Patient Satisfaction

Some practices use patient satisfaction surveys as part of their internal marketing program to improve their existing levels of service or create new services or improvements. The office manager uses patient satisfaction survey results to monitor, assess, analyze, and improve upon levels of expectation and perceived quality of care reported by patients.

Patient satisfaction is measured using a variety or combination of survey tools including telephone surveys, face-to-face surveys, email surveys, and mail-in surveys. Dental office managers must also monitor satisfaction review Websites such as Yahoo and Dr. Oogle along with many other "review" Websites. Dissatisfied patients often use these sites because they provide anonymity and this can be especially frustrating to the dental staff. Dental office managers should encourage satisfied patients to add their comments on these Websites as a part of marketing the practice.

Read the reviews and comments objectively to determine if indeed a problem does exist. For example: a comment might say "great doctor and staff but they are always running late so expect to have to wait"; if this is true, adjustments to the current scheduling may be warranted. The only thing worse than being made aware of a problem on a public review forum is not addressing and resolving it.

Focus groups

Another method some practices use to improve levels of patient satisfaction or to determine new services the patient population may be interested in is periodic focus groups. A focus group is a small group or representative cross-section of the patient base.

The function of a focus group is to obtain valid feedback and suggestions from a cross-sectional representation of patients. The office manager uses this opportunity to record patient perceptions and impressions of the practice and to obtain specific suggestions for improvement in services or office amenities. On the dentist's direction, the office manager selects and schedules focus groups that meet as often as monthly or as occasionally as one or two times annually. These patients could receive a small reward or incentive for their time as long as there is no expectation beyond honest feedback.

In larger practices, the focus group may be directed by an outside marketing organization in which an independent moderator asks patient-specific questions about the practice and solicits suggestions for improvement.

Event Marketing

Event marketing is a form of marketing that acknowledges specific events or occasions according to information contained in the patient's personal profile. The office manager uses this information to acknowledge the special event in the patient's life or reason for celebration. Examples of event marketing might include patient birthdays and anniversaries within the practice, graduations, job promotions, and retirement.

A practice may use other types of event marketing to promote itself with celebrations such as an annual office open house to celebrate a specific number of years in practice. If an office undergoes a transition, such as a purchase or sale or entering into a partnership, this may also be announced and celebrated through an event-marketing program.

Some practices use these occasions to make special promotions or offers either to existing patients or others in the community who may be interested in becoming patients. Examples of special marketing promotions include rewards to existing patients for referring new patients or incentive services to new patients such as complimentary x-rays or exam at their first visit.

External Marketing

External marketing is another form of practice marketing. As the name implies, it is the opposite of internal marketing and encompasses specific targeted promotions to people outside of the practice or prospective patients, for example, those people who may, as a result of receiving marketing messages targeted directly to them, inquire about becoming patients.

External marketing encompasses a number of methods for contacting prospective patients, including radio and television spots either through advertisements or public information segments, notices in telephone directories and community newspaper columns, participation at health fairs, press releases, or articles about the practice published in the newspaper.

Some dental practices use outside mailing houses or independent marketing services to distribute external marketing flyers, mailing inserts, or other notices to new residents in the neighborhood. For maximum impact, mailings are selected using predetermined local zip codes within a specific radius of the practice. Some dentists also use list management services for new move-in information from local mailing services, and direct-mail organizations to send get acquainted mailings or welcome to the neighborhood greetings to new residents.

Public Speaking

Public speaking is a form of external marketing often used by dentists to gain community exposure and referrals of new patients. Public speaking is an excellent opportunity for the dentist to address a particular aspect of the practice or available services, such as pit and fissure sealants, cosmetic bonding, prevention of dental and periodontal disease, or prevention and treatment of sports-related mouth injuries.

Public speaking presentations should be geared to the specific target audience for the best effect. When addressing parent groups, for example, the dentist may speak on the development of children's teeth, the benefits of pit and fissure sealants, fluoride, chewing tobacco awareness, or preventing sports-related injuries. When speaking to a more mature target audience, the dentist may choose topics such as crown and bridge, prevention and treatment of periodontal disease, or dental implants.

Because people in the audience often have questions about specific dental procedures, the dentist can use a speaking engagement as a marketing opportunity by providing appointment or business cards, practice pamphlets, or other helpful handouts. Additional effective presentation and teaching tools include educational videos and personalized patient education brochures.

Tracking Marketing Results

To analyze the effectiveness of marketing promotions or campaigns, the office manager must track the results and report periodically to the dentist and team members. The office manager can track marketing campaign results using a variety of methods. If the practice is trying to attract new patients, the office manager can simply ask all new patients, "Who may we thank for referring you to our practice?" The office manager maintains a record of referral sources that includes patient's name, the source of referral, and when appropriate how the referral was acknowledged.

The office manager may also track results by compiling a report listing the number of new patients enrolled in the practice as a result of direct mailing to new residents in nearby zip codes. The office manager should also track all specific procedures completed and note increasing or decreasing trends.

When an office is using marketing to increase the number of crowns being done, the office manager can track the total number of crowns and compare the tally with the previous monthly number. For example, if the previous monthly total was 35 units and the practice's goal was to increase this to 40, the office manager can track this month's total and note an increase to 42 units; this indicates the practices goal was exceeded.

Many practices include monthly or quarterly bonuses paid to staff for meeting or exceeding production goals.

Referral Source Analysis

Referrals represent a significant source of practice growth. In fact 80 percent of new patients are referred by 20 percent of the practice's existing patient base. Many practices use referral source analysis as a method for monitoring the source of new patients, the number of dollars generated as a result, and increases in demand for specific types of dental procedures or services. The office manager maintains and prints out referral source analysis reports from the computer that provide information on the source of referrals and the total fees generated as a result. Referral tracking using practice management software is covered in Section VI.

Thanking Referral Sources

Under the dentist's direction, the office manager uses the information from the referral source analysis to send thank you cards or letters to patients, professional colleagues, or associates of the dentist who refer new patients to the practice. In addition to thank you cards and letters, many practices show their appreciation for new patient referrals by sending flowers, gift certificates, or tickets to theater or local sporting events.

Using a variety of marketing strategies and campaigns, the practice can increase new patient referrals and the demand for additional services.

Dental Office Website

An office Website has become a critical part of practice marketing. Prospective patients rely on a Website to supply information about the doctor, staff, and location of the practice. Websites can be simple and inexpensive or elaborate, interactive, and pricy.

When planning the office Website, the dental team, under the guidance of the dentist and office manager, needs to decide what they want to include on the Website, the budget, and the amount of time needed to keep it current. They may also want to consider if additional staff training will be needed.

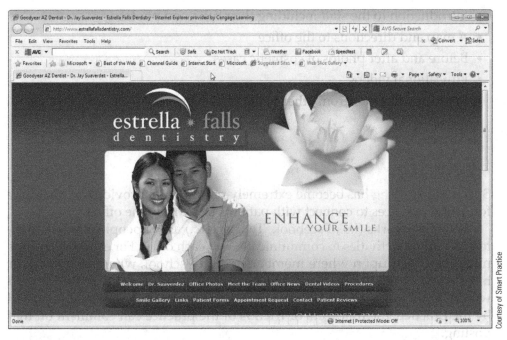

Courtesy of Smart Practice

FIGURE 6-2 A practices Website can serve to attract new patients as well as provide a resource for current patients.

A simple and economical Website can be done with a template from many different dental suppliers. These follow a fill in the blank format and do not require an experienced person for setup or maintenance. Although these are simple, they can still include multiple tabs with information and patient education information as seen in Figure 6-2.

Some practices hire a professional to create a unique custom Website that contains the same basic information but also might include patient acquaintance forms that can be completed and submitted online or even allow the patient to access their appointment and account information.

Regardless of whether the Website is designed by a template or customized, it must be kept current for maximum effectiveness. When a patient opens the practice Website and sees 4th of July in December or a newsletter from two years ago, they will question the attention to detail within the practice. Patients have no real way of evaluating the actual quality of materials and technique of the dental services they have received; they rely on the overall experience and the things they can see regarding the practice such as its Website. The contents for a practice Website may include:

- Welcome to the Practice
- Introduction to the dentist highlighting education, experience, and a photo

THINK Green

Even a simple Website not only promotes the practice but allows you to post newsletters and even give patients access to previous newsletters. Depending on your practice some patients may still want the newsletter as hard copy but many patients prefer just to view it online saving paper.

- Introduction to the staff including their roles and photos
- A map and directions to the office
- Before and after photos of cosmetic cases
- Educational videos
- Recommendations from other patients in the practice

Social Networking

Social networking has become extremely popular and provides another way for dental practices to connect with patients away from the office.

Social networks (i.e., Facebook, Twitter, etc.) allow people who share interests and/or activities to communicate with each other. For example, groups might be based upon where members went to school, where they work or have worked, or simply friends in common. In this case, the shared thread would be the dentist/dental practice. When something of interest is posted by the practice, the followers or friends of the practice can comment on that posting.

Dental offices might use a social network to promote the non-dental as well as dental side of the practice. A dental team might post volunteer work they are doing in the community or activities they are involved with away from the office, such as sports. Because non-patients can view what the office is doing it is another way of marketing the practice. To make the practice's social networking sites easy to find, the practice's social media pages can be linked directly to the practice webpage.

To be effective, social networks must be monitored and kept up to date. As comments can be added by patients, staff, and prospective patients, comments need to be checked frequently to make sure they are appropriate. To be an effective tool, social networking sites need to be updated on a regular basis. Maintaining a social network involves a commitment by the dentist and staff. Patients and prospective patients will stop visiting if nothing is happening. HIPAA applies to patients' privacy in regard to anything *posted by your office* on websites or social networking sites.

Things to consider before getting started in a social network:

- Does social networking reach the target audience of patients and prospective patients?
- Do we have time to maintain our network with the same high quality as our dentistry?
- Does this fit within our mission and office philosophy?

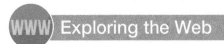

Exploring the Web

Dental Economics — Practice Management Magazine
www.dentaleconomics.com

Skill Building

These optional activities and exercises are designed to help the student put into practice information learned in the chapter.

1. Divide into groups and choose a team leader within each group; every team member will be assigned to contact (call or visit) a different office in the area to determine what type of marketing programs the office uses and to request samples of their marketing materials. In a later designated class, each team member will give a five-minute presentation of the offices marketing programs and show examples of the marketing materials. The class will discuss what marketing efforts it thinks would be most effective and give reasons why.

2. Find direct-mail companies that are promoting dental office marketing materials online. Bring ideas to the classroom and discuss ways these materials could be used in a dental practice.

3. Invite a local dental office to send a representative (for example the doctor, the office manager, or the entire team) to make an office marketing presentation to the class. Be prepared to ask questions such as "how did you determine this was the most effective marketing for your practice?" "What would you do differently?" "What would you include in your next marketing campaign?"

Challenge Your Understanding

Select the response that best answers each of the following questions. Only one answer is correct.

1. The need for dental offices to engage in marketing campaigns has evolved because of all of the following except:
   a. Changes in dental practice patterns
   b. An increase in the birth rate
   c. Reduction of dental insurance benefits
   d. Increase in the dental school enrollments

2. Practiced ethically, marketing concepts can be successfully used to:
   a. Increase the number of new patients
   b. Increase in demand for services from the existing patient base
   c. Generate referrals
   d. All of the above

3. Marketing is the promotion of products or services available from a specific business organization through a variety of media.
   a. True
   b. False

4. Forms of media the dental practice may use for marketing include:
   a. Radio and television broadcasting
   b. Billboards, newspapers, and magazines
   c. Advertisements in telephone directories
   d. Any or all of the above

5. Dental practices may ethically promote their services using a variety of _____ and _____ strategies.
   a. Internal/external
   b. Formal/informal
   c. Exogenous/intravenous
   d. Ethical/unethical

6. On average, U.S. dental practices spent about _____ percent of their total overhead on marketing.
   a. 5
   b. 8
   c. 10
   d. 12

7. Examples of event marketing include:
   a. Patients' birthdays
   b. Anniversaries in the practice
   c. Patient attributes
   d. Both a and b

8. Patient satisfaction may be measured through:
   a. Telephone surveys
   b. Face-to-face surveys with patients
   c. Patient focus groups
   d. Any or all of the above

9. External marketing may include target mailings to new residents in the neighborhood according to zip code numbers.
   a. True
   b. False

10. The results of any marketing promotion or campaign are incomplete without tracking the results.
    a. True
    b. False

11. Referral source analysis reports created by the office manager provide information that:
    a. Pinpoints referrals sources who recommended new patients
    b. Reports the total fees generated from these new patients
    c. Reflects the results of patient satisfaction surveys
    d. All of the above

12. In addition to sending thank you cards and letters, some practices show their appreciation for new patient referrals with:
    a. Complimentary dinners
    b. Flowers sent to the refers place of business
    c. Tickets to the theater or local sporting events
    d. All of the above

13. The key elements to a successful dental marketing campaign include all of the following except:
    a. Creating a need
    b. Demonstrating expertise
    c. Emphasizing overall expense
    d. Offering convenience

14. Psychological correlation to elevated self-esteem, increased self-confidence, any youthful appearance or preservation of the patient's natural smile are marketing benefits often used to create a need for services in the mind of the patient.
    a. True
    b. False

15. To be measurable, goals must be definable.
    a. True
    b. False

16. A dentist recently purchased a new laser and wants to market the benefits of laser treatment to patients. Which of the following represents the best measurable goal that can be tracked?
    a. To inform and educate our patients about the benefits of laser treatment
    b. To inform and educate our patients about the benefit of laser treatment and to schedule 10 laser appointments per month during the first quarter of the year
    c. To compare our laser treatment figures to those of another practice in the building
    d. All of the above

17. The practice website might contain all of the following, *except*:
    a. New patient forms
    b. The practice newsletter
    c. Fees for office procedures
    d. Photos of the practice and dentist

18. Social network marketing connects patients and prospective patients in a fun online setting.
    a. True
    b. False

Printed Communications

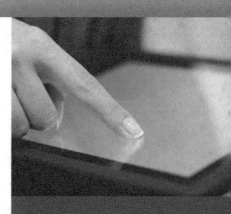

CHAPTER OUTLINES

- **Printed Communication**
  The Logo Sets the Practice Tone
  Letterhead Stationery
  Business Cards
  Appointment Cards
  Practice Statements
  Practice Brochures and Information Packets
  Cards as Practice Builders
  Practice Surveys
- **Business Letters**
  Business Letter Styles
  Welcome to the Practice Letter
  Thank You for the Referral Letter
- **Other Printed Communication from the Practice**
- **Email**
  Basic Rules for Using Email

LEARNING OBJECTIVES

Upon completion of this chapter, the reader should be able to:

1. Describe the importance of a logo in practice identity.
2. List the components of letterhead stationery.
3. Describe the reasons for all staff members to have practice business cards.
4. List the necessary information contained on an appointment card.

KEY TERMS

appointment card
business card
email
information packet
letterhead stationery
logo
newsletter
patient education
   brochures
practice brochure
practice survey
recall card
referrals
statement

5. List the components of a practice statement.

6 Describe the importance of the practice brochure and introductory information packet.

7. List the ways patient education brochures are used effectively in practice communications.

8. Describe important components of a practice newsletter and the role of an office manager in newsletter organization and production.

9. Describe the importance of recall cards in retaining patients.

10. Describe how birthday cards and other holiday cards are used as an effective marketing tool in the dental office.

11. List the components of a well-written business letter.

12. Discuss the elements and uses of email within the dental practice.

Printed Communication

The dental office manager is the primary communications director for the practice. As such, it is her or his responsibility to see that all communications, whether printed, electronic, or verbal, are in keeping with the doctor's standards and the philosophy of the practice. This chapter addresses the primary components of printed communications sent from the dental office.

The Logo Sets the Practice Tone

A logo is a design or symbol that represents a business, or in this case the dental practice. The practice logo may consist of a visual graphic such as a picture or symbol, letters, words, the name of the practice or the doctor's name, or all of these elements (Figure 7-1).

Great care and thought must be used when designing or changing a practice logo, as this is the symbol patients, other professionals, and members of the community recognize as representing the dentist and the office.

A logo reflects the tone or philosophy of the practice, and may be as simple as a single tooth or letter and may be friendly and casual in nature. The logo may reflect the type of practice (general or specialty) and specific services offered.

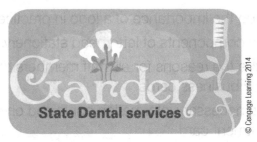

FIGURE 7-1 A well designed logo will be well recognized within the practice community.

Once established, the logo appears on all printed communications of the practice. These may include, but are not limited to, stationery, business cards, appointment cards, recall notices, monthly statements, uniforms and scrubs, checks, envelopes, practice brochures, information packets, newsletters, recall cards, the practice Website, and imprinted giveaways.

Letterhead Stationery

Office **letterhead stationery** is a key component in printed communication to patients, other doctor's offices, and professional contacts. It contains all pertinent information required to contact the doctor or the doctor's practice, including the name of the practice or the doctor's name, professional credentials and other designations such as DDS, DMD, PC, FAGD, the type of practice, the office address telephone number, email address, and Website information.

Stationery should include standard size business paper, 8.5" x 11", with matching envelopes. It may also include additional blank pages that are used for second pages of letters, smaller notecards called monarch size with matching envelopes and/or notepads. All pieces of letterhead stationery are printed with identical practice information and the logo. Many dentists also have their prescription pads printed with the letterhead information and logo, as well as, other pertinent information required for writing prescriptions such as license or Drug Enforcement Agency (DEA) number.

Business Cards

The **business card** is also a key component of the practice's printed communication (Figure 7-2). It is essentially a marketing device that contains all of the information found on the letterhead stationery in a condensed size.

Business cards are given out to promote the practice and as a convenient means for patients of record, prospective patients, or other professionals to contact the office.

THINK Green

When purchasing letterhead or other paper products, look for the highest amount of post–consumer recycled material.

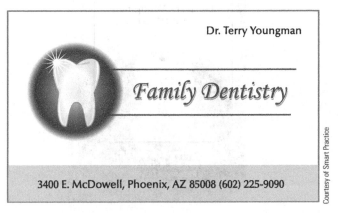

Dr. Terry Youngman

Family Dentistry

3400 E. McDowell, Phoenix, AZ 85008 (602) 225-9090

Courtesy of Smart Practice

FIGURE 7-2 Business cards are a method used to help promote the practice.

Many practices also provide individual business cards for all of their staff members. Individual business cards promote self-esteem and provide staff members the opportunity to promote the practice to prospective patients. A business card from a staff member can also encourage patients to call the practice after appointments with treatment questions or concerns.

Appointment Cards

The primary use of the **appointment card** is a courtesy to remind patients of their next dental visit. One appointment card style contains the business card information on one side and the specifics of the appointment on the reverse (Figure 7-3). Like a business card, the appointment card provides all of the necessary information to contact the office.

Some practices have a self-adhesive appointment card where the appointment information can be peeled off and attached to a desk or wall calendar as a reminder of the appointment.

Practices using practice management software to schedule appointments can print an appointment reminder slip when the appointment is scheduled. Using the directions in Chapter 23 (Communication Using Practice Management Software; Section VI) and the Dentrix Learning CD at the back of the book, you can print appointment reminders and attach the next appointment information directly from the appointment book to statements or walkout information.

Specific appointment information includes the patient's name, the day of the week, the date, and time. Including a year is a good idea because appointment cards often get buried in purses, wallets, or drawers for extended times. In a practice with multiple doctors, the appointment card may also indicate the name of the specific doctor or hygienist that will be treating the patient.

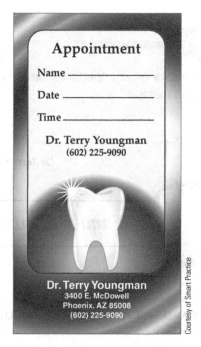

Appointment

Name _____

Date _____

Time _____

Dr. Terry Youngman
(602) 225-9090

Dr. Terry Youngman
3400 E. McDowell
Phoenix, AZ 85008
(602) 225-9090

Courtesy of Smart Practice

FIGURE 7-3 An appointment card serves as a reminder to patients.

Most appointment cards also contain an office policy statement requesting that the patient contact the office 24 hours in advance if a change of appointment is necessary. This is a courtesy to the office that prevents lost production time because of failed or broken appointments. It is a policy of some practices to assess a charge for broken appointments. Because this charge is almost always less than the fee the patient would have paid for treatment, preventing broken appointments is a goal of using appointment cards in the dental practice.

Practice Statements

The practice statement is the primary means by which the practice receives compensation from patients for services provided. Thus, statements are an important form of printed communication from the practice. The practice statement contains all information provided in the office letterhead. It also contains the name of the patient, responsible party (if different from the patient), the type of service rendered, the fee or fees for services rendered, the history of the account (how many days the balance has been owed to the practice), and the balance due (see Chapter 13: Managing Accounts Receivable, for additional information on patient statements.)

The practice statement may also be used to communicate information or new services available, extended office hours, holiday greetings, or to introduce new staff members.

Practice Brochures and Information Packets

Distributing information about the office may also be done with practice brochures, information packets, patient education brochures, and newsletters.

The Practice Brochure

A practice brochure, sometimes referred to as a "Welcome to the Practice," brochure introduces the practice philosophy and policies to new patients. A practice brochure can

- increase recognition of the practice's name among prospective patients;
- reinforce information about the practice to existing patients;
- communicate the practice's mission statement and philosophy;
- provide information about the practice, including the location, office hours, payment plans, acceptance of insurance and other third-party payment systems, and the types of services available for patients; and
- indicate education and level of experience of the dentist, hygienist, dental assistant, office manager, and receptionist.

THINK Green

Most offices collect co-pays or payments at the time of treatment and provide a receipt or walkout statement showing the payment and the amount the patient should expect the insurance company to pay. This reduces printing and mailing costs, as well as, accounts receivable.

The practice brochure can be used

- as a marketing piece to attract new patients;
- to reinforce the practice to patients of record;
- as a referral communication device for other professionals;

The Practice Information Packet

The practice information packet provides a number of pieces of information about the practice. It is often used in conjunction with the practice brochure to describe, in detail, amenities, services, and the policies of the office such as children's play area, handicapped access ramps and parking, and referral to specialists.

The practice information packet may additionally contain

- an enlarged map inset and printed directions to the office;
- a description of public transportation and parking amenities;
- the doctor's educational training and background, areas of expertise, a brief history of the practice, and the doctor's personal philosophy and hobbies or outside interests;
- an introduction of staff members and the respective roles in the practice;
- financial policies and general fee information;
- information for new patients about what to expect;
- the individualized types of services offered; and
- request for referrals.

Patient Education Brochures

Patient education brochures help inform patients about oral conditions and the need for preventive, restorative, postoperative, or corrective treatment. They can save valuable chairside time explaining procedures and reinforcing information given by the doctor during chairside consultations or formal case presentations.

Patient education brochures are available in a wide variety of topics and help answer most commonly asked prevention and treatment questions of the patients. Patient education brochures also serve as a reminder to the patient when explaining proposed treatment to a family member following the conclusion of the appointment.

Patient education brochures should be imprinted or stamped with the office name or doctor's name, address, and telephone number. This information readily assists patients who wish to call the office with additional questions about treatment or postoperative care.

Many offices have a display rack featuring a variety of patient education printed material in the reception area. These may be purchased from the American Dental Association (ADA) or one of many dental supply companies.

The Practice Newsletter

Many practices send out a newsletter to households of patients of record and to referring colleagues. The office newsletters communicate information about the practice and the services it provides. The newsletter may also provide interesting developments in dental techniques and treatments and offer professional advice to patients.

Newsletters may be prepared by the doctor or staff or they may be prepared by an outside professional newsletter service. Most often it is the office manager's responsibility to prepare the production schedule and arrange content of the newsletter, ensure it is printed, the labels are printed, and it is mailed out in a timely manner. If the office has transitioned to an online newsletter, the process of preparation is basically the same as it is for a traditional newsletter; just the delivery system has changed.

Newsletter content is most often determined by specific columns or topics of interest, such as a letter from the dentist, clinical or treatment updates, puzzles, games, healthful recipes, staff news, or practice changes. The newsletter may also be used to announce specific practice events or promotions such as a smile contest, share news of the doctor and staff visiting a local school, or to promote oral hygiene and regular dental visits at a local health fair, as well as inform readers of postgraduate and continuing education courses completed by the doctor and/or staff.

Each issue of the newsletter should also carry a seasonal theme or event, such as "back-to-school checkup time" or "sealed with a smile" to promote pit and fissure sealants.

Cards as Practice Builders

Many practices also use cards to communicate with patients. The most commonly sent include recall notices, birthday cards, and anniversary cards.

Recall Notices

Returning patients, called "recall or recare patients," represent a significant lifeline to the practice. A recall card is a printed reminder of the need for a preventive dental care visit, usually issued every six months, although some periodontal patients may require more frequent appointments.

Many practices make patient appointments for a six-month cleaning and exam when patients are in the office and then mail the recall card one to two weeks prior to the appointment as a reminder. Other practices prefer to wait until the patient is due for the recall appointment and contact patients with a phone call or send a printed recall card inviting the patient to schedule an appointment.

Birthday Cards

Practices include date of birth in individual patient data files. In recording this information for medical and insurance purposes, many practices also use it to send out birthday cards (Figure 7-4). These can be printed out at the end of the previous month and circulated around the office so the whole staff can sign

THINK Green

Some offices are using email as a replacement for the traditional recall card sent by mail. This eliminates the paper card and ink and may be more reliable for people who are connected to computers and smart phones.

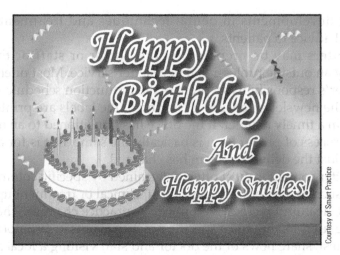

Courtesy of Smart Practice

FIGURE 7-4 Birthday cards are a nice way for a practice to stay in touch with patients.

them. For maximum effectiveness they should be sent near the patient's actual birthday. An easy way to do this is by writing the birth date under where the stamp will go then send them throughout the month.

Practices also send cards or letters for special occasions, such as congratulations on a new baby or new job. Some practices also recognize the special achievements of their school-age patients in sports, drama, dance, art, or other activities.

Practice Surveys

The practice survey or patient satisfaction survey is another way to communicate with patients. This type of written communication enables the practice to improve existing services and amenities, extend office hours, and make improvements in communication with patients. The practice survey may be designed to be completed anonymously by the patient and either placed into a survey box located in the reception area or mailed back to the practice with a stamped, self-addressed return envelope.

Practice surveys are a key measure in assessing the patient's level of satisfaction with service or treatment. They provide information in areas where improvements can be made in efficiency, delivery of services, and courtesy.

Business Letters

The responsibility for developing well-written business letters most often belongs to the office manager. A well-written letter includes a structure that conveys a message with clarity and professionalism. A business letter contains the following components: (see Figures 7-5 and 7-6)

1. The date
2. The address of the recipient
3. Salutation or greeting to the recipient
4. The body or content of the letter
5. The complimentary close

6. Signature
7. Typed signature
8. Reference initials
9. The enclosure (optional)

Business Letter Styles

Business letters are written in different styles, depending on the type of letter and the doctor's preference.

- **Full block style:** there are no indentations; all copy begins at the left margin.
- **Block I style:** the inside address is flush with the left margin; the date and complimentary close are slightly off center and aligned with each other.
- **Block II style:** this style uses block form with no indentations or punctuation after the salutation or complimentary close. Both the right and left margins are justified.
- **Semi-block style:** the inside address is blocked; the first line of each paragraph is indented; the date and complimentary close are slightly to the right of the center page. This letter contains a subject line.
- **Official style:** there is no subject line and each paragraph is indented; the date and complimentary close are at the center of the page.

Welcome to the Practice Letter

Because new patients are a vital key to continue practice growth, one of the most common types of letters written to patients is a welcome to the practice letter. Figures 7-5 and 7-6 are examples of new patient letters using different letter styles.

Thank You for the Referral Letter

Referrals represent a significant form of practice building for all professionals, another important letter from the dental office to another practitioner or a patient is a "thank you for the referral" letter. A referral is a recommendation made by one person to another. Usually the referral is from a patient in the practice to a new person seeking a dentist but not always. Dental practices welcome referrals from all sources.

Other Printed Communication from the Practice

The practice may use additional printed communications for promotional efforts to patients of record and to prospective patients. These include, but are not limited to, imprinted practice giveaways such as pens, pencils, toothbrushes, tote bags, magnets, key chains, and mugs. The purpose of imprinted practice giveaways is to generate referrals and to make it easy for patients to contact the office by having the doctor's name and telephone number readily available.

Philip R. Richardson, DDS
401 Main Street
Morrison, UT 84076
(222) 224-0560
www.richardsondental.com

① Month, Day, Year

② Mrs. Janice Larson
793 West Wishing Well Lane
Morrison, UT 84076

③ Dear Mrs. Larson,

Thank you for choosing us as your dental team. We are delighted to welcome you to our family dental practice.

We are committed to excellence and providing you the finest quality dental care available. Our goal is to help you attain and keep a beautiful smile for a lifetime.

④ We are looking forward to your first visit on Monday, April 7th, at 10:00 am. You may visit our website at www.richardsondental.com, print the acquaintance form and health history to complete at your convenience. Make sure you bring any insurance information that will assist us in filing your dental claim.

Enclosed is a brochure to acquaint you with our office. If you have any questions about your first visit or need directions to our office, please call us at (222) 224-0560.

⑤ Sincerely,

⑥

⑦ Phillip R. Richardson, DDS

⑧ PR/cl

⑨ Enclosure

FIGURE 7-5 Sample business letter.

Email

One popular form of printed communication is electronic mail or **email**. It is received immediately and can contain additional attached documents. Because of its ease of use, email has quickly become the preferred form of internal communication with businesses including dental practices. Increasingly patients are also requesting email for everything from confirmation of appointments to statements of their account.

Email is still written office correspondence and must be treated like all other professional correspondence. It can be printed and saved in a patient chart or saved as an electronic file. Simply deleting it doesn't make it disappear.

Philip R. Richardson, DDS
401 Main Street
Morrison, UT 84076
(222) 224-0560
www.richardsondental.com

① Month, Day, Year

② Mrs. Janice Larson
793 West Wishing Well Lane
Morrison, UT 84076

③ Dear Mrs. Larson,

Welcome To Our Practice

④   Thank you for choosing us as your dental team. We are delighted to welcome you to our family dental practice.

    We are committed to excellence and providing you the finest quality dental care available. Our goal is to help you attain and keep a beautiful smile for a lifetime.

    We are looking forward to your first visit on Monday, April 7th, at 10:00 am. You may visit our website at www.richardsondental.com, print the acquaintance form and health history to complete at your convenience. Make sure you bring any insurance information that will assist us in filing your dental claim.

    Enclosed is a brochure to acquaint you with our office. If you have any questions about your first visit or need directions to our office, please call us at (222) 224-0560.

⑤ Sincerely,

⑥

⑦ Phillip R. Richardson, DDS

⑧ PR/cl

⑨ Enclosure

© Cengage Learning 2014

FIGURE 7-6 Sample business letter.

Basic Rules for Using Email

- Email requires use of proper grammar, punctuation, and upper and lower case letters.
- Business email should contain appropriate abbreviations only and save emoticons or smiling/frowning faces for personal email.
- Personal email should not be sent from the email address of a business.
- The email should include a subject in the subject line that is relevant to the email.
- All Health Insurance Portability and Accountability Act (HIPAA) guidelines apply to email; therefore don't send personal health information.

- Never send personal financial information via email.
- Use caution in emailing anything that could be used as part of legal action.
- Avoid sending email when angry or upset.
- Business email should not be used to forward jokes or cute/pretty photos.
- Do not forward email from unknown sources.
- Spell check and reread all emails before sending!
- Answer email promptly.

It is a good idea to have an office signature attached at the bottom that contains the same contact information as the office letterhead.

 ## Exploring the Web

Writing Business Letters
> www.writingcenter.unc.edu
> www.owl.english.purdue.edu

Marketing Materials
> www.smartpractice.com

 ## Skill Building

These optional activities and exercises are designed to help the student put into practice information learned in the chapter.

1. You are the office manager in a busy practice. Dr. Jones has invited a new partner, Dr. Brown, to join the practice and wants you to update the practice brochure, introducing the new partner and the practice's policies. Make up the office address, telephone number, office hours, policies, and information about Dr. Brown. This practice exercise can be limited to creating parts of a brochure or expanded to the entire brochure.

2. Dr. Garcia just completed an extensive crown and bridge case for Mrs. Dorothy Collins who resides at 514 Willow St., Chicago, IL 60611. He has asked you to write a letter thanking her for being an exceptionally cooperative patient and complimenting her on her new smile. He would like you to include a welcome to her friends, family members, co-workers to become patients, if they are looking for a new dentist. Write this letter using three different styles.

 ## Challenge Your Understanding

Select the response that best answers each of the following questions. Only one response is correct.

1. The practice logo may consist of:
   a. A visual graphic
   b. Letters and words
   c. The name of the practice or the doctor's name
   d. All of these elements

2. The practice logo:
   a. Is a symbol patients, professionals, and members of the community come to recognize as representing the dentist
   b. Reflects the mood and philosophy of the practice
   c. Reflects the type of practice
   d. All of the above

3. Patient education brochures:
   a. Inform the patients of oral conditions and the need for specific types of treatment
   b. Reinforce the information given by the doctor during chair side consultations or in formal case presentations
   c. Save valuable chairside time taken to explain procedures
   d. All of the above

4. Which of the following is not a feature of the practice survey?
   a. A way to communicate with patients
   b. A way to improve existing services and amenities
   c. A method of collecting overdue accounts
   d. Suggestions to help make improvements in the practice

5. For best results, a practice survey should be done anonymously.
   a. True
   b. False

6. Which of the following is not a necessary component of a well-written business letter?
   a. An enclosure
   b. Today's date
   c. Address and salutation
   d. Body

7. The practice survey is a key measure in assessing patients' levels of satisfaction with service in treatment:
   a. True
   b. False

8. _____ is the primary communications director for the practice.
   a. The dental hygienist
   b. The dental lab technician
   c. The dental supply representative
   d. The dental office manager

9. The practice's letterhead stationery features:
   a. The name of the practice
   b. The doctor's name and credentials
   c. The office address, telephone number, and Website or email
   d. All of the above

10. Prescription pads printed with the letter head and practice logo may also include:
    a. The office hours
    b. The dentist's DEA (Drug Enforcement Agency) license number
    c. The date and time of the patient's next appointment
    d. Patient's known drug allergies

11. The practice statement contains:
    a. The name of the responsible party
    b. The fee for service rendered
    c. The amount already paid
    d. All of the above

12. A letter written in full block style has:
    a. No indentations
    b. All copy beginning at the left margin
    c. The date and complimentary close slightly off center page
    d. a and b

13. Appointment cards may contain an office policy statement requesting the patient contact the office 24 hours in advance when a change of appointment is necessary. This:
    a. Is a courtesy to the office
    b. Prevents lost production time because of failed or broken appointments
    c. May result in assessment of a broken appointment charge to the patient
    d. All of the above

14. The practice statement may be used to communicate:
    a. Information on new services available
    b. Extended office hours and holiday greetings
    c. Introduction of new staff members
    d. All of the above

15. Which of the following is good office email etiquette?
    a. Forwarding things you think are cute or pretty
    b. Sending person financial information to save paper
    c. Abbreviating dental terms because the patient won't understand them anyway
    d. Avoid sending emails when angry or upset

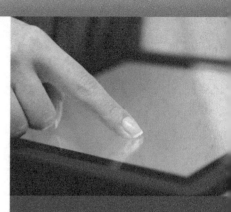

CHAPTER 8

Business Office Equipment

CHAPTER OUTLINES

- **Practice Communication Equipment**
- **The Telephone**
  Telephone Features
  Speaker
  Headset
  The Conference Call
  Voice Mail
  Answering Service
  Office Cell Phone
  Tone of Service
  Telephone Courtesy
  Telephone Etiquette
- **Printer, Copier, Scanner, Fax Machine**
- **The Practice Computer**
  Computer Hardware
  Information Storage
  Portable Computers
  Computer Software
  Computer Terminology
- **Selecting Practice Management Software**
  Managing Patient Information
  Appointment Scheduling Features
  Fee Calculations
  Reports
- **Internet in the Office**

KEY TERMS

bridge
compact disc (CD)
central processing
  unit (CPU)
digital versatile disc
  (DVD)
file extension
flash drive
hardware
link
modem
scanner
software
tone of service
voice mail
wireless

LEARNING OBJECTIVES

Upon completion of this chapter, the reader should be able to:

1. Describe the importance of the telephone as a primary communication contact between patients and the office.
2. Be familiar with the different types of telephone messaging systems, on-hold systems, and conference calling.
3. Differentiate between computer hardware and software components and describe their functions.
4. List the features of dental practice management software.
5. List five important rules of telephone etiquette.
6. Discuss ways an office can handle after hours emergency calls.

Practice Communication Equipment

Running a modern dental practice efficiently requires the same expertise and high-tech equipment as other fast-paced businesses. The office manager may already be familiar with many of the basic components of an automated practice; however, constant upgrading of applications requires continuous learning and retraining.

The Telephone

The telephone is the voice of the practice. It represents the office's personality to the community and is the first and primary point of contact with patients in the introduction to the practice.

The minimum for most dental practices is two incoming lines into the main number. Depending on the size of the practice there may be additional incoming lines and a private line designated for outgoing calls to be used by the doctor in his or her private office. Some practices have call waiting or call forwarding features that allow messages to be picked up from another number.

Most commonly, the telephone at the front desk is wired for the office manager to receive all incoming calls, including personal calls for the dentist. The line on which a specific call is received is associated with the light on the key panel, alerting the office manager to the incoming line to allow him or her to extend the proper greeting.

Telephone Features

Many dental practices use a telephone system with some form of caller ID. This is a digital panel that displays the name and number of the calling party. Most dental office phones also feature a hold button, which plays music from a radio station, prerecorded music, or a specifically recorded message for the holding caller often featuring new products and services of the practice. Your phone system may also allow you to place the call on hold for a specific person so if the patient is holding to make an appointment they don't get directed to a person who specializes in insurance claims. Some hold buttons have a timer that goes from a slow flash to a rapid flash after a designated period of time so patients don't linger on hold forever. The goal is not to have patients hold at all; no one likes to be put on hold.

Speaker

Commonly dental office phones feature a built-in speaker that allows the user to engage in a conversation without having to pick up the receiver. A benefit of built-in speakers is to enable a group of people in the same room to hold a conference call using one telephone. If the speaker feature is being used, caution must be taken to preserve the privacy of the caller in compliance with HIPAA.

Headset

Most dental office telephones can be adapted for a headset. Some office managers prefer to wear a headset to maintain a more comfortable posture and for greater efficiency leaving both hands free to schedule appointments and enter new information into the computer system (Figure 8-1).

The Conference Call

Another popular option of the dental office telephone system is conference calling capability, which allows the user to add additional lines to an existing call. For example, the dentist, the patient, and a dental specialist could discuss proposed treatment together from different locations on a conference call.

For better service with larger conferences "more than three participants" it will be necessary to schedule a call through a conference call service. The office manager does this by calling the company that provides conference call services to the practice. The conference call service creates a voice bridge that permits a number of callers to call a phone number, enter an access code, and join the conference call. The dental office is billed for the call by the service provider.

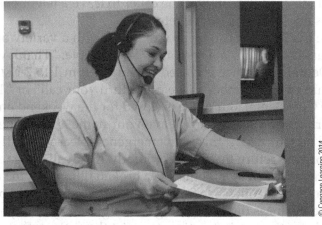

FIGURE 8-1 A headset allows the office manager to have her hands free to attend to paperwork of typing while on the phone with a patient.

Conference Call Etiquette

The appropriate etiquette for a conference call is for the office manager to introduce everyone participating. Everyone on the call should be aware of anyone listening in on the call to avoid an awkward or embarrassing situation. For example, the office manager says "Hello, Jane. This is Shannon from Dr. James Olson's office. Also on the line are Dr. Olson, Charlene Roberts, his hygienist, and our patient Daniel Smith, who we are referring to Dr. Donaldson for periodontal surgery."

If the office manager has not yet added the patient to the call, he or she should announce the intention to do so. For example, "if there are no questions, I would like to add Mr. Smith to the line for information and questions about his surgery and directions to your office." If there are no questions, the office manager can say, "I'm leaving the line briefly while I add Mr. Smith."

When the patient answers, the office manager tells him, "Mr. Smith, I have Dr. Olson, Dr. Donaldson, his scheduler Jane, and Dr. Olson's hygienist Charlene holding on a conference call. Would you like to join us for a brief review of your scheduled surgery and directions to Dr. Donaldson's office?"

The office manager presses the conference button again, adding the second line to the conference call and announces that Mr. Smith has joined them on the line.

If it becomes necessary or convenient for one of the parties to disconnect, it is courteous to inform the others. The office manager can say, "Excuse me, Dr. Olson and Dr. Donaldson, if there are no further issues regarding the appointment time or place, I am going to say goodbye to complete Mr. Smith's paperwork. Mr. Smith, I will be following up with Jane and she will take care of your insurance claim for the surgery."

Voice Mail

Another telephone feature in many dental offices is voice mail, a recorded message service that intercepts the line after a set number of rings and asks the caller to leave a message. With this capability, if a caller dials the office when all lines are busy, the system automatically answers a call with a recorded message rather than transmitting a busy signal. The system announces that the call is being answered by the messaging system and that the office is unavailable to take the call at the moment but will return the call as soon as possible. The recorded message then invites the caller to leave a telephone number and detailed message so the call can be returned.

The voice mail system can be programmed with a variety of messages so the caller hears an appropriate response. For example: "Thank you for calling Smile City Dental, our office is closed for lunch from 1 to 2 P.M. Please leave your name and phone number so we can return your call" or "Thank you for calling Smile City Dental, our office is closed for the weekend and will reopen Monday morning at 8 A.M. Please leave your name and phone number and your call will be returned. If this is an emergency, please call 501-888-OUCH."

It is a priority to return these calls promptly. If the call is regarding a patient with an emergency such as a toothache, a broken filling etc., the call should be returned as soon as the message is received. Other calls should be returned by the end of the business day. Returning calls right away is to your advantage because you have the maximum time to assist the patient. For example: Mike needs to reschedule his appointment for tomorrow. A delay in returning his call gives you less time to find a patient on your "will call" list that wants that appointment.

Answering Service

Some dental practices engage a professional answering service to ensure all emergencies are addressed according to policy. The answering service personnel can be scripted to manage after hours or forwarded calls in a manner consistent with specific circumstances.

Usually the office phone can be programmed to forward calls to the answering service as the office manager chooses. The answering service can be instructed to handle calls differently when the doctor is out of the office from those the practice receives during times with an unusually heavy volume of calls or after office hours when the doctor would be handling the office emergencies personally.

Some offices exercise the maximum amount of control over varying situations by employing an answering service as backup to the electronic answering options of the phone system.

Depending upon the complexity of the options available on the office phone, it may be necessary for the office manager to spend some time examining the instructions, programming the appropriate functions, and practicing the accurate use of all systems features. The credibility and professionalism of the practice is jeopardized if the office manager accidentally disconnects parties to a conference call, connects callers to the wrong dentist, or answers multiple phones with the wrong greeting. These errors can be avoided by studying the system and practicing function commands ahead of time.

Office Cell Phone

One popular way to maintain very personal patient contact is to have an emergency cell phone that rotates among staff members. The number for the cell number is the office emergency number and every member of the dental team takes a turn being responsible for it.

When the cell phone rings it is answered with the same response the office phone would be answered. Patients often recognize the staff member they are speaking with and are immediately reassured by the personal contact. The staff member evaluates the emergency and can often solve simple problems or answer questions. For more severe problems, the staff member can call the doctor at home or take the patients information and return the call as soon as the office reopens.

Tone of Service

A professional, courteous, pleasant telephone manner is worth measurable revenue and public relations value to the practice. Some consultants call these qualities tone of service, a phrase that encompasses timely resolution of all callers' issues, accuracy of all information dispensed to callers, and personality traits projected to callers, such as friendliness and helpfulness, concern, and patience. Good grammar and diction are also essential.

Some office managers "shop" their offices regularly asking other professionals to call the practice anonymously to critique the quality of the phone response. It is every team member's responsibility to maintain the highest possible standards of practice communication and patient education. A great deal of communication in the office occurs via phone contacts and it is a reflection of the professionalism of the office.

Telephone Courtesy

As with all forms of communication, extreme courtesy must be exercised by the office manager when talking with patients and other callers. The office manager should answer the phone with a greeting specified by the doctor such as, "Good morning or good afternoon, Dr. Marks office this is Mary, how may I assist you?"

The conclusion of the phone call must also follow the doctors required close such as "Thank you for calling, Mrs. Jackson." When the office manager initiates the call, he or she should conclude with "thank you." Other standard courtesies used when speaking face-to-face should be used when speaking on the telephone.

Telephone Etiquette

Basic rules of telephone etiquette include the following:

1. Speak clearly and with a smile on your face. Even though the caller cannot see you the cheerfulness of your smile will come across (Figure 8-2).
2. Always focus on the call instead of things happening around you.
3. Use your normal tone of voice and speak into the phone. You do not need to shout but speak loudly enough so the caller can hear you.

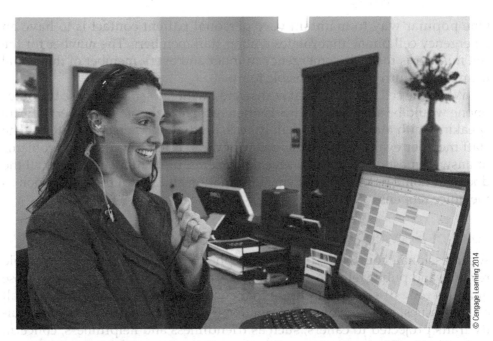

FIGURE 8-2 Speaking with a smile on your face projects a positive, friendly attitude to the caller.

Sample Telephone Checklist

☐ Answer calls appropriately and pleasantly

☐ Remain patient and sympathetic toward a confused caller

☐ Handle refusal to quote fees with positive phrases

☐ Attempt to schedule new patients for a diagnostic consultation

☐ Handle a caller who owes money with positive phrases

☐ Remain calm and professional with an abusive caller

☐ Resolve complicated scheduling problems quickly

☐ Convert an angry patient to a happy patient

☐ Invite prospective patients to visit the office for a complimentary tour

☐ Politely discourage suspected drug abusers from attempting to obtain prescriptions

☐ Avoid the temptation to diagnose over the phone

☐ Always let the caller hang up first

© Cengage Learning 2014

4. Listen, listen, and listen. Do not interrupt the caller. Don't guess why they have called.

5. Do not use slang such as "hang on" or "yeah."

6. Do not eat or drink when you are at the front desk answering phones.

7. Address the caller properly by name. If it is a patient you are unfamiliar with, err on the side of formality. Instead of guessing how Mrs. Jane Smith would like to be addressed, call her Mrs. Smith.

8. Be patient and helpful. If a caller is irate or upset, listen to what the caller has to say and then refer the caller to the appropriate resource. Avoid getting into an argument on the phone.

9. Always ask if you can put the caller on hold and wait for a response.

10. If you are helping a patient, let another dental team member answer a call or let it go to the voice mail system. The most important patient is the one in front of you.

Printer, Copier, Scanner, Fax Machine

Most offices find multifunctional pieces of equipment (printer, copier, and scanner) important to running an efficient dental practice.

With most dental offices engaging in heavy computer use, a printer is essential when documents must be printed on letterhead and for general printing needs. Today's printers also act as copiers to duplicate existing materials and as scanners as well.

Scanners have become particularly valuable with the increase in electronic storage of documents. Materials received by mail or other modes can be scanned and stored electronically in the patients' chart or in an office file. For offices with high scanner usage, additional stand-alone scanners may be extremely helpful.

Telephone lines into the office are also utilized for another form of electronic communication, fax (facsimile) machines. Although these machines are declining in popularity, documents can still be faxed, saving time and postage. Most requests for written materials can be answered by an offer to fax the information immediately. Caution must be taken not to expose personal health information protected under HIPAA.

The Practice Computer

Most dental offices rely on computers for many of their routine functions, such as insurance claims, billing, recall, word processing, and marketing communications. A growing number of offices are moving away from traditional patient charts and are using a computer to store patient histories and treatment information.

The computer consists of two parts: the hardware and the software (Figure 8-3).

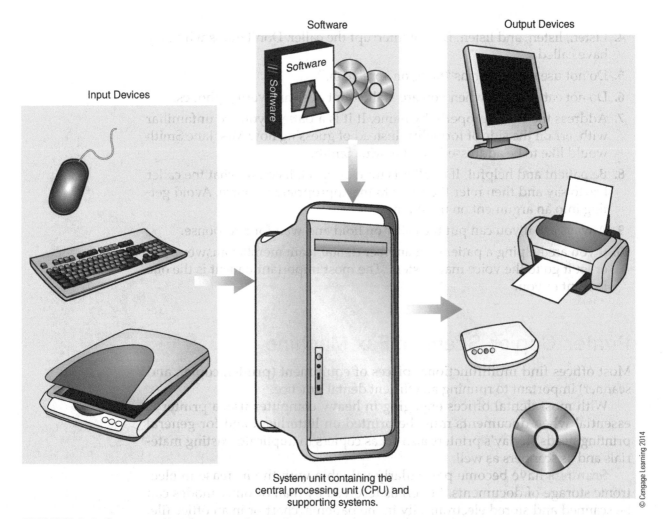

FIGURE 8-3 Components of a computer system.

Computer Hardware

The physical or visible computing equipment is called the hardware .

- *System unit*: The system unit is the core of the computer system. Usually it's a rectangular box placed on or underneath a desk. Inside the box are many electronic components that process information. The CPU (central processing unit) is the brain of the computer. The RAM (random access memory) stores information that the CPU uses. Almost every other part of the computer connects into the system unit using cables or a wireless connection; hardware that connects into the system unit is sometimes called a peripheral device.

- *Monitor*: A monitor is an output device that displays information in visual form, using text and graphics. The portion of the monitor that displays the information is called the screen. Like a television screen, a computer screen can show still or moving pictures.

- *Keyboard*: A keyboard is an input device used mainly for typing text into the computer. Like the keyboard on a typewriter, it has keys for letters and numbers, but it also has special keys:

  - The *function keys*, found on the top row, perform different functions depending on where they are used.
  - The *numeric keypad*, located on the right side of most keyboards, allows the user to enter numbers quickly.
  - The *navigation keys*, such as the arrow keys, allow the user to move positions within a document or webpage.

- *Mouse*: The mouse is also an input device that allows movement within the workspace and documents. Mice come in many shapes; the typical mouse does look a bit like an actual mouse. It's small, oblong, and connected to the system unit by a long wire that resembles a tail. Some newer mice are wireless.

- *Modem*: To connect the computer to the Internet, a modem is needed. A modem is an output device that sends and receives computer information over a telephone line or high-speed cable. Modems are sometimes built into the system unit, but they can also be separate components. Modems can be wireless and broadcast a signal that users access with a code or wired where the user accesses the modem through a cable.

Information Storage

A computer has one or more disk drives—devices that store information on a disk. The disk preserves the information even when the computer is turned off.

Hard Disk Drive

A computer's hard disk drive stores information on a hard disk, a rigid platter or stack of platters with a magnetic surface. Because hard disks can hold massive amounts of information, they usually serve as the computer's primary means of storage, holding almost all computer programs and files. The hard disk drive is normally located inside the system unit.

CD and DVD Drives

Nearly all computers today come equipped with compact disc (CD) or digital versatile disc (DVD) drives that are usually located on the front of the system unit or the side of a laptop computer. CD drives use lasers to read or retrieve data from a CD, and many CD drives can also write or record data onto CDs. If a recordable disk drive is installed, copies of files can be stored on blank CDs. A CD drive can also be used to play music CDs on a computer. DVD drives can do everything that CD drives can, plus read DVDs. A DVD drive, allows the user to watch movies on a computer. Many DVD drives can record data onto blank DVDs.

Portable Computers

Portable computers are often referred to as "laptop" or "tablet computers."

- A full-size *laptop* is large enough to accommodate a "full size" keyboard. The minimum width of 11 inches is required for a full-size laptop.
- A *netbook* is a smaller, lighter laptop. It is often less expensive than a full-size laptop but it also has fewer features and less computing power along with a smaller keyboard that can be difficult to operate.
- *Tablet computers* are a type of mobile computer that uses a touch screen or pen-enabled interface instead of a traditional keyword (Figure 8-4). These devices are gaining in popularity.

Computer Software

Software refers to the instructions that direct the CPU to process information. These instructions are called programs. The two main groups of software are system software and application software.

System software programs or operating systems control the hardware capabilities of the computer. They organize user commands to function, call up, and start up the appropriate application software, and manage the data as its input and output. In most cases, the system software is built in by the manufacturer and must be brand-compatible. Examples of operating systems are Windows XP, Vista, and Windows 7 and 8. Operating systems are constantly being updated.

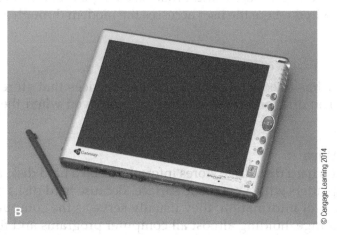

FIGURE 8-4 Tablets are gaining in popularity on practice.

Application software can be purchased commercially from numerous vendors. Software can be written for very specific applications. If the practice uses a scheduling, insurance management, practice promotion, an accounts payable tracking program, or any combination of the above, the software used would be written specifically for a dental practice.

Computer Terminology

When working with technology there are numerous terms that are helpful to be familiar with including several that are important when evaluating and selecting a software package.

- *File extension*: A **file extension**, usually just referred to as an extension, is the suffix at the end of a filename that indicates what type of file it is. For example: in the filename "productionreport.txt," txt is the file extension. It tells you that the file is a text document. When shopping for software knowing what an extension is would be important when discussing reports and storage.

- *Link*: Most of us work with links all the time. Whenever you see a highlighted or underlined word you are probably looking at a **link**. By clicking on the link you can immediately "jump" to a new web page providing additional information. Learning to use links is helpful when investigating different types of dental practice management software.

- *Bridge*: A **bridge** connects two or more local networks together. The data uses the bridge to move to and from different areas of the network. Bridges typically transfer data very rapidly. Dental software uses bridges for digital imaging, automated calling systems, and some charting applications and computerized fabrication systems that are used to produce crowns or other lab work.

- *Flash drive*: A **flash drive** has many names—jump drives, thumb drives, or pen drives. Regardless of the name they are a small data storage device. A flash drive uses flash memory and a USB connection to store data. This type of data storage is very portable because of its size and would enable a doctor to easily take diagnostic data to a specialist when referring a patient. The ability to use this type of flexible storage would be helpful when choosing software for the office.

Selecting Practice Management Software

Purchasing or updating dental software is a big decision. If the office manager is delegated to choose or assist in choosing a dental software program, it is advisable to try several different programs and to request demonstrations and visit offices currently using them. Narrowing the choices to two or three favorites based on price, features, support, and ease of use and then asking for the assistance of the dental team can be helpful. Many times office staff has had previous experience with a variety of software and their opinion can be very valuable.

Managing Patient Information

The primary reason for a practice to invest in dental practice management software is to organize patient information and make it easily accessible. All dental software enables the office to create patient profiles. When a practice chooses software they need to determine how they want to use that information.

Appointment Scheduling Features

Appointment scheduling is an example of a software function normally set up by the user. The office manager must input all the relevant information about the way the practice schedules according to procedures, operators, and dentist preferences. The most common feature to look for in a scheduling program is a series of prompts that leads the user through this task. The software system presents a selection menu, and then offers the capacity to add additional procedures as needed. The program should be able to schedule multiple treatment rooms, with prompts that guide the user through simple choices.

Some scheduling programs also offer a default time requirement. This allows the office manager the flexibility to allot specific times for each appointment or procedure automatically.

Another common feature is scheduling the entire treatment series or sequence. This allows the office manager to enter the treatment plan at the time the patient accepts it. The program automatically appoints the inclusive plan, including the next recall visit, and prints out a treatment calendar for the patient showing all the visits, the duration, the associated fees, the payment schedule including interest if any. The automatic scheduling feature also can be used to pre-book hygiene appointments in advance.

In researching a dental software program, the office manager should also look for a program that automatically enters the comments into the days treatment notes if they are flagged as clinical.

Most scheduling programs automatically track the production of each day's patient load, in such a way that is not visible on the printed schedule, but can be printed out separately. The production can be included on the schedule that is posted in the dentist's private office only, or in another private area such as the instrument sterilization room.

Fee Calculations

The office manager should also ensure that the program calculates fee changes based on a percentage increase including all fees, the percentage increase on a specified procedure, or an item by item change of a set or variable amount. The program should reflect the percentage of the practice composed of demographics, fee-for-service procedures, or referrals. The office manager may command a series of reports reflecting how the practice would be impacted by an increase in fees. The software program can assist the office manager in sorting capabilities to reflect several different ways to recover costs, either by raising all fees by a certain percentage or by adding a set surcharge to all procedures or to certain procedures.

Reports

Report lists are commonly used to track recall patients, referral sources, or even the day's surgery and restorative patients, with phone numbers for postoperative telephone courtesy calls.

Another way in which report lists are used is to command the system in merging a letter or printing mailing labels. Targeting specific patients for the purpose of informing them of recall visits, mailing thank you letters or welcoming new patients to the practice can be done with report lists.

Reports alert the office manager and administrative staff to the number of patients who were 30 days, over 60 days, over 90 days delinquent on financial arrangements. These lists are calls to action, as these patients require immediate attention to collect their outstanding balances.

Many accounts receivable programs generate a series of appropriate collection letters automatically, based on criteria entered by the office manager through a series of prompts. Reports retrieve the names and address of delinquent accounts directly from the aging account application, incorporating an electronic calendar (a timing device built into the hardware that does not rest when the computer is turned off) and merges it with a letter.

The account aging capabilities generate a report that reflects the percentage of improvement over the accounts receivable balance for the same quarter the previous year, over the past quarter in the current year, or a group by term of delinquency (30, 60, or 90 days).

Internet in the Office

With the advantages to the practice of having Internet with access to email and websites comes the potential of viruses infecting the office computer system and employee distraction. Often those two things go hand in hand. The office manual, discussed in Chapter 3 (Legal and Ethical Regulations in Dental Office Management) should include specific guidelines for using the practice computer system even during breaks or lunch. Some offices ask employees not to access the Web to check personal email or to look up personal information. Other offices grant some access to the Internet for employees during nonscheduled time or permit restricted use such as checking personal email but no Web searches.

Even with excellent virus protection, accessing the Web can be an invitation for viruses to infect the computer system. Employees should be instructed that email from unknown or suspicious sources should not be opened. This includes mail not only received on a personal account but also on the practice email account. Although having an outside source gain access to confidential records is a concern of many practices, good security makes the risks minimal. Practice management software companies are aware that offices must be in compliance with HIPAA so additional steps have been taken to preserve patient privacy.

In the course of doing business, the dental practice will probably do some Web searches particularly when purchasing supplies or referring patients. All employees should use caution and avoid opening sites that are unfamiliar. The same applies for employees who are allowed to use the computer for person business. Dealing with a virus can take valuable staff time so the goal is to avoid inviting one into the system.

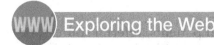

Exploring the Web

Dentrix
www.dentrix.com

Eaglesoft
www.eaglesoft.net

PracticeWorks
www.carestreamdental.com

QSI, *Cloud-based software*
www.qsii.com

Dental Bridge Software
www.opendental.com

Automated Voice Messaging
www.televox.com

Computer Terminology
www.techterms.com/

Email Etiquette
www.office.microsoft.com/en-us/outlook-help/12-tips-for-better-e-mail
-etiquette-HA001205410.aspx

Skill Building

These optional activities and exercises are designed to help the student put into practice information learned in the chapter.

1. Divide into groups. Each group should select a leader. The leader directs each member to contact a minimum of three area dental practices to determine the following information. What dental computer software program they currently use? What features do they especially like about it? What additional applications or features would they want if they were available? In one week, each member of the group reports to the team leader. The team leader provides a consensus from his or her group as to the most beneficial computer programs in software applications.

2. If possible, arrange for the class to visit a dental practice in the area and request a demonstration of its computer system.

Challenge Your Understanding

Select the response that best answers each of the following questions only one response is correct.

1. Telephone automation has made personal "tone of service" less important in modern practices.
   a. True
   b. False

2. Caller ID provides:
   a. A video camera image or an image of the caller
   b. Camera images of both the caller and the person who answers
   c. A digital display of the number of the calling party
   d. A light that corresponds to the area code of calling party

3. Which of the following may patients hear when on hold?
   a. Digitally recorded music
   b. A local radio broadcast
   c. A recorded message
   d. Any of the above

4. Because of new telephone technology, only one incoming line is now necessary regardless of the number of doctors in the practice.
   a. True
   b. False

5. Which of the following is true of telephone conferencing?
   a. Three-way conferences can be accessed internally
   b. Conferences can be prearranged with a conference call service
   c. The conference call service can create a voice bridge for caller dialed conferences
   d. All of the above

6. If the practice uses a sophisticated on-hold system with a personalized message, it would not be necessary to hire an answering service as well
   a. True
   b. False

7. Which of the following is the main precaution regarding fax transmissions?
   a. Is very expensive
   b. Faxes are usually not legal documents
   c. Confidentiality has to be carefully guarded
   d. It is not considered professional

8. What do the initials CPU stand for?
   a. Computer processing unit
   b. Central processing unit
   c. Control pendulum utilization
   d. Computer pod unit

9. Primary storage is also called:
   a. CD
   b. DVD
   c. Brain
   d. Memory

10. The typical dental management software system performs all of the following except
    a. Schedule appointments
    b. Delete inactive files automatically when memory is used up

   c. Create insurance forms

   d. Ages accounts and generate state statements

11. Which is not an appropriate use of the Internet in a dental office setting?

   a. Communication with patients

   b. Communication with other professionals

   c. Communication with friends and relatives

   d. Professional search

12. Which is/are a serious concern of Internet users?

   a. Is very expensive

   b. Files are bulky and use a lot of electricity

   c. Information is often obsolete

   d. Information is not secured cannot be kept confidential

13. The CPU:

   a. Executes programs

   b. Performs calculations

   c. Temporarily stores data and programs

   d. All of the above

14. To access the Internet, a modem is required.

   a. True

   b. False

15. When choosing software for a dental office, which of the following is most important?

   a. How the software will be used in the practice

   b. Features the sales person says you will need

   c. The computer expertise of the dental team

   d. Program graphics

16. Scanners can be used to:

   a. Add documents to a patient's chart

   b. Send information to a referring doctor

   c. Add photos to the patient chart

   d. All of the above

SECTION III

Clinical Records Management

CHAPTER 9

Dental Nomenclature and Related Terminology

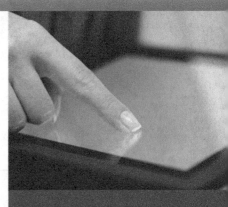

CHAPTER OUTLINES

KEY TERMS

anterior
bicuspid/premolar
buccal
canine/cuspid
cementum
deciduous/primary
  dentition
dentin
distal
edentulous
enamel
facial/labial
foramen
incisal
incisor
lingual
mandible
maxilla
mesial
midline
molar
occlusal
occlusal plane
periodontal ligament
periodontium
permanent dentition
posterior
pulp
quadrants
sextants
temporomandibular joint
  (TMJ)

Dental Nomenclature

The dental office manager must be thoroughly familiar with dental nomenclature (names of the teeth) and related terminology. This is essential to interpret the dentist's, hygienist's, or chairside assistant's charting or related treatment records, and to provide patients with accurate information in determining treatment costs. Knowledge of terms is also essential in educating patients about existing dental conditions and recommended treatment, as well as creating case presentations or billing patients and third-party payers accurately for treatment performed.

Dental Arches

The skull is made up of the cranium and the face. The cranium, made up of eight bones, houses and protects the brain. The face consists of 14 bones including the maxilla and mandible that make up the oral cavity or mouth. The maxilla and mandible are commonly called jaws but are also known as dental arches.

The occlusal plane is an imaginary line that distinguishes the upper and lower arches. It is the point where the teeth come together when biting.

Mandibular Arch

The mandible is the only movable bone in the face and has a horseshoe shape curving upward at the back on both sides to a posterior projection called a condyle. The condyle of the mandible is attached to the temporal bone by a movable joint called the temporomandibular joint (TMJ). The mandible is the lower jaw and contains all of the lower teeth in bone called the alveolar process.

Maxillary Arch

The maxilla or upper jaw is two bones that are joined together at the median suture to form the roof of the mouth or hard palate. This suture fuses as a person ages. The maxilla extends from below the eye, forms the sides of the nasal cavity and the alveolar process. The maxilla is the upper jaw and contains all of the upper teeth supported in the alveolar process.

Quadrants and Sextants

The oral cavity is divided into four **quadrants** and has six **sextants**. The quadrants are determined by an imaginary vertical line, the **midline**, dividing the front of the face into right and left halves. This line runs from between the eyes to the middle of the chin. The occlusal plane divides the mouth into upper and lower.

The four quadrants ("quad" means four) are the maxillary right, maxillary left, mandibular right, and mandibular left (Figure 9-1).

The mouth is also divided into **anterior** (front) and **posterior** (back) teeth. The anterior sextants comprise the six anterior teeth contained in the mandible and maxilla. The posterior teeth include all remaining teeth (Figure 9-2).

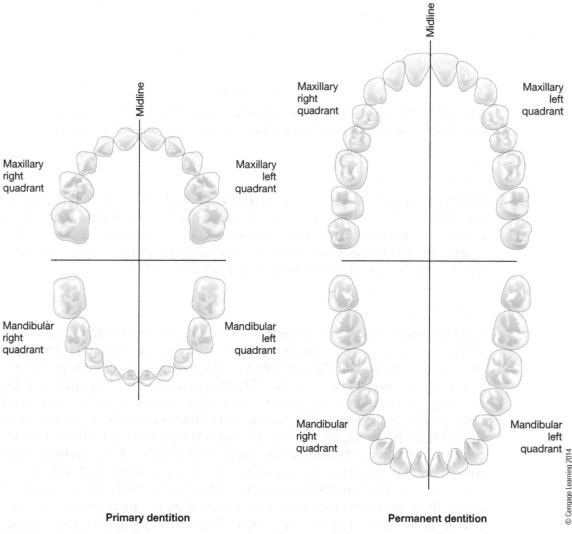

Primary dentition

Permanent dentition

© Cengage Learning 2014

FIGURE 9-1 Dental arches of (A) primary (deciduous) dentition and (B) permanent dentition divided into quadrants with the midline identified.

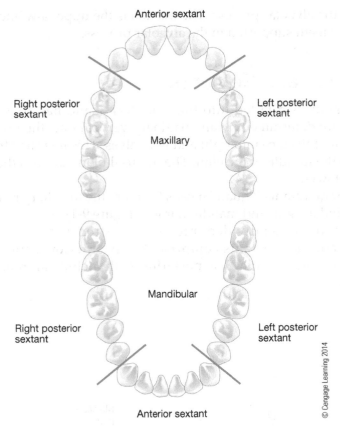

Anterior sextant

Right posterior
sextant

Left posterior
sextant

Maxillary

Mandibular

Right posterior
sextant

Left posterior
sextant

Anterior sextant

© Cengage Learning 2014

FIGURE 9-2 Permanent dentition divided into sextants. The maxillary and mandibular arches each have two posterior sextants and one anterior sextant.

Tooth Composition

Each tooth is imbedded in the respective jaw, attached by surrounding tissue called the periodontium. *Perio* means around and *odont* means tooth. Each tooth is composed of hard and soft tissues. The periodontium consists of the gingiva or gum tissue, periodontal ligaments/fibers, and the alveolar process, which is the bone that holds the teeth in place (Figure 9-3).

Hard Structures

Hard tissues of the tooth include enamel, dentin, and cementum (Figure 9-4). The anatomical crown is the part of the tooth covered by enamel. The clinical crown is the part of the tooth that is seen when looking into the mouth. In a tooth that is just erupting, the clinical crown could be very small and for an older person with some gum recession the clinical crown could extend onto the root of the tooth. The clinical root of the tooth is the portion beneath the gumline; however, the anatomical root is the part of the tooth covered by cementum and would normally be beneath the gumline. For a variety of reasons, it is not unusual to see some of the anatomical root exposed and visible.

Enamel is the hardest substance in the human body. It is composed primarily of inorganic materials and is shaped by prismatic rods. The function of the enamel is to protect the tooth. Enamel ranges in color from shades of white to yellow to gray to brown and covers only the anatomical crown of the tooth.

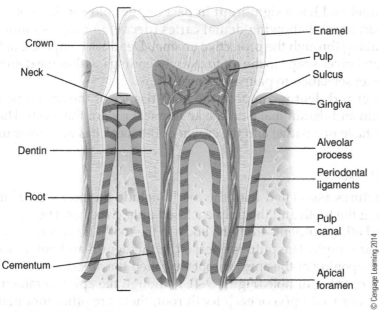

Crown

Neck

Dentin

Root

Cementum

Enamel

Pulp

Sulcus

Gingiva

Alveolar process

Periodontal ligaments

Pulp canal

Apical foramen

© Cengage Learning 2014

FIGURE 9-3 Structures of the periodontium and tooth.

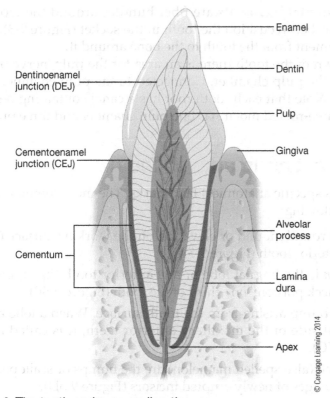

Dentinoenamel junction (DEJ)

Cementoenamel junction (CEJ)

Cementum

Enamel

Dentin

Pulp

Gingiva

Alveolar process

Lamina dura

Apex

© Cengage Learning 2014

FIGURE 9-4 The tooth and surrounding tissues.

Cementum is the yellowish-white outer covering of the root portion of the tooth that is normally below the gumline. It is softer than enamel and has a rough, textured surface that permits the periodontal fibers to attach to the tooth. Cementum can rebuild its tissue, forming secondary cementum.

Dentin comprises the majority of the tooth and is under the enamel and cementum on both the crown and root portion of the tooth. It is yellower than enamel and has a significant impact on the color of the tooth. It is also softer than enamel allowing dental caries (decay) to progress more rapidly after breaking through the protective enamel. Dentin is composed of S-shaped tubules and gives shape to the tooth. Nerves endings within the dental tubules also register sensation to pain and temperature.

Enamel and dentin compose the hard tissues of the anatomical crown. Cementum and dentin make up the anatomical root of the tooth. The roots of the tooth have no enamel and the crown of the tooth has no cementum.

Soft Structures

Soft structures associated with the tooth include the periodontal ligaments supporting the tooth and the pulp enclosed pulp chamber. The pulp provides blood and other nutrients from the body to the tooth. It is composed of nerve, blood, and lymph. The pulp is encased in the dentin and enters each tooth at a small opening at the apex or root tip called the apical foramen. Foramen means an opening or hole (Figure 9-4). Although the apical foramen is found at the apex or root tip(s) of each tooth root, there are other foramen that are part of the maxilla and mandible allowing nerves to pass through the bone (e.g., mental foramen, lingual foramen, and incisive foramen).

The periodontal ligaments are fiber bundles around the tooth that act as a shock absorber to cushion the tooth in the socket (Figure 9-3). They also provide attachment from the tooth to the bone around it.

In the crown of the tooth there is an area for the pulp/nerve of the tooth referred to as the pulp chamber. Connected to the pulp chamber is/are the pulp canal(s). Note that each tooth root has a canal containing nerve tissue. Therefore, a three-rooted molar has one pulp chamber and three pulp canals.

Anatomical Landmarks of Teeth

Each tooth has specific anatomical landmarks. The most common landmarks include the following:

- A *cusp* is a round mound or elevation on the working surface of a cuspid or any posterior tooth (Figure 9-5A).
- A *cingulum* is the lingual lobe of any anterior tooth that appears on the cervical "neck portion" one-third of the tooth (Figure 9-5B).
- A *lobe* is a bump arising from the tooth surface. When a lobe arises from the lingual side of the maxillary anterior teeth, it is called a *cingulum* (Figure 9-5C).
- A *mammelon* (also spelled mamelon) are the bumps or scalloped edges on the incisal edges of newly erupted incisors (Figure 9-5D).
- A *ridge* is any linear elevation of the tooth surface named according to its location, for example, "marginal" ridge (Figure 9-5E).
- A *marginal ridge* is a rounded border of enamel that forms the tips of the cusp on the posterior teeth toward the center of occlusal surfaces (Figure 9-5F).
- A *transverse ridge* is formed by two triangular ridges that meet and cross the occlusal surface of any posterior tooth (Figure 9-5G).
- An *oblique ridge* is one that runs across the occlusal surface of maxillary molars in diagonal direction (Figure 9-5H).

- A *pit* is a very small depression on a tooth surface, most often located at the end of a groove, or where two or more grooves join (Figure 9-5I).
- A *fissure* is a linear fault that occurs along a developmental groove between tooth lobes (Figure 9-5J).
- A *fossa* is an irregular depression on a tooth surface (Figure 9-5K).
- A *developmental groove* is a shallow groove or line on the surface of a tooth (Figure 9-5L).

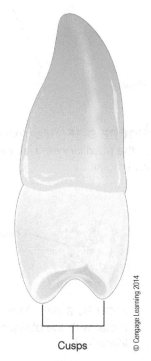

Cusps

FIGURE 9-5A Maxillary second premolar with the cusps identified.

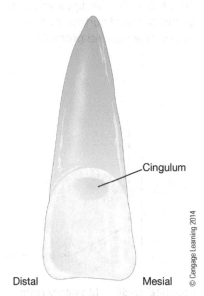

Cingulum

Distal   Mesial

FIGURE 9-5B Lingual surface of a central incisor with the cingulum shaded.

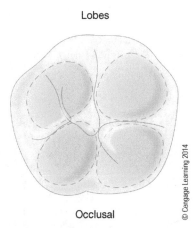

Lobes

Occlusal

FIGURE 9-5C Occlusal view of the maxillary first molar showing the lobes and how they come together.

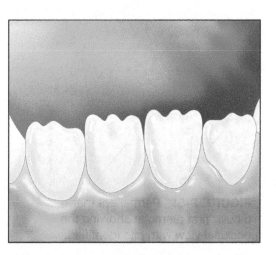

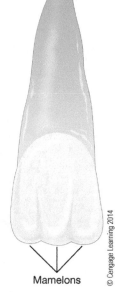

Mamelons

FIGURE 9-5D (A) Newly erupted maxillary incisors and laterals showing the three bulges on the incisal edge, called mamelons. (B) Mamelons shown on the anterior of the maxillary dentition.

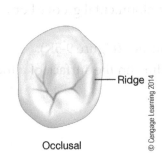

FIGURE 9-5E Ridge identified on the occlusal surface of the mandibular second premolar.

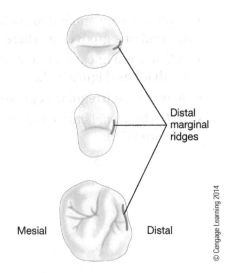

Distal marginal ridges

Mesial   Distal

FIGURE 9-5F Marginal ridges of the maxillary central, premolar, and molar.

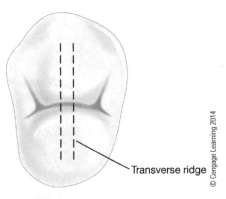

Transverse ridge

FIGURE 9-5G Maxillary right first premolar occlusal view showing transverse ridge.

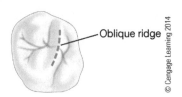

Oblique ridge

FIGURE 9-5H Maxillary first molar with the oblique ridge identified.

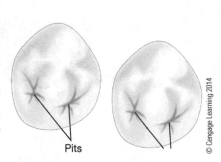

Pits

FIGURE 9-5I Permanent mandibular first premolar showing the occlusal view with pits identified.

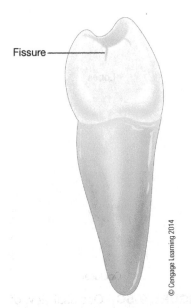

Fissure

FIGURE 9-5J Mandibular second premolar showing the imperfect union or fissure on the occlusal surface.

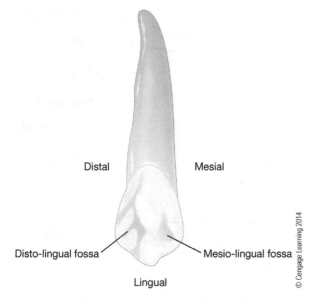

© Cengage Learning 2014

FIGURE 9-5K Lingual view of a maxillary canine with the mesiolingual fossa and distolingual fossa shaded.

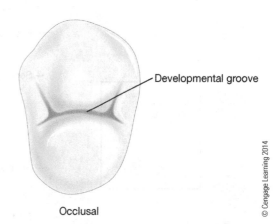

© Cengage Learning 2014

FIGURE 9-5L Developmental groove on the occlusal surface of the maxillary first premolar where lobes were united.

Types and Functions of Teeth

Teeth have three main purposes: chewing food, aiding in speech, and enhancing appearance or esthetics.

The human dentition has four types of teeth:

- **Incisors** are used for biting and cutting food.
- **Cuspids** or **canines**, also known as eye teeth, are used to tear and break off food.
- **Premolars** or **bicuspids** are used to break up and mash food.
- **Molars** are used to grind and pulverize food before swallowing.

Tooth Identification: Deciduous Dentition

The first set of teeth or baby teeth is termed the deciduous or primary dentition because this set of teeth is eventually lost and replaced by the permanent or secondary teeth.

The deciduous or primary dentition consists of 20 teeth: 10 in each arch with 5 in each quadrant. Starting from the midline and moving toward the back of the mouth, the teeth that comprise the deciduous dentition in each quadrant are: one central incisor, one lateral incisor, one cuspid (also referred to as a canine), one first deciduous molar, and one second deciduous molar (Figure 9-6A).

Tooth Identification: Permanent Dentition

The second set of teeth is termed the **permanent dentition** because these teeth comprise the final set of natural dentition. They are sometimes referred to as the secondary teeth because they follow the primary dentition.

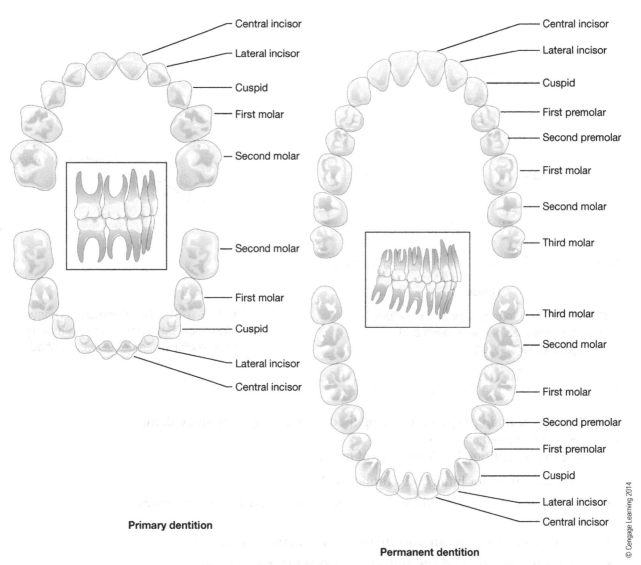

Primary dentition

Permanent dentition

FIGURE 9-6 (A) Deciduous dentition, identifying each tooth by name.
(B) Permanent dentition, identifying each tooth by name.

The permanent dentition consists of 32 teeth, 16 in each arch with 8 in each quadrant. Starting from the midline and moving toward the back of the mouth, the eight teeth that comprise the permanent dentition in each quadrant are: one central incisor, one lateral incisor, one cuspid (canine), one first premolar (bicuspid), one second premolar (bicuspid), and one each first, second, and third molars (Figure 9-6B).

The permanent first and second molars are also referred to as the "six-year" and "twelve-year" molars because they erupt into the oral cavity at approximately those respective ages. The third molar is sometimes referred to as a "wisdom tooth" because it is the last to appear in the oral cavity and is associated with coming of age.

The adolescent who has both primary and secondary teeth in the mouth concurrently is said to have a mixed dentition.

A patient with no natural teeth is said to be **edentulous**.

Tooth Surfaces and Edges

Each tooth is unique in its shape, morphology, and anatomical landmarks. The following is a description of the *surfaces* and *edges* of the human teeth (Figure 9-7). In dentistry, classification of caries and restorative procedures are defined in terms of the surfaces or edges involved. The office manager is responsible for correctly noting restorative procedures to be billed by the *number of surfaces* treatment planned and completed. Incorrectly identifying surfaces could result in under or overbilling.

Mesial Surface

Each tooth has a mesial surface. **Mesial** means *toward the midline* of the mouth.

Distal Surface

Each tooth has a distal surface. **Distal** means *away from the midline* of the mouth.

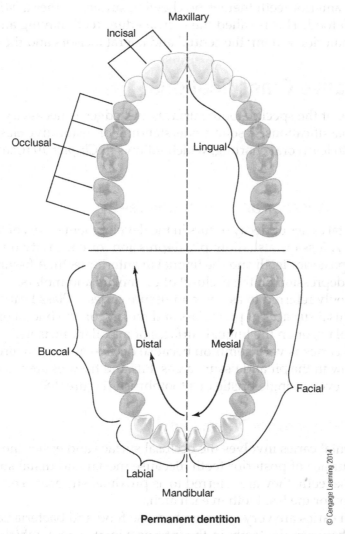

FIGURE 9-7 Surfaces of the teeth identified on the dental arches in a permanent dentition. Posterior teeth colored in blue.

Facial/Labial/Buccal Surface

In the anterior sextant, each tooth has a facial or labial surface. The terms *facial* and *labial* are used interchangeably. On the anterior teeth, this surface faces *toward the face or lips*.

On the posterior or back teeth, which are the premolars and molars, the surface of the tooth *facing the cheeks* is called the buccal surface. The name buccal comes from the buccinator or chewing muscle in the cheek that is adjacent to these tooth surfaces.

Lingual Surface

Each tooth has a lingual surface. Lingual means tongue and the lingual surface of the tooth that *faces toward the tongue*.

Occlusal Surface/Incisal Edge

On the posterior teeth, the chewing surface is referred to as the occlusal surface. Teeth having an occlusal surface are the premolars and molars.

On the anterior teeth there is no chewing surface, rather a *biting edge* used to shear off food. This is called the incisal edge. Teeth having an incisal edge are in the anterior sextant; the central and lateral incisors and the cuspids.

Restorative Classifications

Knowledge of the specific tooth surfaces and edges is necessary to define restorative classifications. A solid understanding of restorative classifications is necessary to learn oral charting, which follows in *Chapter 10 (Charting the Oral Cavity)*.

Class I — Anterior and Posterior Teeth

Class I dental caries or decay occurs in the developmental area of tooth fissures and fossa. A fossa is a shallow pit, depression, or concavity on the occlusal surface of posterior teeth and the lingual of anterior teeth. A fissure is a groove or natural depression on the occlusal of premolars and molars.

Commonly referred to as "pit and fissure caries," Class I caries may occur on the occlusal surfaces of premolars and molars, on the buccal or lingual surfaces of molars, or on the lingual surfaces of maxillary incisors.

Class I caries is very common because decay-causing anaerobic bacteria tend to grow in the pit and fissure areas. Pits and fissures are too narrow to be cleaned by even a single bristle of a toothbrush (Figure 9-8).

Class II — Posterior Teeth Only

Class II dental caries involves the occlusal surface and either the mesial and/or distal surface of posterior teeth. Because mesial and distal surfaces are in between the teeth, they are referred to as proximal surfaces. This is true of all teeth except for the last tooth in each arch.

Class II caries are very common because food and bacteria easily become impacted between the teeth, in the interproximal spaces, which are difficult for the patient to clean. Flossing is the most effective method to remove food particles and debris from interproximal spaces (Figure 9-9).

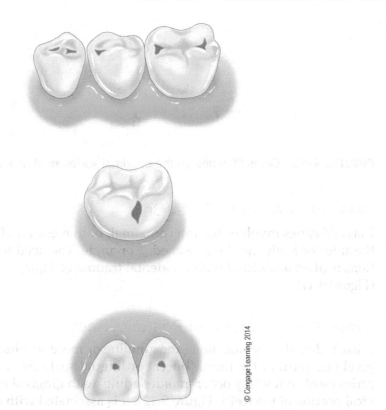

FIGURE 9-8   Class I caries on the (A) occlusal surfaces of the premolars and molars, (B) buccal surface on the molar, and (C) lingual surface on the maxillary incisors.

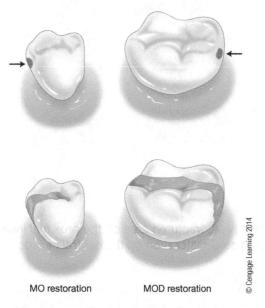

MO restoration   MOD restoration

FIGURE 9-9   (A) Class II caries on the proximal surface of a premolar and a molar and (B) restorations on the MO surface of a premolar and the MOD surfaces of a molar.

Class III — Anterior Teeth Only

Class III caries involves the proximal, mesial, or distal surfaces of the anterior teeth (Figure 9-10).

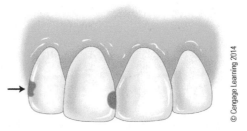

FIGURE 9-10 Class III caries on the proximal surfaces of an incisor and a cuspid.

Class IV — Anterior Teeth Only

Class IV caries involves the interproximal, both mesial and distal surfaces, of the anterior teeth and the incisal edge or angle. The need for Class IV restorations is often associated with accidental trauma or injury to the face or mouth (Figure 9-11).

Class V — Anterior and Posterior Teeth

Class V dental caries are along the gumline or more specifically along the gingival one-third of the facial/buccal or lingual surfaces of the tooth. Class V caries most commonly occur in older adults with gingival recession at the cervical portion of the teeth (Figure 9-12). It is associated with dry mouth.

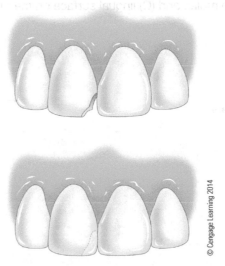

FIGURE 9-11 Class IV (A) fractured area on the proximal incisal surface of the incisor and (B) a completed restoration on the central incisor.

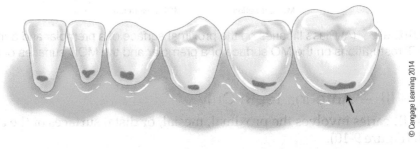

FIGURE 9-12 Class V caries on the gingival buccal areas of the teeth.

Class VI — Posterior Teeth and Cuspids

Class VI decay involves the incisal edges or cusp tips of teeth. It is associated with enamel erosion (Figure 9-13).

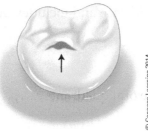

FIGURE 9-13 Class VI caries on the occlusal surface of a mandibular incisor due to abrasion.

 Exploring the Web

American Dental Association
www.ada.org

Web Search Terms: dental terminology, classification of dental caries, primary dentition, permanent dentition, and dental anatomy.

 Skill Building

These optional activities and exercises are designed to help the student put into practice information learned in the chapter.

1. Divide into groups and in a laboratory setting examine each other's mouths. This will require PPE, including gloves, masks, and safety glasses. Note restorations of different classifications, number and type of teeth present, and tooth surfaces. At home you may be able to use a family member as your patient to make these observations.

2. Using a mouth model called a typodont, identify the tooth surfaces, names of the teeth, and upper/lower jaws. If you have access to a human skull model, you can also observe the temporomandibular joint (TMJ) and other anatomical landmarks.

 Challenge Your Understanding

Select the response that best answers each of the following questions. Only one response is correct.

1. The office manager must be thoroughly familiar with dental nomenclature to:
   a. Interpret the dentist's, hygienist's, or chairside assistant's charting and treatment related records
   b. Provide patients with accurate information in predetermining treatment
   c. Bill patients and third-party payers accurately for treatment performed
   d. All of the above

2. The maxilla is attached to the skull by a movable joint called the temporomandibular joint (TMJ):
   a. True
   b. False

3. The maxilla is part of the face and includes the hard palate and the maxillary teeth:
   a. True
   b. False

4. All of the following are oral quadrants *except*:
   a. Maxillary right
   b. Mandibular left
   c. Temporomandibular joint
   d. Mandibular left

5. Which of the following teeth comprise the anterior sextants?
   a. Central incisors
   b. Lateral incisors
   c. Cupids (canines)
   d. All of the above

6. The quadrants are determined by an imaginary vertical line, the midline, that divides the face into right and left sides.
   a. True
   b. False

7. The periodontium consists of all of the following except:
   a. The gingiva
   b. Periodontal ligament
   c. The pulp chamber
   d. The alveolar process

8. Which of the following is/are true of enamel? It:
   a. Is the hardest substance in the human body
   b. Is composed of primarily inorganic materials and is shaped by prismatic rods
   c. Protects the tooth
   d. All of the above

9. Which of the following is/are true of dentin? It:
   a. Comprises the bulk of the tooth
   b. Determines tooth color
   c. Registers sensation to pain and temperature
   d. All of the above

10. All of the following are true of cementum except:
    a. It is the yellowish-white outer covering of the anatomical crown portion of the tooth

    b. It has a porous, rough, textured surface that permits the periodontal fibers to attach

    c. It can rebuild itself, forming secondary cementum

    d. It covers the anatomical root of the tooth

11. The dental pulp:
    a. Provides the blood and other nutrients from the body to the tooth
    b. Is composed of nerve, blood, and lymph
    c. Enters the tooth through the apical foramen
    d. All of the above

12. The periodontal ligament acts as a shock absorber to cushion the tooth in the socket and provides attachment to the jawbone.
    a. True
    b. False

13. The pulp in the root of the tooth is contained in the pulp chamber.
    a. True
    b. False

14. A cingulum is the lingual lobe of any posterior tooth appearing on the cervical (neck portion) one-third of the tooth.
    a. True
    b. False

15. A developmental groove is a shallow groove or line on the surface of a tooth.
    a. True
    b. False

16. The permanent dentition consists of :
    a. 16 teeth in each arch
    b. 5 teeth in each quadrant
    c. 38 teeth in total
    d. a and b only
    e. All of the above

17. The deciduous or primary dentition consists of :
    a. 10 teeth in each arch
    b. 5 teeth in each quadrant
    c. A total of 20 teeth
    d. All of the above

18. Commonly referred to as "pit and fissure caries," Class I dental caries may occur on all of the following except:
    a. The occlusal surfaces of premolars and molars
    b. The buccal or lingual surfaces of molars
    c. The mesial and/or distal surface of posterior teeth
    d. The lingual surfaces of maxillary incisors

19. Class V dental caries involves the gingival one-third of the facial/buccal or lingual surfaces of the teeth and is most commonly seen in older adults with gingival recession.
    a. True
    b. False

20. Class III dental caries involves the incisal edges or cusp tips of teeth and is associated with enamel erosion.
    a. True
    b. False

Charting the Oral Cavity

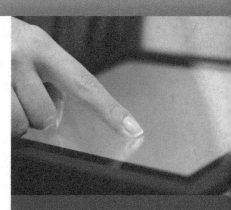

CHAPTER OUTLINES

KEY TERMS

abutments
amalgam
anatomical dental chart
caries
composite/resin
crown
extraction
Fédération Dentaire
   Internationale System
geometric dental chart
impacted
Palmer System
Periodontal
pontic
porcelain-fused-to-metal
   crown
Universal System

LEARNING OBJECTIVES

Upon completion of this chapter, the reader should be able to:

1. Explain the importance of accurate charting records.

2. Describe and differentiate the three most commonly used tooth numbering systems and how they are used in charting: The Universal System, Palmer System and Fédération Dentaire Internationale System.

3. Be familiar with manual, electronic, and voice-activated charting.

4. Demonstrate accurate charting of existing dental restorations, caries, and required treatment using accepted charting symbols, terms, and abbreviations.

5. Demonstrate knowledge in interpreting charted dental information to communicate planned treatment information accurately to other team members and to educate patients about the dentist's recommended treatment plan, as well as treatment completed.

The Importance of Accurate Clinical Records

Accurate clinical records are the mainstay of the dental practice. The dental office manager should be able to review a patient's chart, and then understand, explain, and interpret the patient's planned treatment, as well as treatment already completed. Clinical records are generated either manually or electronically using a system of words, numbers, letters, symbols, or commands that comprise the practice's charting system. Before proceeding with this chapter, make sure you have a good understanding of the information in Chapter 9 (Dental Nomenclature and Related Terminology).

Thorough understanding of charting includes knowledge of the individual names of the teeth in the primary and secondary dentitions, familiarity with the names of related oral structures and their use and function, knowledge of the names of the surfaces and edges of the teeth, knowledge of the six cavity classifications, and abbreviations of various terms used in preparing and completing patients' records.

Once familiar with this information, the office manager is able to accurately interpret the dentist's planned treatment and to present this information to patients and insurance carriers using both layman's terms and professional terminology appropriately. She or he also uses this information to process manual and electronic claims accurately to third-party carriers/insurance companies. Finally, the office manager must be able to interpret and understand chart notations and accurately describe treatment completed.

The dental chart is a permanent record of the patient's oral conditions, existing restorations, and diagnosed need for treatment. The dentist's diagnosis is based upon clinical visual examination, review of diagnostic records including radiographs and study models, the patient's health history, and any symptoms or complaints reported by the patient.

As addressed in Chapter 3 (Legal and Ethical Regulations in Dental Office Management), keeping accurate, detailed, and up-to-date clinical records is the first line of defense in reducing the risk of malpractice suits. Neither the office manager nor any other member of the dental team should ever attempt to falsify or alter clinical charting and/or notations.

If done manually, charting and other clinical notations must be made in ink. If an error is to be corrected or a change made in the chart notations, a single line should be drawn through the error with the initials of the person entering the notation and the correction made immediately beside it.

Records are the property of the practice and the information contained in them is confidential. Information should not be released except when requested in writing by the patient, another treating dentist, a third-party insurance carrier, or when subpoenaed by an attorney or State Board of Dental Examiners. Sharing information must be done in compliance with HIPAA. When forwarding records, the office manager should always send duplicates, never the originals!

The Complete Dental Chart

The complete dental chart provides additional information about the patient, including clinical examination notes and a diagram of the teeth that indicates carious lesions to be repaired and existing restorations. Typically, information included on the clinical chart includes the following:

- *The patient's personal information*, including name, address, and home and work telephone numbers.
- *Specific medical history*, with notations of importance to the dentist, such as known allergies, current medications prescribed by the physician, blood pressure reading, and the patient's family physician.

Note: The office manager should update this information at each recall visit or at least annually.

- *The charting area*, a tooth chart with space for additional notations related to the clinical findings.
- *Treatment entry area*, indicating dates of service, treatment, or procedure performed, and the types of impression, restorative materials, and anesthetic used. The patient's financial documentation should never be included in the treatment information.
- *The remarks area*, indicating teeth to be watched or other clinical or treatment notations made by the dentist.

Note: Personal remarks or observations about the patient should not be made in this area. If non-dental observations or anecdotal information is added, it should be entered on a separate piece of paper included in the file jacket and never entered into the clinical records. This is to prevent embarrassment to the practice should records be transferred to another office or should they be subpoenaed.

Tooth Numbering Systems

Charting is based upon tooth numbering systems. Three accepted dental numbering systems are used for dental charting in the United States with most dentists using the system they used in dental school. Although dental practices may use slightly different charting methods, the following are the most commonly used numbers, symbols, terms, and abbreviations.

It is important for the office manager to remember that dental charting is performed as though facing the patient, that is, left and right are reversed when charting notations are entered. Starting with the last tooth in the patient's upper right quadrant, charting entries begin on the upper left of the dental chart or computer screen. Visually the dental chart is from the prospective of looking into the patient's mouth.

Universal Numbering System

The Universal System was adopted by the American Dental Association in 1968 as a uniform way for dental practitioners, insurance carriers, and other professionals to communicate using the same language. This numbering system is the overwhelming favorite among American dentists. The intent of the Universal System is to avoid confusion by assigning each tooth in the permanent dentition its own number, from #1 to # 32. Each tooth in the deciduous dentition has its own letter, from A to T.

Permanent Dentition

In the permanent dentition, the teeth are assigned a number starting with the upper right third molar, which is tooth #1. The numbers follow from #1 through #16 sequentially around the entire maxillary arch to the upper left third molar, which is #16. Next, the Universal System drops down to the mandibular arch, starting directly below #16 with the lower left mandibular third molar, which is #17. The Universal System continues from the lower left third molar all the way around the mandibular arch to the lower right third molar. The mandibular arch includes teeth #17 through #32 (Figure 10-1).

When a tooth is missing, it still has the number assigned to the tooth in that position but the notation is made that it is not present. For example, Susan has had all of her wisdom or third molars removed. The charting would begin by stating that tooth #1 is missing and tooth #2 would be the first tooth on Susan's chart for any notation regarding observations.

Deciduous Dentition

The designations of the Universal System for deciduous or primary teeth follow the same pattern. Starting with the upper right second deciduous molar, the letters begin with A and continue all the way around the maxillary arch to the upper left second deciduous molar, which is letter J. The Universal System drops down to the mandibular arch, starting with the lower left second deciduous molar, which is letter K, and follows all the way around the mandibular arch to the lower right second deciduous molar, which is the letter T (Figure 10-1).

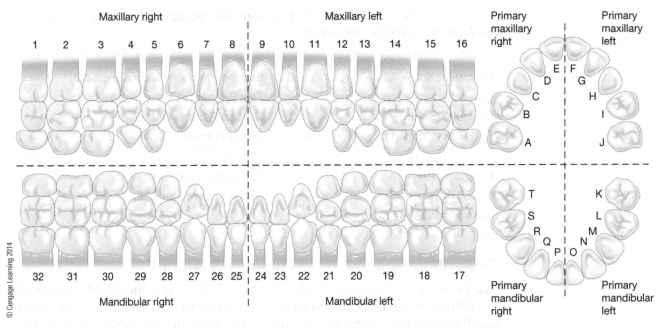

FIGURE 10-1 Universal numbering system for both permanent and deciduous teeth with identifying numbers and letters.

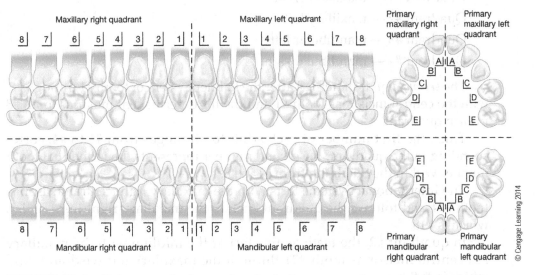

FIGURE 10-2 Palmer numbering system for both permanent and deciduous teeth with identifying numbers and letters.

Palmer System

Prior to the acceptance of the Universal System, many dentists used the Palmer System of tooth numbering and lettering. Today, some family practices use it and it is especially popular with orthodontists.

In the Palmer System, each tooth in the *quadrant* has a designated number and a *bracket* indicating its quadrant. Starting with the central incisor and working back in each quadrant to the third molar, the teeth in the adult permanent dentition are designated from the central incisor as #1 to the third permanent molar #8. A bracket designates the quadrant (Figure 10-2 and Table 10-1).

TABLE 10-1 **Palmer System** The following table represents tooth numbers by *quadrant*, using the Palmer System.

Adult (Permanent) Dentition:	
Central Incisor — #1	Second Premolar (second bicuspid) — #5
Lateral Incisor — #2	First Permanent Molar — #6
Canine (Cuspid) — #3	Second Permanent Molar — #7
First Premolar (first bicuspid) — #4	Third Permanent Molar — #8
Primary (Deciduous) Dentition:	
Central Incisor — A	First Deciduous Molar — D
Lateral Incisor — B	Second Deciduous Molar — E
Cuspid (canine) — C	

Fédération Dentaire Internationale System

The Fédération Dentarie Internationale System is a modified version of the Palmer System for the adult permanent teeth. Brackets are replaced by quadrant numbers, representing the *first digit* of the numbering system. The quadrants of the permanent mouth are numbered as follows:

Quadrant #1 — maxillary right

Quadrant #2 — maxillary left

Quadrant #3 — mandibular left

Quadrant #4 — mandibular right

The *second digit* is patterned after the Palmer System of tooth #1 through #8, with the central incisor as tooth #1 and the third permanent molar as tooth #8 in each quadrant.

Thus, the first number of each adult tooth ranges from #1 to #4, corresponding to the quadrant; the second number represents the individual tooth number within the quadrant, from #1 to #8.

The International System starts with the maxillary right central incisor as tooth #11 and follows the quadrant back to the maxillary right third molar, which is #18.

In quadrant #2, the teeth again start at the midline with the maxillary left central incisor as tooth #21 through the maxillary left wisdom tooth, which is #28.

In quadrant #3, the teeth start at the midline with the mandibular left central incisor, which is #31 and goes back to the mandibular left third molar, which is #38.

In quadrant #4, the teeth start at the midline with the central incisor as tooth #41 to the mandibular right third molar, which is tooth #48 (Figure 10-3).

In the Fédération Internationale System, the primary dentition uses quadrant #5 through #8 as follows:

Quadrant #5 — maxillary right

Quadrant #6 — maxillary left

Quadrant #7 — mandibular left

Quadrant #8 — mandibular right

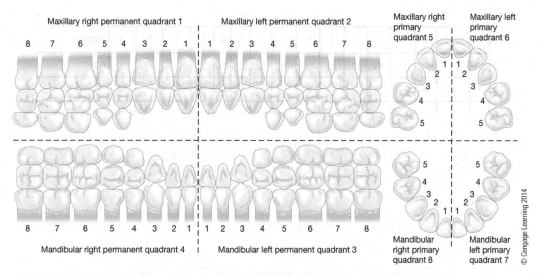

FIGURE 10-3 International Standards Organization (ISO) Designation System/Fédération Dentaire Internationale numbering system for both permanent and deciduous teeth with identifying numbers and letters.

The deciduous teeth are numbered with the quadrant number as the first digit and the tooth number as the second digit, starting with the central incisor in each quadrant as #1 and the second deciduous molar as tooth #5.

The teeth in the maxillary right quadrant start with #5 representing the quadrant number and the second number to indicate the tooth in the quadrant. Thus, the teeth in the maxillary right quadrant comprise #51 through #55, starting with the upper right deciduous central incisor and ending with the maxillary right second deciduous molar, #55.

In the maxillary left quadrant tooth designations start with #6 representing the quadrant number, the teeth began with the maxillary left deciduous incisor, tooth #61, and in with the maxillary left second deciduous molar, tooth #65.

In the mandibular left quadrant tooth designation start with #7 representing the quadrant number, the teeth start with the mandibular left central incisor, #71, and the end with the mandibular left second deciduous molar, tooth #75.

In the final quadrant, the mandibular right, it is designated by the number #8 and begins at the right central incisor, tooth #81, and ends with the mandibular right second deciduous molar, tooth #85.

Figure 10-4 compares all three tooth numbering systems.

Charting Symbols and Abbreviations

Having familiarity with tooth numbering systems, the office manager must also become familiar with charting symbols and other abbreviations used in charting the oral cavity.

There are different types of dental charts, supplied by a variety dental suppliers and dental software providers. The two general types of charts are anatomic and geometric.

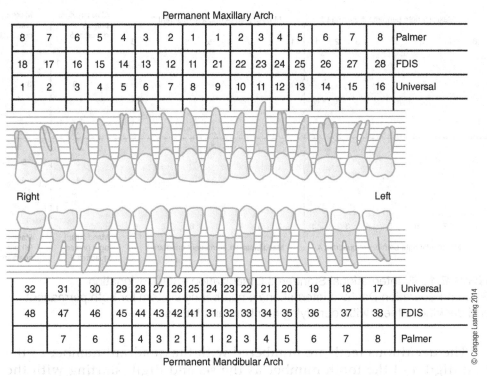

Permanent Maxillary Arch

8	7	6	5	4	3	2	1	1	2	3	4	5	6	7	8	Palmer
18	17	16	15	14	13	12	11	21	22	23	24	25	26	27	28	FDIS
1	2	3	4	5	6	7	8	9	10	11	12	13	14	15	16	Universal

Right   Left

32	31	30	29	28	27	26	25	24	23	22	21	20	19	18	17	Universal
48	47	46	45	44	43	42	41	31	32	33	34	35	36	37	38	FDIS
8	7	6	5	4	3	2	1	1	2	3	4	5	6	7	8	Palmer

Permanent Mandibular Arch

FIGURE 10-4a Comparison of tooth numbering systems.

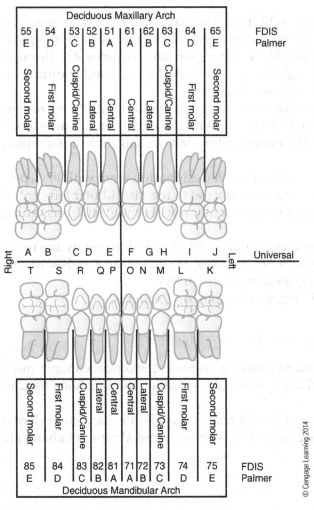

Deciduous Maxillary Arch

55	54	53	52	51	61	62	63	64	65	FDIS
E	D	C	B	A	A	B	C	D	E	Palmer
Second molar	First molar	Cuspid/Canine	Lateral	Central	Central	Lateral	Cuspid/Canine	First molar	Second molar	

Right   Left

A	B	C	D	E	F	G	H	I	J	Universal
T	S	R	Q	P	O	N	M	L	K	

Second molar	First molar	Cuspid/Canine	Lateral	Central	Central	Lateral	Cuspid/Canine	First molar	Second molar	
85	84	83	82	81	71	72	73	74	75	FDIS
E	D	C	B	A	A	B	C	D	E	Palmer

Deciduous Mandibular Arch

FIGURE 10-4b

Anatomic Chart

The **anatomic dental chart** depicts the teeth and related oral structures as they generally appear upon clinical examination that is with the cusps, grooves, pits, and other landmarks. Some anatomic charts depict a portion or all of the tooth roots. When charting, the chairside dental assistant fills in the surfaces on the corresponding anatomic areas as directed by the dentist (Figure 10-5).

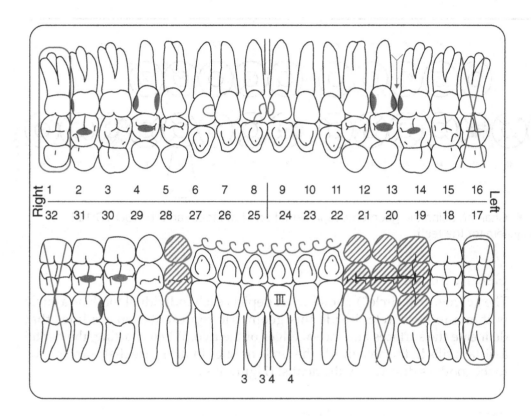

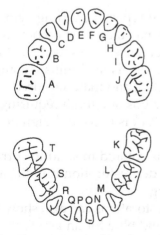

FIGURE 10-5 Charting using the anatomical teeth and the Universal/National System for numbering.

© Cengage Learning 2014

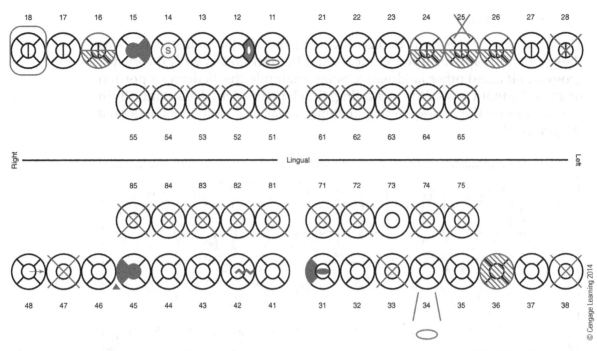

FIGURE 10-6 Charting using the geometric representation of the teeth and the ISO TC 106 designation system for the teeth.

Geometric Chart

The **geometric** ("circle") **dental chart** depicts each individual tooth as a circle within another circle. Inside this geometric representation are lines that delineate the surfaces and incisal edges of the two. When charting, the dental assistant fills in the area inside the circle or lines in the space that corresponds to the tooth as directed by the dentist (Figure 10-6).

Office Systems and Color Charting

Although there are different types of charting symbols and ways to indicate specific findings, the office manager must become accustomed to the method the dentist prefers. Many practices use specific colors in the charting area to designate clinical findings. This is to eliminate confusion between treatment required, treatment completed, and materials used.

Red indicates carious lesions or a tooth requiring treatment, *Blue* indicates existing restorations, and *Black* is used to designate restorations done by this practice.

An area of new **caries** is colored in solid to correspond with the area; recurrent caries around an older restoration is indicated by a *Red* outline of the existing restoration or filling.

Blue used for existing restorations can also show the type of material used, with the area filled with solid blue for an **amalgam** restoration, the area outlined for a composite/resin or tooth colored restoration, and crosshatching to indicate a gold restoration.

Many offices like to use *Black* to indicate the work that they have done for a quick reference. In that case, black would be used in the same manner that blue is used for existing work.

Symbols may vary slightly between offices so it is important for office managers to become familiar with those variations and ask for clarification when unsure about a charting symbol.

Charting Terms and Abbreviations

It is helpful for all members of the dental team to use a standard set of abbreviations and symbols with charting. This enhances communication and assists the office manager when explaining required treatment to the patient, especially in numbers of surfaces requiring restoration, in developing payment estimates, and when filing third-party claims for reimbursement (Table 10-2).

TABLE 10-2 Common Dental Terms and Abbreviations Used for Charting

Abscess	Abs
Adjustment	Adj
Amalgam	Amal
Anesthetic	Anes
Anterior	Ant
Bitewing	BW or BWX
Bridge	Br
Buccal	B
Cement	Cem
Composite	Com
Consultation	Cons or Consult
Crown	Cr or CRN
Deciduous	Dec or Decid
Delivery	Del
Denture	Dent
Diagnosis	Diag or DX
Distal	D
Examination	EX or Exam
Extraction	Ext or Exo
Estimate	Est
Facial	F
Fluoride	Fl
Fixed Bridge	Fix Br
Fracture	FX
Full Gold Crown	FGC
Full Lower Denture	FLD
Full Mouth X-rays	FMX
Full-Upper Denture	FUD
Gold	G
Gold Inlay	GI
Gold Onlay	GO
Impaction	Impac

(continues)

TABLE 10-2 *(continued)*

Implant	IMPL
Impression	Imp
Incisal	I
Laser	LS
Lidocaine	Lido
Lingual	L or Li
Mesial	M
Missing	X
Nitrous Oxide	N$_2$O
Occlusal	O
Onlay	On
Oral Health Instruction	OHI
Panorex	Pano
Partial Lower Denture	PLD
Partial Upper Denture	PUD
Periodontal Screening Record	PSR
Permanent	Perm
Pit and Fissure Sealants	PFS
Porcelain	Porc
Porcelain Fused to Gold	PFG
Porcelain Fused to Metal	PFM
Porcelain Jacket Crown	PJC
Posterior	Post
Postoperative	PO
Preventive Oral Hygiene	POH
Prophylaxis	Pro or Prophy
Proximal	Prox
Removable	Rem
Root Canal Therapy	RCT
Seat (final cementation)	St
Shade	Sh
Study Models	SM
Temporary	Temp
Treatment	TX
Treatment Plan	TxPl
Xylocaine	Xylo
Zinc-oxide eugenol	ZOE
Zinc oxyphosphate	ZnP

Some abbreviations are used together in describing multiple surfaces of teeth. For example, when compound surfaces of caries are involved, as in a mesial-occlusal-distal restoration, the names of the surfaces are combined and referred to as an M-O-D. Each letter is pronounced individually. When tooth surfaces are combined and spoken the "al" is dropped from all but the last surface and replaced with an "o," such as mesio-occluso-distal.

The most common abbreviations of combined tooth surfaces are as follows:

- Mesio-occlusal or MO pronounced "M"-"O"
- Disto-occlusal or DO pronounced "D"-"O"
- Mesio-occlusal or MO pronounced "M"-"O"
- Disto-incisal or DI pronounced "D"-"I"
- Disto-lingual or DL pronounced "D"-"L"
- Bucco-occlusal or BO pronounced "B"-"O"
- Linguo-occlusal or LO pronounced "L"-"O"

With practice, all members of the dental team quickly learn to use consistent terminology and abbreviations.

Common Charting Symbols

Following are the commonly used charting symbols. It is important for the dental office manager not only to know how to enter these symbols onto a chart (either manually or electronically) but also to be able to interpret them. Various charting symbols are presented in Figure 10-7.

Caries

Caries or dental decay is always charted in red because it stands out as work that needs to be done. It is illustrated as accurately as possible and includes all the surfaces involved. Recurrent decay around an existing restoration shows that restoration outlined in red.

Existing Restorations

Existing restorations are outlined in blue and filled in to indicate the material used. The area inside the outline is empty to indicate a tooth color restoration (composite/resin), it is colored solid blue to show an amalgam restoration, and with crosshatching to indicate it is gold.

Missing Tooth

A missing tooth is one that has been extracted or never formed. A tooth that never formed is called congenitally missing. A missing tooth is designated by an X in blue through all of it or in some practices the root only.

Tooth to Be Extracted

A tooth scheduled for extraction or removal because of advanced caries, impaction as in the case with many third molars, or at the request of the orthodontist is designated with two vertical lines in red.

Impacted Tooth

An impacted tooth is covered with bone, soft tissue, or both and there is some interference with normal eruption; it is not visible in the mouth. An impacted tooth is indicated with a circle around it and an arrow to indicate the direction of the impaction.

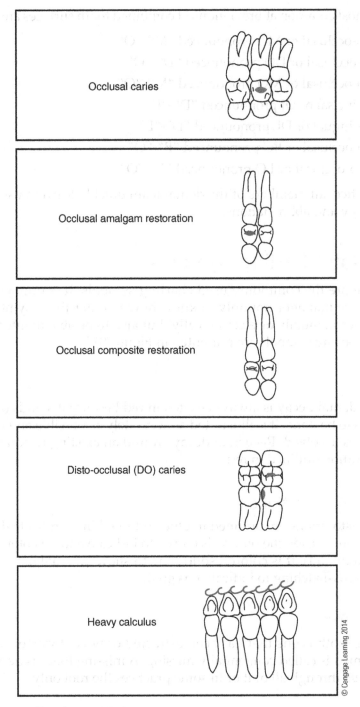

FIGURE 10-7a Charting symbols.

Drifted Tooth

A tooth that has moved from its original position in the oral cavity, usually a result of other missing teeth or periodontal disease, is described as having drifted. A tooth may drift downward, upward, forward (mesially), or backward (distally) as indicated with an arrow in the direction of the drift. Teeth that have drifted downward in the maxilla and upward in the mandible are called hyper-erupted, meaning they have erupted past the occlusal plane, the point that the teeth would normally bite together. This occurs when the

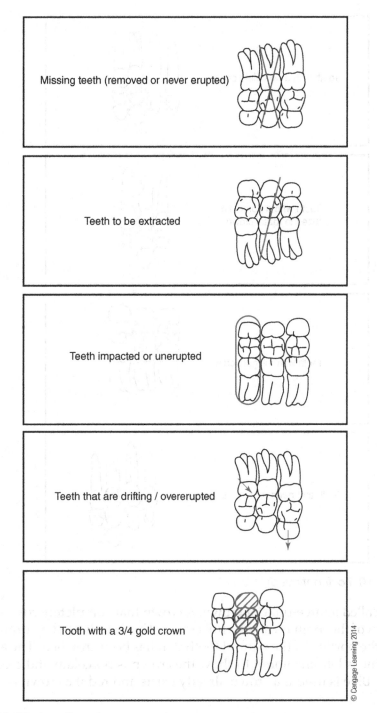

Missing teeth (removed or never erupted)

Teeth to be extracted

Teeth impacted or unerupted

Teeth that are drifting / overerupted

Tooth with a 3/4 gold crown

© Cengage Learning 2014

FIGURE 10-7b (*continues*)

opposing tooth is missing. Blue would be used because this is a description of clinical appearance; red would be used for treatment if any was indicated.

Crown

When a tooth has had the clinical portion of the natural enamel reduced and replaced with an artificial covering, the replacement is called a crown. Some patients may also refer to this as a cap. A crown that covers three-quarters of a

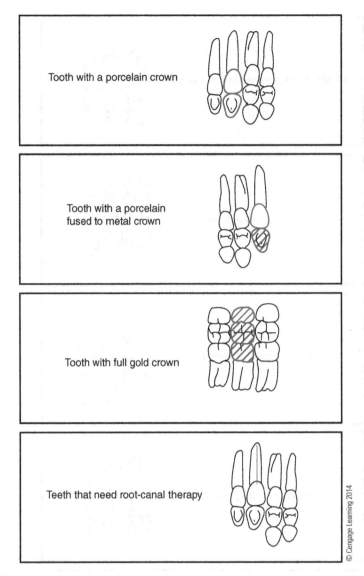

© Cengage Learning 2014

FIGURE 10-7c *(continued)*

tooth is called a three-quarter crown. A crown that completely covers the clinical crown of the tooth is called a full crown. This is indicated by drawing a line around the portion of the natural tooth that has been crowned. The area inside the outline is left uncolored to show the crown is porcelain and crosshatched for gold. Blue is used if a crown already exists and red if a crown is needed.

Porcelain-Fused-to Metal Crown

A crown that is made of porcelain fused to metal in the laboratory is called a porcelain-fused-to metal crown. Draw a line around the portion of the natural tooth that has been crowned and parallel diagonal lines to indicate the portion of the metal.

Fixed Bridge

A fixed bridge contains a minimum of one abutment (anchor tooth) and one pontic (a false tooth that replaces a missing natural tooth). To chart a fixed bridge, draw an X through all the missing natural teeth. Indicate the abutments by outlining them and drawing parallel diagonal lines through all the teeth that comprise the bridge.

Fractured Tooth

Sometimes teeth become fractured, usually due to physical trauma or sometimes due to advanced decay, biting force, or desiccation (drying out) as the result of root canal therapy. Draw a single jagged line on the chart through the area of the tooth fractured.

Periapical Abscess

A periapical abscess forms around the apex (tip) of the root portion of the tooth. On a radiograph, it often appears as a darkened round mass. To chart a periapical abscess, draw a small red circle around the tip of the abscessed root.

Root Canal

A tooth that has a root canal is one that has received endodontic treatment. Indicate a root-canal-treated tooth by drawing a single straight vertical line through each root of the tooth. Blue indicates the root canal has been completed; red indicates the root canal is yet to be completed.

Periodontal Charting

In addition to charting of the treatment needed and restorations present during the clinical examination, dentists also chart the periodontal health of the patient. This is done by measuring the sulcus around each tooth. The sulcus extends from the top of the gingiva to the point where the gingiva and tooth attach. An instrument called a periodontal probe is used to measure the sulcus depth in millimeters; this sulcus depth is called a periodontal pocket. In healthy tissue this space would be 1–3 mm, with deeper measurements indicating periodontal or gum disease, which is the leading cause of tooth loss. As these pockets become deeper because of bacterial accumulations, the bacteria that thrive in these deep pockets create even deeper pockets and eat away at the bone that supports the tooth.

Periodontal pocket depths are measured at six points around each tooth. Three measurements are done on the buccal/facial of each tooth at the distal, buccal midpoint, and mesial; these same measurements are done on the lingual of each tooth at the distal, lingual midpoint, and mesial (Figure 10-8). This process is known as a periodontal screening record (PSR).

As part of the periodontal charting, notations are made regarding bleeding of surrounding tissue and tooth mobility.

Manual Charting

Traditionally, dental charting has been accomplished by the dentist's oral dictation of clinical findings to the chairside assistant or hygienist. The assistant or hygienist recorded this information onto the clinical record or chart, which

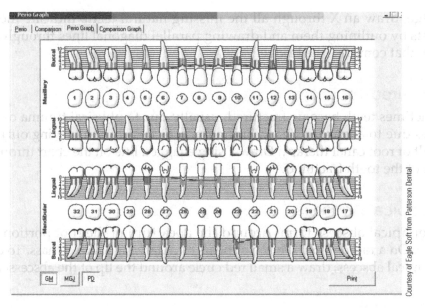

FIGURE 10-8 Periodontal chart includes probing depth, bleeding index, notation for any furcation involvement, level of gingival margin, tooth mobility, and the attachment level for both arches.

was then filed in the office. Manual charting is still done in many practices today, although the trend is rapidly moving toward computerized charting and paperless practices. Regardless of the method used the basics are always the same.

Computer-Assisted Charting

The computer may be used to store and retrieve information collected regarding the clinical observations made by the dentist during an oral examination. Once the information is entered the computer stores this diagnostic information. Some dental software programs can also compare information collected during successive office visits. One advantage of computer stored information is that it is faster, more legible, and potentially more accurate than manual charting. Also the amount of paper is reduced and patient charts are retrieved more easily. Voice recognition software is available to assist with charting, leaving the clinician free to record information without moving between the patients mouth and keyboard. This software also aids in eliminating cross contamination of the treatment area.

Computer software programs can assist the dentist in planning and initiating treatment. Patients without appointments that need treatment can quickly be located and it can also be helpful in educating patients about their treatment progress.

The computer can also generate graphic representations, for example, of a patient's periodontal condition. This information may include periodontal pocket depths, gingival bleeding scores, plaque scores, and/or tooth mobility. Visual graphics of periodontal disease are helpful to the dentist and the office manager in providing patient education, explaining treatment plans, and making comparisons of oral health improvement from appointment to appointment.

Exploring the Web

Dental Charting
   Search dental charting on **www.youtube.com**

ADA Charting
   http://www.ada.org/sections/professionalResources/pdfs/dentalpractice
   _abbreviations.pdf

Skill Building

These optional activities and exercises are designed to help the student put into practice information learned in the chapter.

1. Divide into groups of patient-clinician-assistant and wearing appropriate PPE, take turns practicing charting.

   Using the Universal System, the clinician starts at the patient's last tooth on the upper right quadrant. The clinician calls out existing restorations by tooth number and surface. The operator also calls out any missing teeth. The chairside assistant records the information onto the patient's chart using a blue pencil or pen.

   When you have completed the oral charting have an instructor verify the results. Each student should take a turn being the clinician dictating the charting and assistant entering it into the patient record. Be kind to your classmates as you assume the different roles; remember it will soon be your turn to be in that position.

2. Have someone dictate oral charting to you. Complete the charting using symbols, letters, and abbreviations. It is helpful for the person doing the dictation to vary speed and if possible add distraction to simulate the dental office environment.

Challenge Your Understanding

1. Clinical records are generated either manually or electronically; using a system of words, numbers, letters, symbols, or commands that comprise the practice's charting system.
   a. True
   b. False

2. Thorough understanding of charting includes:
   a. Familiarity with names of related oral structures and their use and function in the oral cavity
   b. Knowledge of the names of the surfaces and edges of all teeth
   c. Knowledge of the six cavity classifications
   d. All of the above

3. The office manager must understand charting to do all of the following accurately *except*:
   a. Interpret the dentist's planned treatment
   b. Present planned treatment information to patients and insurance carriers using both layman's terms and professional terminology
   c. Make a proper diagnosis of the patient's oral condition
   d. Accurately process manual and electronic claims to third-party carriers

4. The dental chart is a permanent record of:
   a. The patient's oral condition(s)
   b. Existing restorations
   c. Diagnosed need for treatment
   d. All of the above

5. The dentist's diagnosis is based upon all of the following except:
   a. Clinical visual examination
   b. The insurance company's recommendations
   c. Review of diagnostic records
   d. The patient's health history and any symptoms or complaints reported by the patient

6. When forwarding records, the office manager always sends the originals to ensure accuracy.
   a. True
   b. False

7. Information contained in the clinical chart should include:
   a. The patient's personal information and medical history
   b. A chart to illustrate existing and needed treatment
   c. An area to enter treatment notes
   d. All of the above

8. Personal remarks about a patient should be entered in the "remarks" area of the clinical chart.
   a. True
   b. False

9. Starting with the last tooth in the upper right quadrant, charting entries begin on the upper left of the dental chart or computer screen.
   a. True
   b. False

10. Using the Universal system, the upper right adult central incisor is tooth:
    a. #1
    b. #16
    c. #8
    d. #11

11. Using the Universal System, the lower left first deciduous molar is tooth letter/number:
    a. K
    b. 74
    c. B
    d. S

12. Using the Palmer System:
    a. Each tooth in the quadrant has a designated number or letter
    b. Each tooth's quadrant is designated by a bracket
    c. Each tooth's quadrant is designated by the first digit
    d. a and b only

13. Using the Palmer System, the second premolar in any quadrant is tooth:
    a. #1
    b. #5
    c. #4
    d. #13

14. In the Fédération Dentaire Internationale System, the mandibular right third molar is tooth:
    a. #16
    b. #8
    c. #48
    d. #58

15. The anatomic dental chart:
    a. Depicts the teeth and related oral structures as they generally appear upon clinical examination
    b. Depicts the teeth as circular graphics with lines to depict the surfaces and edges of the teeth
    c. Provides cusps, grooves, pits and other oral landmarks, including some or all of the roots
    d. a and c only

16. When marking chart entries, many offices use different colors of pencil or ink to eliminate confusion between treatment required and treatment completed.
    a. True
    b. False

17. As treatment is completed, the areas charted in blue are colored over using red to indicate the required treatment was completed.
    a. True
    b. False

18. The charting abbreviation for full-mouth X-rays is:
    a. BWX
    b. FX
    c. FMX
    d. FUD

19. A missing tooth is indicated on the dental chart by:
    a. Drawing a circle around the tooth
    b. Drawing an X through the tooth
    c. Drawing an arrow in the space the tooth used to occupy
    d. Drawing a circle around the tooth and filling in the space with parallel diagonal lines

20. Periodontal pockets are:
    a. Measured in millimeters
    b. Considered healthy when measurement is more than 3.
    c. Measured with a sulcular depth preceptor (SDP)
    d. All of the above

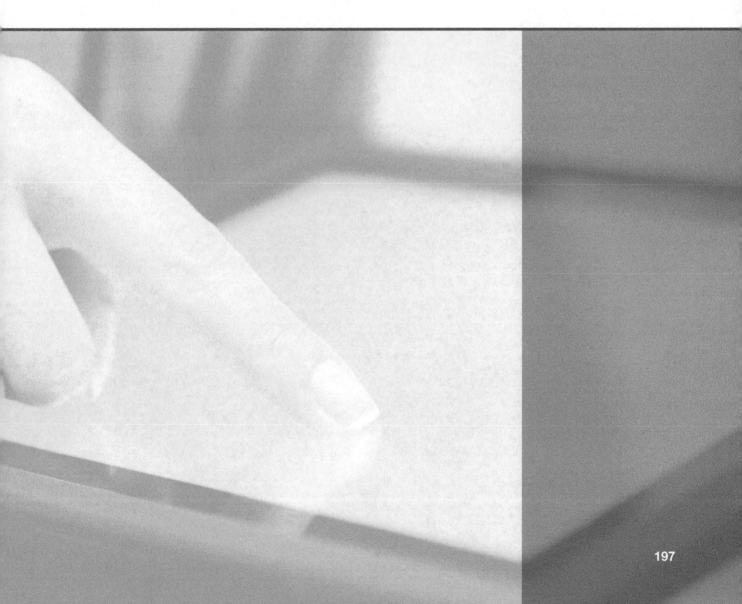

SECTION IV

Business and Financial Records Management

CHAPTER 11

Patient Records, Diagnosis, and Treatment Planning

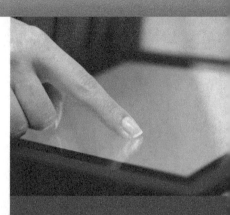

CHAPTER OUTLINES

KEY TERMS

1. Describe types of filing systems and the role of the office manager in utilizing and maintaining them.

2. Be familiar with alphabetization and its importance in maintaining patient records.

3. Describe the types of clinical, financial, and medical/dental history forms required in the dental office, and the role of the office manager.

4. Describe ownership and confidentially of patient records and the legal implications.

5. Describe the steps in diagnosis, treatment planning, and case presentation, and the role of the office manager related to them.

6. Be familiar with the most commonly used types of dental radiographs and new technological advances in digital radiography, as well as necessary steps to protect the operator and patient from radiation.

7. Understand the concept of patient referral to a specialist under the direction of the dentist.

8. Describe the office manager's role in maintaining a recall system.

9. List the nine parts of a pharmaceutical prescription and have an understanding of commonly used prescription terms and their meanings.

10. Understand the necessity of a dental laboratory prescription (work order) and the information most commonly required as directed by the dentist.

11. Understand the importance of maintaining a lab case tracking system.

Records Management

The role of the dental office manager in setting up and maintaining dental files and patient records is essential. To function smoothly, the well-run dental business office must have sound records management, whether the system is traditional with paper files or computer-based and paperless.

To ensure the continued smooth running and efficiency of the dental business office, one person in the practice, usually the office manager, should be responsible for all files and related information. A second dental team member should be cross-trained in records management to ensure continuity in the event of illness or staff turnover.

Filing Systems

Whether the office uses traditional paper files and filing cabinets or electronically stores and retrieves patient records, the philosophy and format of filing systems are similar. Patient files may be alphabetic, numeric, or chronological. Alphabetic is the most common.

If using traditional paper files, the filing system may be either horizontal or vertical. Stickers are affixed to the side or top of the file or jacket, indicating a range of letters that begin the last name, such as "Ja-Jg" or "Jh-Ju." The labels may also be color coded to assist the office manager in finding a specific patient by range of letters in the last name and the associated color (e.g., "Ja-Jg" may be red and "Jh-Ju" in green; (Figure 11-1). If the office manager were looking for Mr. Jones' file, he or she would rapidly scan the file for a green label with the "Jh-Ju" marker.

In the past additional stickers or labels were adhered to the outside of the folder to communicate other information understood within the office. Under HIPAA personal health information, these could constitute a breach in the patient's privacy, so all information should be contained inside the chart. These stickers when adhered to the inside of the chart form a color-coded communication having meanings such as "penicillin allergy," "special needs patient," "pre-medicate," "insurance," "prefers nitrous oxide," and so on. Placing stickers inside the chart or jacket ensures patient confidentiality.

Alphabetized Filing

Knowing proper alphabetization is essential for the office manager to quickly access patient records. Alphabetization is in the following order: the surname (last name), the given name (first name), the middle name or initial, and the patient's title or degree last (Mr., Mrs., Miss, Ms., or Dr.).

The standard rule is *"nothing comes before something."* As such, "Smith, J." is filed before "Smith, John."

When the patient's last name is hyphenated, such as George S. Martin-Jenkins, the hyphenated last name is treated as one name.

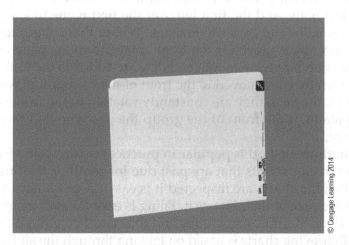

FIGURE 11-1 An example of a traditional paper file showing the tabbing system.

When filing the chart of a married woman, her record is filed by her name, not her husband's. Thus she is "Smith, Charity" and neither "Mrs. Frank T. Smith" nor "Smith, Mrs. Frank T."

If there are two Charity Smiths in the practice, the one with no middle initial is filed first. If there are two Charity Smiths with different middle names, the one with the middle initial or name closer to the beginning of the alphabet is filed first. For example, "Smith, Charity" is filed before "Smith, Charity C." If two Mrs. Smiths list themselves as "Charity C. Smith" and "Charity Catherine Smith," respectively, the Mrs. Smith with the C. initial is filed ahead of the Mrs. Smith with the full middle name.

Numeric Filing

Another option for filing charts is to arrange them by patient number. With this system patient charts are filed according to a number assigned to the patient when they enter the practice. Many dental management software programs, including Dentrix (see Section VI), will automatically assign numbers to patients. If the practice uses paper charts, this number can be displayed along the side of the chart using stickers similar to the lettered stickers used when filing alphabetically.

A negative with this filing method is that when a patient calls before a chart can be found the patient number must be located in the computer. The computer can find the patient by name and then a chart is retrieved by the patient number.

A positive of numerical filing is it maintains the privacy of the patient because the patient name is not displayed on the chart where it might be visible to others in the office. The filing accuracy and speed is also improved because using only 10 digits is less confusing than 26 letters.

An example of this filing method would be that Smith, James with patient number 04456 would be filed before Adams, Alice whose number is 05644.

Chronological Filing

Chronological filing using the date of a patient's last visit is another method of filing. The benefit of this filing system is to keep the charts you are actively using within easy reach while drawing attention to the patients who have not been seen recently. This method commonly combines using the first letter of the last name and the first letter of the first name to keep the groups of patients smaller and easier to manage. Within that subgroup, the patient seen most recently is moved to the front of the group. As patients are seen in the current calendar year, a month and date are added to the visible size of the chart and then they are moved to the front of their subgroup. As patients are seen through the year, they are constantly rotating to the front of the group, with the patient at the front of the group the one who had the most recent appointment.

This charting method is popular in practices that rely on visual chart inspection to track patients that are past due for recall or treatment appointments. When the charts are inspected it is easy to see patients with stickers indicating the date of their last visit. Filing is easy for staff members because charts are divided into small groups and the chart being filed simply goes to the front. Retrieving charts is based on looking through the alphabetized subgroup assisted by knowing about when the patient was last seen.

An example of this charting is Johnson, Barbara 10/12 would be filed before James, Bob 8/12. Both are in the JB group and then arranged by most recent date of visit.

Filing Safety Rules and Courtesy

The office manager should follow commonsense safety rules when using a mechanical file. These rules include the following:

- Never leave a file drawer open; this could cause accidental bruising, tripping, or falling.
- Never pull out more than one drawer at a time; this could force the file cabinet to fall over, causing injury.
- Always return the file promptly to its proper position and location.
- If you don't have time to file it properly, don't file it at all. Most offices have a designated area for "to be filed" charts. This assures patient privacy without forcing a staff member to put the file away so quickly it could be misplaced.

Under HIPAA personal health information must be protected and never left out in the open where other people may read the contents. The name and contents should always be kept confidential.

Contents of the Patient File

The patient file must contain the patient's name usually with the last name listed first, the clinical record, financial responsibility form, informed consent form, medical/dental history form, and necessary dental radiographs.

Other personal information, such as non-clinical notes about the patient, should be compiled on a separate sheet of paper or on a separate computer document. Non-clinical notes may include personal information such as hobbies, information about the patient's personal preferences, family life, or business or civic affiliations. Personal information should never be part of the clinical or financial record.

Active Files

Active files are those charts of patients of record who have been treated in the office within the past 12 months and/or who owe outstanding fees. But some offices extend their active files longer than 12 months.

Inactive Files

Inactive files are those charts for patients of record who have not been treated or have not contacted the office for 12 or more months prior and have no outstanding balance. Charts for patients that have moved from the area or passed away would also be filed as inactive. Most practices conduct routine computer searches or manual audits of patient files. This is to keep patients from becoming lost mid-treatment; to see the patients who may have canceled appointments without reappointing; patients that need to schedule recommended treatment; and to ensure that patients are notified of all the recall appointments when due.

It is the office manager's job to contact and reschedule those patients who have incomplete treatment or who are past due for their recall appointment. Maintaining contact with patients is important because patient abandonment is a serious offense. Dental offices must call patients or notify them by mail then document those contacts until the patient meets the criteria for filing as inactive.

Types of Patient Records

Whereas all dental offices function with slight differences between them, the following are the most commonly used types of dental forms, patient records, and diagnostic aids.

Clinical

Before proceeding, it is recommended the student has reviewed Chapter 10 (Charting the Oral Cavity). The information covers common components of the clinical record, dental charting, and related terms. The clinical record contains pertinent information resulting from the oral examination conducted by the dentist, the patient's report of pain or other complaints, if any, and the treatment required or completed.

Each chart entry must be legible, dated, and initialed by the person making the entry.

Financial Responsibility

All patients, both those of record or new, must complete a financial responsibility form. This information includes the name, address, and phone numbers of the patient and the responsible party, if different, specific insurance information such as name of the carrier, the insured's group and/or policy number, and expiration date.

Additional information required includes the responsible parties' Social Security number and place of employment. Often a signature is required by the responsible party agreeing to pay fees not covered by insurance.

The financial responsibility form may also contain specific information about availability of financial payment plans and the office's policy regarding assessment of interest on extended or late payments.

Note the financial records are *not* part of the clinical record. Information on insurance and statements of financial responsibility are often found on the welcome form (Figure 11-2).

For additional information on insurance coverage and completing financial forms, refer to Chapter 13 (Managing and Accounts Receivable).

Informed Consent

Prior to initiating treatment, the dentist should have a signed informed consent form as part of the patient's complete permanent record. Informed consent is addressed in Chapter 3 (Legal and Ethical Regulations in Dental Office Management).

Welcome

We are pleased to welcome you to our practice. Please take a few minutes to fill out this form as completely as you can. If you have questions we'll be glad to help you. We look forward to working with you in maintaining your dental health.

Patient Information

Name _____ Soc. Sec. # _____
  Last Name   First Name   Initial

Address _____

City _____ State _____ Zip _____ Home Phone _____

Cell Phone _____ Email _____

Sex ☐ M ☐ F Age _____ Birthdate _____ ☐ Single ☐ Married ☐ Widowed ☐ Separated ☐ Divorced

Patient Employed by _____ Occupation _____

Business Address _____ Business Phone _____

Business Email _____

Whom may we thank for referring you? _____

Notify in case of emergency _____ Home Phone _____

Cell Phone _____ Business Phone _____

Email _____

Primary Insurance

Person Responsible for Account _____
         Last Name   First Name   Initial

Relation to Patient _____ Birthdate _____ Soc. Sec. # _____

Address (if different from patient) _____ Home Phone _____

City _____ State _____ Zip _____

Cell Phone _____ Email _____

Person Responsible Employed by _____ Occupation _____

Business Address _____ Business Phone _____

Business Email _____

Insurance Company _____ Phone _____

Insurance Email _____

Contract # _____ Group # _____ Subscriber # _____

Name of other dependents under this plan _____

Additional Insurance

Is patient covered by additional Insurance? ☐ Yes ☐ No

Subscriber Name _____ Relation to Patient _____ Birthdate _____

Address (if different from patient) _____ Soc. Sec. # _____

City _____ State _____ Zip _____ Home Phone _____

Cell Phone _____ Email _____

Subscriber Employed by _____ Business Phone _____

Business Email _____

Insurance Company _____ Phone _____

Insurance Email _____

Contract # _____ Group # _____ Subscriber # _____

Name of other dependents under this plan _____

Please complete both sides.

Courtesy of Smart Practice

FIGURE 11-2 Sample Welcome form. (*continues*)

Dental History

What would you like us to do today? _____ Are you in dental discomfort today? _____

Former Dentist _____ Address _____

Dentist's Email _____ Phone _____

Date of last dental care _____ Date of last x-rays _____

Check (✓) yes or no if you have had problems with any of the following:

☐ Y ☐ N Bad breath	☐ Y ☐ N Food collection between teeth	☐ Y ☐ N Periodontal treatment	☐ Y ☐ N Sensitivity to sweets
☐ Y ☐ N Bleeding gums	☐ Y ☐ N Grinding or clenching teeth	☐ Y ☐ N Sensitivity to cold	☐ Y ☐ N Sensitivity when biting
☐ Y ☐ N Clicking or popping jaw	☐ Y ☐ N Loose teeth or broken fillings	☐ Y ☐ N Sensitivity to hot	☐ Y ☐ N Sores or growths in mouth

How often do you brush? _____ Floss? _____

How do you feel about the appearance of your teeth? _____

Have you ever experienced an adverse reaction during or in conjunction with a medical or dental procedure? ☐ Y ☐ N

Other information about your dental health or previous treatment _____

Medical History

Physician's Name _____ Phone _____

Date of last visit _____ Have you had any serious illnesses or operations? ☐ Y ☐ N

If yes, describe _____

Are you currently under physician care? ☐ Y ☐ N   If yes, describe _____

Have you ever had a blood transfusion? ☐ Y ☐ N   If yes, give approximate dates _____

Have you ever taken Fen-Phen/Redux? ☐ Y ☐ N

Women: Are you pregnant? ☐ Y ☐ N   Nursing? ☐ Y ☐ N   Taking birth control pills? ☐ Y ☐ N

Check (✓) yes or no whether you have had any of the following:

☐ Y ☐ N AIDS/HIV Positive	☐ Y ☐ N Cough, persistent	☐ Y ☐ N Jaw pain	☐ Y ☐ N Shingles
☐ Y ☐ N Anaphylaxis	☐ Y ☐ N Cough up blood	☐ Y ☐ N Kidney disease or malfunction	☐ Y ☐ N Shortness of breath
☐ Y ☐ N Anemia	☐ Y ☐ N Diabetes		☐ Y ☐ N Skin rash
☐ Y ☐ N Arthritis, Rheumatism	☐ Y ☐ N Epilepsy	☐ Y ☐ N Liver Disease	☐ Y ☐ N Spina Bifida
☐ Y ☐ N Artificial heart valves	☐ Y ☐ N Fainting	☐ Y ☐ N Material allergies (**latex**, wool, metal, chemicals)	☐ Y ☐ N Stroke
☐ Y ☐ N Artificial joints	☐ Y ☐ N Food allergies		☐ Y ☐ N Surgical implant
☐ Y ☐ N Asthma	☐ Y ☐ N Glaucoma		☐ Y ☐ N Swelling of feet or ankles
☐ Y ☐ N Atopic (allergy prone)	☐ Y ☐ N Headaches	☐ Y ☐ N Mitral valve prolapse	
☐ Y ☐ N Back problems	☐ Y ☐ N Heart murmur	☐ Y ☐ N Nervous problems	☐ Y ☐ N Thyroid disease or malfunction
☐ Y ☐ N Blood disease	☐ Y ☐ N Heart problems Describe _____	☐ Y ☐ N Pacemaker/ Heart surgery	
☐ Y ☐ N Cancer		☐ Y ☐ N Psychiatric care	☐ Y ☐ N Tobacco habit
☐ Y ☐ N Chemical dependency	☐ Y ☐ N Hemophilia/ Abnormal bleeding	☐ Y ☐ N Rapid weight gain or loss	☐ Y ☐ N Tonsillitis
☐ Y ☐ N Chemotherapy		☐ Y ☐ N Radiation treatment	☐ Y ☐ N Tuberculosis
☐ Y ☐ N Circulatory problems	☐ Y ☐ N Herpes	☐ Y ☐ N Respiratory disease	☐ Y ☐ N Ulcer/Colitis
☐ Y ☐ N Cortisone treatments	☐ Y ☐ N Hepatitis	☐ Y ☐ N Rheumatic/Scarlet fever	☐ Y ☐ N Venereal disease
	☐ Y ☐ N High blood pressure		

Is patient currently taking any medications? If yes, list all:

_____

_____

_____

Does patient have drug allergies? If yes, list all:

_____

_____

_____

Authorization

I have reviewed the information on this questionnaire, and it is accurate to the best of my knowledge. I understand that this information will be used by the dentist to help determine appropriate and healthful dental treatment. If there is any change in my medical status, I will inform the dentist.

I authorize the insurance company indicated on this form to pay to the dentist all insurance benefits otherwise payable to me for services rendered. I authorize the use of this signature on all insurance submissions.

I authorize the dentist to release all information necessary to secure the payment of benefits. I understand that I am financially responsible for all charges whether or not paid by insurance.

Signature _____ Date _____

Payment is due in full at time of treatment, unless prior arrangements have been approved.

©Smartpractice™   #80–679 R1

FIGURE 11-2 (continued)

Medical/Dental Health History

Prior to examining a patient or initiating treatment, it is essential to have the patient, parent, or guardian complete or update a medical/dental health history form. This is to alert the dentist to prescribed drugs currently being taken by the patient, the name and telephone number of the patient's family physician, recent hospitalizations or surgeries, current medical conditions (such as a history of heart disease, diabetes, hypertension, hepatitis, or HIV), and any known allergies. The health history form should also contain the name and telephone number of a responsible party to contact in case of an emergency.

It is important that any allergies are noted in the health history. Anaphylaxis is an allergic reaction to a food or drug. Anaphylactic shock is a severe reaction to a particular allergen that is life-threatening. Once the allergen is in the blood stream the body produces large amounts of histamine and other chemicals, causing the blood pressure to drop, the airway to become restricted, and the tongue and throat to swell. This reaction can occur in the dental office with local anesthesia.

> **Note:** With the recent rise in latex sensitivity reported by health care workers and anaphylaxis reported by patients, it is important to question patients about any known sensitivity to latex products.

The medical/dental history form provides an excellent opportunity to note the patient's feelings and attitudes about his or her teeth, to list current dental complaints, and to record goals for improved oral health.

When necessary, the office manager should assist the new patient in completing this and all other forms and no blank spaces should be left on the form (Figure 11-3). If there is no answer to a question, indicate that by writing *no answer* or with the abbreviation *N/A* rather than leaving a blank.

Ownership of Patient Records

The HIPAA Privacy Rule grants patients access to their personal records, including medical and dental records. The question occasionally arises, "Who owns the records?" Although the patient has the right to review records or obtain copies of them, the practice owns the records.

Transfer of Patient Records

When a patient changes dentists or relocates, he or she may request copies of his or her records be transferred to the new treating dentist. The new dental practice may also request copies of the patient's records. The office manager should ask the patient or new dentist to send a written, signed, and dated request for transfer of records. Upon the patient's signed request, the records may be released either to the new dentist or to the patient. The office manager should send legible, high-quality duplicates of the records and never the originals. Many practices charge a small fee for duplication and mailing costs.

Patient Number _____ **A B C** **HEALTH HISTORY & REGISTRATION**

PATIENT INFORMATION

PATIENT'S NAME Last _____ First _____ Middle Initial _____ SEX: M F BIRTHDATE _____ AGE _____

Soc. Sec. # _____ If Patient is a Minor, give Parent's or Guardian's Name _____ TODAY'S DATE _____

Who May We Thank for Referring You to our Office? _____ Reason for this Visit _____

RESPONSIBLE PARTY INFORMATION

NAME Last _____ First _____ Middle Initial _____ MARITAL STATUS _____

RESIDENCE Street _____ Apt. # _____ City _____ State _____ Zip _____

MAILING ADDRESS Street _____ Apt. # _____ City _____ State _____ Zip _____

HOW LONG AT THIS ADDRESS _____ HOME PHONE _____ CELL PHONE _____

WORK PHONE _____ E-MAIL _____

PREVIOUS ADDRESS (if less than 3 yrs.) Street _____ City _____ State _____ Zip _____ How Long _____

SOCIAL SECURITY # _____ BIRTHDATE _____ DRIVER'S LICENSE # _____ RELATION TO PATIENT _____

EMPLOYER _____ OCCUPATION _____ NO. YEARS EMPLOYED _____

RESPONSIBLE PARTY'S SPOUSE

NAME _____
LAST   FIRST   MIDDLE

EMPLOYER _____ OCCUPATION _____ ( )
NO. YEARS EMPLOYED

SOC. SEC. # _____ BIRTHDATE _____

HOME PH. _____ CELL PH. _____

WORK PH. _____ E-MAIL _____

EMERGENCY INFORMATION: RELATIVE NOT LIVING WITH YOU.

NAME _____ RELATIONSHIP _____

ADDRESS _____ CITY, STATE _____

HOME PH. _____ CELL PH. _____

WORK PH. _____

DENTAL INSURANCE INFORMATION (Primary Carrier)

Insured's Name _____

Insurance Co. _____ E-MAIL _____

Insurance Co. Address _____

Insured's Employer _____

Insured's Soc. Sec. # _____ Group # _____ Local # _____

if you have double dental insurance coverage, complete this for the second coverage.

Insured's Name _____

Insurance Co. _____ E-MAIL _____

Insurance Co. Address _____

Insured's Employer _____

Insured's Soc. Sec. # _____ Group # _____ Local # _____

It is important that I know about your Medical and Dental History. These facts have a direct bearing on your Dental Health. This information is strictly confidential and will not be released to anyone. Thank you for taking the time to completely fill out this questionnaire.

DENTAL HISTORY	YES	NO
HOW LONG SINCE you have seen a dentist?		
Last COMPLETE Dental Exam, Date:		
Last FULL MOUTH X-RAYS, DATE: (16 Small Films or Panoramic)		
Are you having PROBLEMS now?	☐	☐
WHAT?		
Is your present dental health POOR?	☐	☐
Do you wear DENTURES? (Partials or Full)	☐	☐
Are you UNHAPPY with your dentures?	☐	☐
Would you like to know more about PERMANENT REPLACEMENTS?	☐	☐
Are you APPREHENSIVE about dental treatment?	☐	☐
Have you had any PERIODONTAL (GUM) treatments?	☐	☐
Do your gums BLEED, or feel TENDER or IRRITATED?	☐	☐
Are your teeth SENSITIVE to hot, cold, sweets, pressure? (circle)	☐	☐
Are you UNHAPPY with the APPEARANCE of your teeth?	☐	☐
Are you aware of GRINDING or CLENCHING your teeth?	☐	☐
Do you have HEADACHES, EARACHES, or NECK PAINS?	☐	☐
Have you worn BRACES on your teeth (ORTHODONTICS)	☐	☐
Do you have DISCOLORED teeth that bother you?	☐	☐
Would you like your smile to LOOK BETTER or DIFFERENT?	☐	☐
Do you REGULARLY use DENTAL FLOSS?	☐	☐

Name of Previous Dentist:

City: _____ State: _____

How do you feel about your teeth?

Please RANK the following in the order in which they would
KEEP YOU FROM having dental treatment.

FEAR of pain _____ # _____ LACK of concern _____ #

COST of treatment _____ # _____ MISSING work time _____ #

PATIENT Signature(Parent of Child) _____ Date: _____ DENTIST Signature _____

MEDICAL HISTORY	YES	NO
Do you have any CURRENT HEALTH PROBLEMS?	☐	☐
Are you under a PHYSICIAN'S CARE now?	☐	☐
For what?		
What MEDICATIONS are you currently taking?		
Have you ever taken Fen-Phen/Redux?	☐	☐
Are you PREGNANT?	☐	☐
Do you use cigars/cigarettes, pipe or chewing tobacco? (circle)	☐	☐

PLEASE ✓YES OR NO OF THE FOLLOWING WHICH YOU HAVE HAD, OR PRESENTLY HAVE:

	YES	NO		YES	NO		YES	NO
AIDS/HIV Pos.	☐	☐	Fainting	☐	☐	Psychiatric care	☐	☐
Anaphylaxis	☐	☐	Food allergies	☐	☐	Rapid weight gain/loss	☐	☐
Anemia	☐	☐	Glaucoma	☐	☐	Radiation treatment	☐	☐
Arthritis (Rheumatism)	☐	☐	Headaches	☐	☐	Respiratory disease	☐	☐
Artificial heart valves	☐	☐	Heart murmur	☐	☐	Rheumatic/scarlet fever	☐	☐
Artificial joints	☐	☐	Heart problems (please describe)	☐	☐	Shingles	☐	☐
Asthma	☐	☐				Shortness of breath	☐	☐
Atopic (Allergy Prone)	☐	☐	Hemophilia (Abnormal bleeding)	☐	☐	Skin rash	☐	☐
Back problems	☐	☐	Herpes	☐	☐	Spina Bifida	☐	☐
Blood disease	☐	☐	Hepatitis	☐	☐	Stroke	☐	☐
Cancer	☐	☐	High blood pressure	☐	☐	Surgical implant	☐	☐
Chemical dependency	☐	☐	Jaw pain	☐	☐	Swelling of feet or ankles	☐	☐
Chemotherapy	☐	☐	Kidney disease or malfunction	☐	☐	Thyroid disease or malfunction	☐	☐
Circulatory problems	☐	☐	Liver disease	☐	☐	Tobacco habit	☐	☐
Cortisone treatments	☐	☐	Material allergies	☐	☐	Tonsillitis	☐	☐
Cough (persistent)	☐	☐	(latex, wool, metal, chemicals)			Tuberculosis	☐	☐
Cough up blood	☐	☐	Mitral valve prolapse	☐	☐	Ulcer/Colitis	☐	☐
Diabetes	☐	☐	Nervous problems	☐	☐	Venereal disease	☐	☐
Epilepsy	☐	☐	Pacemaker/heart surgery	☐	☐			

ARE YOU ALLERGIC TO OR HAVE YOU REACTED ADVERSELY TO ANY OF THE FOLLOWING MEDICATIONS?

Aspirin Local anesthetic Erythromycin Latex (balloons,
Nitrous Oxide Codeine Penicillin gloves, etc.)

Are your aware of being allergic to any other medications or substances?
If yes, please list:

Is there any other Medical or Dental information that you feel I should know about?

FAMILY PHYSICIAN _____ PHONE _____ E-MAIL _____

FIGURE 11-3 Sample medical/dental history form. (*continues*)

COMPLETED TREATMENT

	1	2	3	4	5	6	7	8	9	10	11	12	13	14	15	16	
A B C D E																	F G H I J

RIGHT   LEFT

T S R Q P																	O N M L K
	32	31	30	29	28	27	26	25	24	23	22	21	20	19	18	17	

INITIAL PERIODONTAL EXAM:

GINGIVAL INFLAMMATION:	☐ Slight	☐ Moderate	☐ Severe
SOFT PLAQUE BUILDUP:	☐ Slight	☐ Moderate	☐ Heavy
HARD CALCULUS BUILDUP:	☐ Light	☐ Moderate	☐ Heavy
STAINS:	☐ Light	☐ Moderate	☐ Heavy
HOME CARE EFFECTIVENESS:	☐ Good	☐ Fair	☐ Poor
PERIODONTAL CONDITION:	☐ Good	☐ Fair	☐ Poor
PERIODONTAL DIAGNOSIS:	☐ Normal	☐ Gingivitis	
PERIODONTITIS:	☐ Early	☐ Moderate	☐ Advanced
MUCOGINGIVAL DEFECTS #s:			

CLINICAL DATA:

OCCLUSION: ☐ Class I   ☐ Class II   ☐ Class III   ☐ Crossbite: _____
T.M.J. EXAM: ☐ Normal   ☐ Popping   ☐ Deviation   ☐ Tooth Wear   ☐ Pain

INITIAL SOFT TISSUE EXAM:

☐ Lips   ☐ Floor of Mouth   ☐ Palate   ☐ Tongue   ☐ Neck & Nodes

PATIENT'S TREATMENT DECISIONS:

☐ DOCUMENTATION OF DENTAL RECORD COMPLETED
☐ PATIENT INFORMED OF TX. RECOMMENDATIONS AND CONSENTS TO TX.
  (ALTERNATIVES DISCUSSED.)
☐ PATIENT WANTS NO TX. OR PARTIAL TX. INFORMED OF CONSEQUENCES
  AND RISKS INVOLVED.

INITIAL X-RAY FINDINGS:

X-RAYS TAKEN: ☐ FM-PAS   ☐ BWX   ☐ PANO: ☐ OTHER _____

	UR	UL	LR	LL
	QUADRANTS			
☐ NO BONE LOSS				
☐ SLIGHT BONE LOSS (04600)				
☐ MODERATE BONE LOSS (04700)				
☐ MAJOR BONE LOSS (04800)				
☐ BEGINNING FURCATION (04700)				
☐ ADVANCED FURCATION (04800)				
☐ OTHER: _____				

SHADE		
Teeth	Upper	Lower
Cents		
Lats		
Cusp		
Posts		

PERIODONTAL SCREENING & RECORDING

SEXTANT	SCORE	MONTH	DAY	YEAR

EXISTING PROSTHESIS:

MAX: _____ DATE PLACED: _____ CONDITION: _____
MAND: _____ DATE PLACED: _____ CONDITION: _____

REFERRALS:

PERIO: _____ ORTHO: _____ ENDO: _____
ORAL SURG: _____ MD: _____ OTHER: _____

NOTES

_____
_____
_____
_____
_____
_____

CONSENT

The undersigned hereby authorizes the Doctor to take X-rays, study models, photographs, or any other diagnostic aids deemed appropriate by Doctor to make a thorough diagnosis of the patient's dental needs. I also authorize Doctor to perform any and all forms of treatment, medication, and therapy that may be indicated. I also understand the use of anesthetic agents embodies a certain risk. I understand that my dental insurance is a contract between me and the insurance carrier, and not between the insurance carrier and the Doctor and that I am still fully responsible for all dental fees. These fees are due and payable at the time services are rendered unless prior financial arrangements have been made. I also assign all insurance benefits to the Doctor. Any payments received by the Doctor from my insurance coverage will be credited to my account, or refunded to me if I have paid the dental fees incurred. I further understand that a late charge will be added to any overdue balance. I understand that where appropriate, credit reports may be obtained.

PATIENT Signature (Parent of Child) _____ Date:_____ DENTIST Signature _____

FIGURE 11-3 (continues)

DIAGNOSIS: MISSING TEETH and EXISTING PROBLEMS

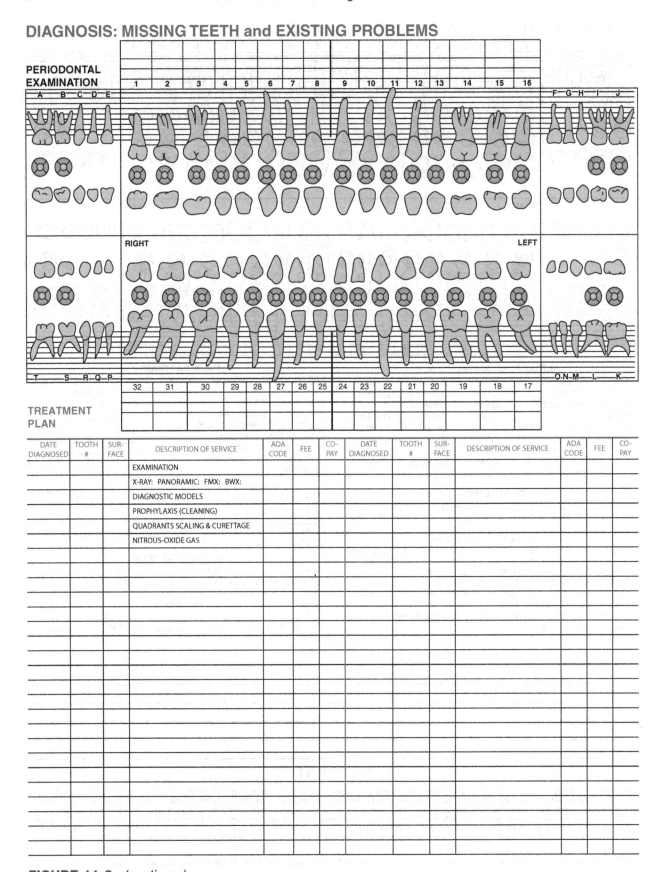

DATE DIAGNOSED	TOOTH #	SUR-FACE	DESCRIPTION OF SERVICE	ADA CODE	FEE	CO-PAY	DATE DIAGNOSED	TOOTH #	SUR-FACE	DESCRIPTION OF SERVICE	ADA CODE	FEE	CO-PAY
			EXAMINATION										
			X-RAY: PANORAMIC: FMX: BWX:										
			DIAGNOSTIC MODELS										
			PROPHYLAXIS (CLEANING)										
			QUADRANTS SCALING & CURETTAGE										
			NITROUS-OXIDE GAS										

FIGURE 11-3   *(continues)*

PERIODIC EXAMINATION HEALTH HISTORY UPDATE

Date: _____ CURRENT MEDICATIONS: _____

Health Changes: _____

Blood Pressure: _____ CANCER EXAM: ☐ Normal ☐ Lesion: _____ Hyg/Asst: _____ Dr. _____

Stain: ☐ No ☐ Lt. ☐ Mod. ☐ Hvy.   TMJ: ☐ Asymptomatic ☐ Symptoms _____   PERIODONTAL SCREENING &
Calculus: ☐ No ☐ Lt. ☐ Mod. ☐ Hvy.   HOMECARE: BRUSH: G F P   FLOSS: G F P   ☐ Maint.   RECORDING
Plaque: ☐ No ☐ Lt. ☐ Mod. ☐ Hvy.   PERIO DIAG: ☐ Normal ☐ Gingivitis ☐ Early Perio ☐ Mod. Perio ☐ Adv. Perio
Bleeding: ☐ No ☐ Lt. ☐ Mod. ☐ Hvy.   INSTRUCTIONS: ☐ Brush ☐ Floss ☐ Perio Aid ☐ Other: _____
RECALL: _____ Months   ☐ Prophylaxis: ☐ Fluoride Tr. ☐ Perio Pro. ☐ Check Next Appt: _____

SEXTANT SCORE   M   D   Y

Patient Signature: _____

Date: _____ CURRENT MEDICATIONS: _____

Health Changes: _____

Blood Pressure: _____ CANCER EXAM: ☐ Normal ☐ Lesion: _____ Hyg/Asst: _____ Dr. _____

Stain: ☐ No ☐ Lt. ☐ Mod. ☐ Hvy.   TMJ: ☐ Asymptomatic ☐ Symptoms _____   PERIODONTAL SCREENING &
Calculus: ☐ No ☐ Lt. ☐ Mod. ☐ Hvy.   HOMECARE: BRUSH: G F P   FLOSS: G F P   ☐ Maint.   RECORDING
Plaque: ☐ No ☐ Lt. ☐ Mod. ☐ Hvy.   PERIO DIAG: ☐ Normal ☐ Gingivitis ☐ Early Perio ☐ Mod. Perio ☐ Adv. Perio
Bleeding: ☐ No ☐ Lt. ☐ Mod. ☐ Hvy.   INSTRUCTIONS: ☐ Brush ☐ Floss ☐ Perio Aid ☐ Other: _____
RECALL: _____ Months   ☐ Prophylaxis: ☐ Fluoride Tr. ☐ Perio Pro. ☐ Check Next Appt: _____

SEXTANT SCORE   M   D   Y

Patient Signature: _____

Date: _____ CURRENT MEDICATIONS: _____

Health Changes: _____

Blood Pressure: _____ CANCER EXAM: ☐ Normal ☐ Lesion: _____ Hyg/Asst: _____ Dr. _____

Stain: ☐ No ☐ Lt. ☐ Mod. ☐ Hvy.   TMJ: ☐ Asymptomatic ☐ Symptoms _____   PERIODONTAL SCREENING &
Calculus: ☐ No ☐ Lt. ☐ Mod. ☐ Hvy.   HOMECARE: BRUSH: G F P   FLOSS: G F P   Maint.   RECORDING
Plaque: ☐ No ☐ Lt. ☐ Mod. ☐ Hvy.   PERIO DIAG: ☐ Normal ☐ Gingivitis ☐ Early Perio ☐ Mod. Perio ☐ Adv. Perio
Bleeding: ☐ No ☐ Lt. ☐ Mod. ☐ Hvy.   INSTRUCTIONS: ☐ Brush ☐ Floss ☐ Perio Aid ☐ Other: _____
RECALL: _____ Months   ☐ Prophylaxis: ☐ Fluoride Tr. ☐ Perio Pro. ☐ Check Next Appt: _____

SEXTANT SCORE   M   D   Y

Patient Signature: _____

Date: _____ CURRENT MEDICATIONS: _____

Health Changes: _____

Blood Pressure: _____ CANCER EXAM: ☐ Normal ☐ Lesion: _____ Hyg/Asst: _____ Dr. _____

Stain: ☐ No ☐ Lt. ☐ Mod. ☐ Hvy.   TMJ: ☐ Asymptomatic ☐ Symptoms _____   PERIODONTAL SCREENING &
Calculus: ☐ No ☐ Lt. ☐ Mod. ☐ Hvy.   HOMECARE: BRUSH: G F P   FLOSS: G F P   Maint.   RECORDING
Plaque: ☐ No ☐ Lt. ☐ Mod. ☐ Hvy.   PERIO DIAG: ☐ Normal ☐ Gingivitis ☐ Early Perio ☐ Mod. Perio ☐ Adv. Perio
Bleeding: ☐ No ☐ Lt. ☐ Mod. ☐ Hvy.   INSTRUCTIONS: ☐ Brush ☐ Floss ☐ Perio Aid ☐ Other: _____
RECALL: _____ Months   ☐ Prophylaxis: ☐ Fluoride Tr. ☐ Perio Pro. ☐ Check Next Appt: _____

SEXTANT SCORE   M   D   Y

Patient Signature: _____

Date: _____ CURRENT MEDICATIONS: _____

Health Changes: _____

Blood Pressure: _____ CANCER EXAM: ☐ Normal ☐ Lesion: _____ Hyg/Asst: _____ Dr. _____

Stain: ☐ No ☐ Lt. ☐ Mod. ☐ Hvy.   TMJ: ☐ Asymptomatic ☐ Symptoms _____   PERIODONTAL SCREENING &
Calculus: ☐ No ☐ Lt. ☐ Mod. ☐ Hvy.   HOMECARE: BRUSH: G F P   FLOSS: G F P   Maint.   RECORDING
Plaque: ☐ No ☐ Lt. ☐ Mod. ☐ Hvy.   PERIO DIAG: ☐ Normal ☐ Gingivitis ☐ Early Perio ☐ Mod. Perio ☐ Adv. Perio
Bleeding: ☐ No ☐ Lt. ☐ Mod. ☐ Hvy.   INSTRUCTIONS: ☐ Brush ☐ Floss ☐ Perio Aid ☐ Other: _____
RECALL: _____ Months   ☐ Prophylaxis: ☐ Fluoride Tr. ☐ Perio Pro. ☐ Check Next Appt: _____

SEXTANT SCORE   M   D   Y

Patient Signature: _____

Date: _____ CURRENT MEDICATIONS: _____

Health Changes: _____

Blood Pressure: _____ CANCER EXAM: ☐ Normal ☐ Lesion: _____ Hyg/Asst: _____ Dr. _____

Stain: ☐ No ☐ Lt. ☐ Mod. ☐ Hvy.   TMJ: ☐ Asymptomatic ☐ Symptoms _____   PERIODONTAL SCREENING &
Calculus: ☐ No ☐ Lt. ☐ Mod. ☐ Hvy.   HOMECARE: BRUSH: G F P   FLOSS: G F P   Maint.   RECORDING
Plaque: ☐ No ☐ Lt. ☐ Mod. ☐ Hvy.   PERIO DIAG: ☐ Normal ☐ Gingivitis ☐ Early Perio ☐ Mod. Perio ☐ Adv. Perio
Bleeding: ☐ No ☐ Lt. ☐ Mod. ☐ Hvy.   INSTRUCTIONS: ☐ Brush ☐ Floss ☐ Perio Aid ☐ Other: _____
RECALL: _____ Months   ☐ Prophylaxis: ☐ Fluoride Tr. ☐ Perio Pro. ☐ Check Next Appt: _____

SEXTANT SCORE   M   D   Y

Patient Signature: _____

FIGURE 11-3 *(continues)*

RECORD OF SERVICES

DATE	TOOTH #	SURFACE	SERVICES RENDERED	PROD. NO.	SERVICE CODE	FEE	RECALL DATE

FIGURE 11-3 (*continued*)

A request for records also occurs when the dentist determines the need for referral to another dentist, most often a dental specialist, for further treatment. For additional information about transfer of records, see Chapter 3 (Legal and Ethical Regulations in Dental Office Management).

Retention of Patient Records

At one time it was thought sufficient to retain patient records for seven years past the last date of treatment. Today it is considered important to retain patient records for 30 years past the last date of treatment or within the statutes of limitation of the state where the practice is located.

If the dentist retires, sells, or transfers the ownership of the practice or the dentist passes away, the records become the property of the new practice owner.

Diagnosis, Treatment Planning, and Case Presentation

Before the dentist can form a treatment plan, he or she must use additional clinical aids to determine a diagnosis. These most often include traditional dental radiographs (x-rays) or digital radiography, and may also include study models either as stone casts or digital images, intraoral images, or other photos.

Intraoral Dental Radiographs

Dental radiographs are a vital aid for the dentist in making a diagnosis. Because radiographs reveal areas between the teeth, structures inside the teeth and below the gingiva, they aid in the detection of significant pathology and other conditions not always apparent upon clinical examination alone.

The most common types of individual dental radiographs used for diagnosis of dental disease are bitewings and periapicals. Bitewings got their name because after they are placed in the patients mouth and the patient bites together to hold the film in place showing both upper and lower teeth on the radiograph. Periapical means around the apical tip of the tooth so those films show the entire tooth from crown to root tip and usually include only one or two teeth in the same arch.

The American Dental Association recommends a full-mouth survey or series of x-rays for adults with teeth once every two years or as needed by the dentist for diagnosis and treatment. A full-mouth survey, commonly abbreviated FMX, traditionally consists of 14–16 periapical films and 4 bitewing films (Figure 11-4). The periapical films are distributed into 7–8 on the maxillary

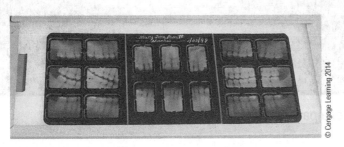

FIGURE 11-4 Sample of a full-mouth radiographic survey properly mounted.

and 7–8 on the mandibular with 1 molar film, 1 premolar film, 1 cuspid film on right and left, and 1–2 anterior films.

Bitewing films show the clinical crowns and interproximal areas of the teeth. They are used primarily for detection of carious lesions (tooth decay) not visible to the naked eye.

Periapical films are used to examine the entire tooth, including the crown, the root structure, and the supporting structures around the teeth. They are used primarily for diagnosis of periodontal disease and assessment of pathological conditions associated with the loss of supportive bone structure, subgingival and interproximal calculus, changes in pulpal health, and abscesses. They also reveal the occlusal effect of the premature loss or the prolonged retention of deciduous teeth and the consequences of losing permanent teeth.

Extraoral Dental Radiographs

Films used to survey the entire oral cavity on one large film are referred to as extraoral because both the film and the source of radiation are outside of the patient's mouth. These panoramic films are not as diagnostically accurate as a full-mouth survey of individual films but they are able to show areas impossible to capture with intraoral films. These extraoral or panoramic films are helpful to the dentist in detecting temporomandibular joint disorders, impactions, orthodontic conditions, supernumerary and unerupted teeth and pathological (disease) conditions (Figure 11-5).

On the direction of the dentist, panoramic x-rays are often used in conjunction with a minimum of posterior bitewing x-rays.

Extraoral dental x-rays include cephalometric films that are common in an orthodontist's office. Cephalometric films show a lateral view of the patient's skull and are used to evaluate the position of the teeth to the face.

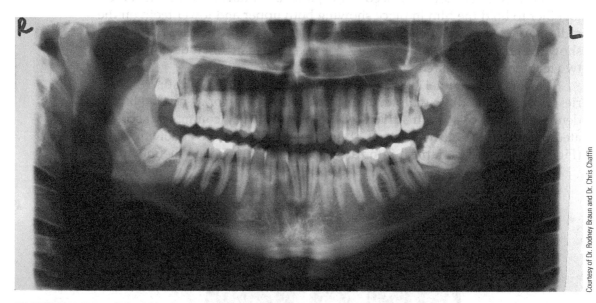

FIGURE 11-5 Sample of a panoramic radiograph.

Radiation Safety

Radiation safety is of primary importance in protecting both dental team members and their patients. Because radiation is cumulative, that is, it builds up over time, repeated exposure may eventually cause harmful side effects. Radiation exposure during pregnancy could cause birth defects by damaging the developing fetal cells. By using safety precautions and modern x-ray equipment, these risks are minimal (Figure 11-6).

Protection of the Operator

The following are steps the dental radiographer should take to protect himself or herself from the effects of radiation.

1. Never attempt to hold a film in a patient's mouth during the radiographic exposure.
2. Never stand in the path of the x-ray beam during exposure.
3. Always stand at a right angle to the x-ray tubehead and a minimum of six to eight feet away from the patient or behind a lead-lined wall or lead shield during exposure.
4. Ensure the x-ray equipment is monitored by an independent examiner according to state laws.
5. Take as few x-rays as possible to achieve a diagnosis. Position film carefully to avoid retakes.

Protection of the Patient

The following are steps the dental radiographer may take to protect patients from radiation.

1. Use a protective lead apron with a collar high enough to protect the thyroid gland on all patients being exposed to radiation (Figure 11-7). When not in use, store the lead apron over a dowel or on a wooden hanger to prevent cracking of the apron. *Note*: Never fold the lead apron or place it over a hook, as this may result in cracking, puncturing, or tearing of the apron.
2. Take only the minimum number of films required by the dentist.

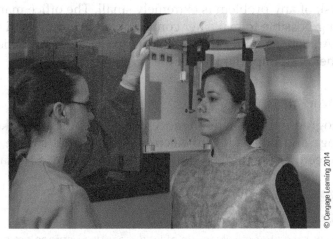

FIGURE 11-6 Modern digital radiographs reduce the exposure to patients.

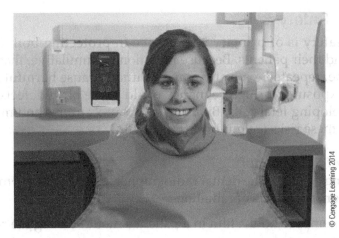

FIGURE 11-7 Patients must wear protective aprons or shields when having radiographs taken.

3. Use proper film positioning, exposure, and processing procedures to reduce the number of retakes.

4. Use the fastest speed film available with the least amount of radiation exposure.

Policy for Protecting Pregnant Patients

An important aspect of exposing the patient to radiation is the possibility of pregnancy and the increased risk to the unborn child. Thus, it is essential that the office manager obtains or updates each patient's medical history at each recall appointment. Many practices display a sign or print a notice on the health history form that indicates *"If you are pregnant or think you may be pregnant, please notify the doctor or staff member."*

Before exposing radiographs for an expectant patient, the dentist may want to consult the patient's obstetrician first. Only absolutely necessary x-rays should be taken for a pregnant patient and then preferably during the second or third trimester when the developing fetus is less susceptible to the effects of radiation.

Every office will experience a phone call from a panicked patient who was in the office recently and had no idea she was pregnant at the time. The office manager can confidently reassure her that because she was wearing the lead apron her risk of any problem is extremely small. The office manager should do everything possible to make her comfortable, including having her talk to the dentist. Anxiety and stress aren't helpful to the pregnant patient, so trying to reassure her is an important job of the dental staff.

Digital Radiography

Digital radiography is a recent advancement in dentistry. It takes the radiographic image and breaks it into electronic pieces that can be viewed on a computer screen. These filmless digital systems employ a reusable intraoral

THINK Green

Not all lead aprons are actually made of lead. Lead-less aprons are available that offer the same protection as the traditional lead apron but can be recycled.

sensor instead of traditional x-ray film. The chairside assistant can use the sensor in conjunction with a traditional x-ray tubehead or with the digital system, which permits automatic activation of the sensor. Digital radiography reduces radiation exposure by 90 percent compared to standard x-ray techniques and also minimizes cross-contamination by eliminating the handling of contaminated film packets.

The benefits of digital radiography include

- reduced radiation exposure for patients and dental team members;
- reduced procedure time because x-ray head and sensor are already prepositioned;
- enhanced diagnostic capability and high resolution;
- color-enhanced image quality;
- reduced storage space and paper costs when images are stored or transferred electronically;
- print-out capability for the patient or a referring dentist/specialist;
- eliminates cost of processing equipment, film, and chemistry (developer and fixer); and
- image enlargement capabilities.

Digital Radiography Technique

The chairside assistant begins by turning on the computer and loading the imaging software then the patient's identification information is entered. Adjustments are made to the settings of the x-ray head to ensure the minimal amount of radiation is used for the patient.,

To expose periapical films, the chairside assistant mounts the sensor covered with a disposable clear plastic sheath into a positioner. The clinician then positions the tubehead by resting the cone against the guide attached to the positioner. Using the paralleling technique, the dental assistant creates parallelism between the long axis of the teeth and the sensor then directs the x-ray beam at a 90° angle to both the teeth and the sensor.

Within a few seconds after activating the timer switch, the image appears on the monitor screen. The image is evaluated for accuracy and can be redone immediately if necessary.

To expose bitewings, the assistant selects the icon for bitewing format. The sensor is sheathed and the flaps are attached to the center of the active side of the sensor. The sensor is placed beside the molars or premolars and the patient is instructed to bite down lightly on the tab to secure the sensor in place. For most adult patients, two bitewings on each side of the mouth are recommended. Only one on each side is recommended for children. The x-ray head is positioned the same way as when taking traditional bitewings. The bitewing image appears on the screen within a few seconds of activating the timer switch.

A full mouth series of x-rays can be completed in about half the time required when using digital radiography instead of conventional methods. Digital radiography requires sliding the sensor to the next location in the mouth unlike traditional x-rays where each new location requires the operator to restart the film loading process. The images are saved and stored on the computer's hard drive eliminating the necessity of traditional patient charts to store hard copies.

THINK Green

The environmental impact of moving to digital radiography is significant. Because there are no chemicals necessary for processing, the caustic chemicals needed for developing and fixing the films are eliminated. Also eliminated are the lead lined film packets necessary for traditional films.

Prevention of Cross-Contamination with the Digital Radiography System

To prevent cross-contamination, the dental assistant places a disposable sheath-barrier on the sensor when used in the mouth. At the end of the procedure, the assistant removes the sheath and disinfects the sensor after every patient according to the manufacturer's recommendation.

Study Models

Study models are a duplicate of the patient's teeth and surrounding structures traditionally in plaster or stone but can also be replicated digitally. Study models are often used by orthodontists prior to treatment or by general dentists and prosthodontist's for crowns and bridges.

Digital study models are gaining in popularity and Invisalign® for orthodontics relies on this technology (Figure 11-8).

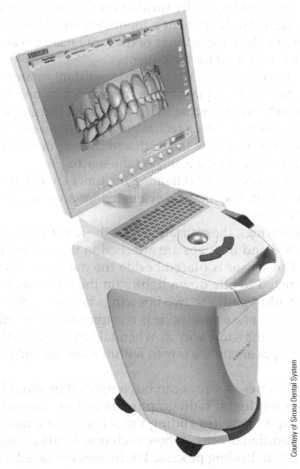

Courtesy of Sirona Dental System

FIGURE 11-8 A CECREC machine takes digital images and can use that data to create a restoration for the patient all in the dental office.

Intraoral Camera

The intraoral camera has improved diagnosis and treatment plan acceptance. Using a wand that contains a small camera attached to a computer and a high-resolution color monitor, the operator freezes enlarged dental images (magnified up to ten times original size) onto the screen. The system uses either a flashing strobe light or fiber-optic light. These images may be printed out instantly as color photographs or saved in the computer database.

Patient acceptance of recommended treatment increases when patients view individual teeth or groups of teeth and see conditions such as:

- Damaged or broken restorations
- Gingival inflammation
- Various stages of periodontal disease
- Failing or discolored restorations
- Gum recession
- Calculus buildup
- Tooth stains and discolorations
- Hairline fractures and cracks in teeth
- Dental caries
- Orthodontic conditions
- Missing or drifted teeth
- Other oral diseases and conditions

Because use of the intraoral camera to record diagnostic photos and images is not an irreversible procedure, the chairside dental assistant may take and record these images to assist the dentist in making a diagnosis.

The Case Presentation

The case presentation is an appointment in which no clinical treatment is performed. With the use of diagnostic aids and charted clinical information, the dentist meets with the patient (often the patient may be accompanied by a person who will be assisting him or her in making treatment decisions) to explain an extensive case. It is the office manager's responsibility to see that all related materials, including the patient's chart, radiographs, study models, intraoral photos, and other demonstration materials such as patient education brochures, or visual aids, are assembled prior to the appointment.

After the doctor explains the diagnosis and recommended treatment plan, if there are treatment options, the doctor can discuss those and the pros and cons of each but leave the financial options to the business staff. Rarely is it a good idea to have the doctor discuss fees with the patient; the doctor's entire focus should be on treatment and the best recommendations for the patient.

The office manager joins the planning session to answer questions regarding treatment, fees, and the time commitment. At the conclusion of the case presentation appointment, the office manager provides the patient with a written treatment plan estimate providing the preferred form of treatment and the alternate treatment as well as different payment options. The patient then makes a decision, often based upon financial resources.

It is the office manager's job to ensure that the treatment plan is accepted, to set up the required number of sequential appointments to complete the treatment, and to make financial arrangements with the patient.

> **Note:** To prevent misunderstandings, complete financial arrangements must be made by the office manager and communicated verbally and in writing prior to commencing the treatment. For additional information on financial arrangements, see Chapter 13 (Managing Accounts Receivable).

Recall Program: Lifeline of the Practice

Recall appointments are addressed in a number of areas throughout this text. A recall program means once a patient has completed current necessary restorative and preventive treatment, he or she will be recalled to the practice in the future for oral examination, prophylaxis, and required radiographs. Additional methods of diagnosis for dental disease may be scheduled as necessary at that recall appointment. Some practices use the term "recare" appointment instead of "recall" appointment.

In most practices, recall duration is six months based on insurance company's payment schedules. For some patients with periodontal conditions, the ideal recall is every three or four months. For patients that need cleaning/prophylaxis more often than six months the office can schedule "prophy only" appointments with the hygienist. The office manager is responsible for maintaining patient records and notifying patients of their recall appointments.

Whether the system is managed manually or by computer, the two most common methods of recalling patients are by pre-booking the next recall or by notifying the patient when the next recall appointment is due, either by mail or telephone. If recalls are handled manually, most office managers use a system where the patient's notice is filed six months from the date of completed treatment. For example, if the patient's restorative treatment is completed in May and he or she is scheduled to be recalled in six months, the office manager files a recall notice behind the November tab of the recall file (Figure 11-9).

If the practice uses a computer system to print out recall notices and/or labels, the office manager inputs the information by month due and prints out the list by month when the notice is due. Recall notices are mailed out informing the patient of an upcoming appointment or letting them know it is time to schedule. Phone confirmation calls are usually done 24–48 hours before a scheduled appointment. For patients who need to schedule but have not done so after receiving the reminder card, a follow-up phone call should be made.

The office manager must be vigilant in contacting patients to prove that patients have not been abandoned. Notes regarding attempted contacts should be included in the patient chart.

Pharmaceutical Prescriptions

The office manager must also understand the importance of the information required when the dentist writes a pharmaceutical prescription for a controlled drug. A controlled drug is one that requires the prescription of a licensed doctor; the drug is not available over the counter in a pharmacy.

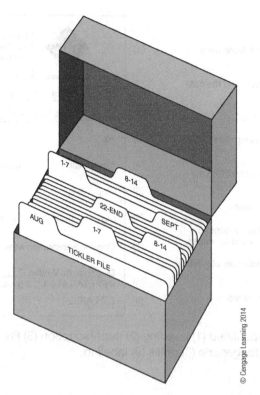

© Cengage Learning 2014

FIGURE 11-9 Tickler files can be used to keep recall appointments organized.

Before writing any prescription, the doctor should double-check the patient's health history for drug interactions, reactions, or allergies reported.

Note: It is illegal for anyone to dispense any drug to a patient without the dentist's consent or to sign a prescription on the doctor's behalf. Any deviation from this may result in the dentist's loss of prescription-writing privileges or other restriction of practice.

In dentistry, drugs are most often prescribed for pain control and infection. Occasionally, they may be prescribed for apprehensive patients to reduce anxiety.

Premedication with prophylactic antibiotics of patients with certain joint replacements, heart valve replacements, mitral valve prolapse, or other cardiac conditions may be necessary after consultation with the patient's physician. This is noted in the patient's chart and also in health alerts on the daily schedule. Prophylactic antibiotics must be taken one hour prior to the appointment. It is the office manager's responsibility to make sure the patient is alerted regarding premedication when confirming the appointment. This is to ensure that the patient picks up the prescription from the pharmacy and takes the medication prior to the appointment.

Parts of a Pharmaceutical Prescription

A pharmaceutical prescription has nine parts (Figure 11-10). The office manager must be familiar with them and be able to interpret their contents and meaning, especially if the patient asks questions regarding their prescription.

Parts of a Prescription

1. The heading includes the dentist's name, address, telephone number, and registration number.

2. The superscription includes the patient's name, address, and the date on which the prescription is written.

3. The *subscription* that includes the symbol Rx ("take thou").

4. The *inscription* that states the names and quantities of ingredients to be included in the medication.

5. The *subscription* that gives directions to the pharmacist for filling the prescription.

6. The *signature* (Sig) that gives the directions for the patient.

7. The dentist's signature blanks. Where signed, indicates if a generic substitute is allowed or if the medication is to be dispensed as written.

8. REPETATUR 0 1 2 3 p.r.n. This is where the dentist indicates whether or not the prescription can be refilled.

9. ☐ LABEL Direction to the pharmacist to label the medication appropriately.

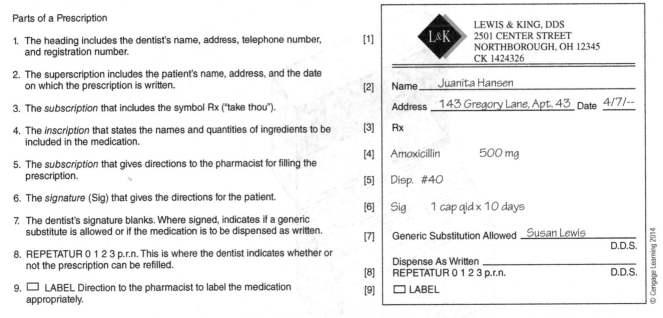

FIGURE 11-10 Prescription with parts identified (1) heading (2) superscription (3) Rx symbol (4) inscription (5) subscription (6) signature (7) signature for generic (8) refills (9) labeling.

1. The **heading** contains the doctor's name, degree (DDS or DMD), office address, and telephone number.

2. The **superscription** includes the date of the prescription, the patient's name, address, and birth date.

3. RX ("take thou")

4. The **inscription** is the portion of the prescription that contains the name of the drug, dosage form, and the amount of the dose. Abbreviations are usually used when writing an inscription, such as *"Penicillin VK 500 mg tabs."* Table 11-1 lists some common abbreviations used on prescriptions.

5. The **subscription** is a portion of the prescription that contains the amount of the drug and directions for preparation of the drug for dispensing. The subscription may include *"dispense #30."* The number indicates the number of tablets or capsules to be dispensed in the bottle. If the prescription is for a liquid, the volume to be dispensed is indicated in this area.

6. The **signature** is derived from the Latin word *Signum*, which is abbreviated *Sig* or *S*; it is followed by specific directions about how the drug is to be taken. The word *signature* directs what is to be printed on the pharmacy label affixed to the container. An example of a signature is *"Sig: tabs 1q4 h,"* which means *"take one tablet every four hours."*

7. The designation for filling the prescription with the **generic equivalent** drug contains the portion of the prescription in which the dentist indicates whether the pharmacist must dispense the prescription as written (when a trade name or brand name is used) or if the generic equivalent may be substituted. Note, not all brand-name drugs have generic equivalents. A generic equivalent drug is non-brand-name protected and is less expensive.

TABLE 11-1 Common Prescription Abbreviations.

Abbreviation	Meaning
ac	before meals
bid	twice a day
caps	capsules
liq	liquid
mg	milligram
pc	after meals
q2h	every 2 hours
q4h	every 4 hours
q6h	every 6 hours
q12h	every 12 hours
qd	daily
qh	every hour
qid	four times a day
prn	as necessary, when necessary
stat	immediately
tabs	tablets
tid	three times a day
tsp	teaspoon

© Cengage Learning 2014

8. The **refill** (Repetatur) is the part of the prescription in which the dentist indicates the number of refills (if any) to be dispensed.

9. The **label** is the part of the prescription that describes the contents. An example of the information is: *"ibuprofen 800 mg."* The label may also contain the dose, for example, 250 mg or 500 mg.

10. The doctor's actual signature and DEA number. The dentist must have a current DEA license to write prescriptions.

The Office Manager's Responsibility Regarding Prescriptions

The office manager must ensure that all information relating to prescription drugs written by the dentist is recorded properly in the patient's chart. Correct written legal documentation will help to avoid confusion later on, and to prevent any misunderstandings and reduce the likelihood of subsequent drug interactions or overdoses.

Many offices use a duplicate prescription pad system in which the top portion is given to the patient and the bottom copy is placed in the patient's permanent file jacket. Numbering of prescriptions is also routinely done in many offices as a tracking system to monitor writing of prescriptions and to reduce the likelihood of stolen or forged prescriptions.

The office manager should take steps to ensure that the dentist prescription pads are not left unattended or in view of patients or visitors in the office.

If the patient calls the office requesting a refill to be issued by the dentist, the office manager must inform the dentist of the request and note it on the patient's chart. Under no circumstances is the office manager to issue, write, or call in to the pharmacy asking for a refill for a prescription without consent of the dentist nor should the dentist sign blank prescriptions for use when he or she is away from the office.

Note: Most dentists arrange for emergency coverage by another dentist in the area during absences from the office.

The Dental Laboratory Prescription

A sometimes overlooked record of the office is the dental laboratory prescription. When the dentist requires lab work done outside the office, the case must be sent with written instructions to be completed by the dental laboratory technician.

A dental lab prescription, sometimes referred to as a work order, is written in duplicate: one copy goes to the lab with the case and the other is retained in the patient's chart. The prescriptions are labeled lab copy, office copy, and doctor's copy.

Many office managers find it helpful to set up a laboratory tracking system to enable the dentist and chairside assistants to know at any given time the location and status of every case sent out of the office (Figure 11-11).

The tracking system may be a notebook, a dry wipe board in the office laboratory, or a tracking system logged into the computer database. The tracking should include the patient's name and all the details of the work ordered as well as when the lab case is due.

It is also essential that the dental office manager keep a schedule of the required number of turnaround working days required for each perspective lab to complete the procedure requested. Appointments requiring lab work should be noted so the appointment is not moved without checking and updating the lab tracking system.

Note: The office manager must allow sufficient time when setting up appointments for the lab to complete the work and return it to the office prior to the patient's next scheduled appointment.

Patient's Name	Date Sent	Lab	Work Ordered	Date Needed	Patient Appt.
Mary Jones	10/3/xx	Smile Dental	PFG 4-unit bridge	10/17/xx	10/24/xx
Harold Johnson	10/5/xx	Dental Works	Denture	10/12/xx	10/20/xx
Ralph Jenko	10/7/xx	Dental Works	Partial framework	10/18/xx	10/20/xx

© Cengage Learning 2014

FIGURE 11-11 Sample tracking system for laboratory prescriptions.

Most dental labs provide their own printed prescription pads for convenience; the following information should appear on the outgoing lab prescription:

- The patient's name (or sometimes a patient's case number)
- The description of the type of lab work required
- The type of material required, such as porcelain or metal
- The shade (tooth color) required by the dentist to match the patient's original or existing dentition and a mold number for denture teeth
- The date required for the case to be returned to the office (usually one to two days prior to the patient reappointment time)
- The dentist's name, address, telephone number, license number, and signature or initials

Note that a member of the dental staff may write dental lab work orders and sign the dentist name or initials, as directed by the dentist.

When the lab case is returned, it should be compared to the original work order or prescription for accuracy and quality. The return case will include a copy of the prescription, which the office manager files to later compare with the monthly statements sent by the various labs with which the doctor works.

 ## Skill Building

These optional activities and exercises are designed to help the student put into practice information learned in the chapter.

1. A patient is undergoing endodontic (root canal) treatment. She calls the office to request an additional refill of pain medication. The dentist is out of town for the next three business days. What are the office manager's options? How can assistance be provided to the patient and stay within legal guidelines? Divide into discussion groups and present at least three ideas of how to handle this situation.

2. The dentist has requested that a young child with extensive decay have bitewing x-rays done. The child is fearful, crying, and uncooperative; today's visit is his first dental experience. The chairside assistant comes to you asking for your help. Divide into discussion groups and present at least three ideas to share with the class regarding how the situation could be resolved.

3. Pretend you are the office manager calling to confirm tomorrow's entire schedule. You notice that a patient is scheduled to have a four-unit bridge cemented tomorrow. You check the lab tracking system and discover the case is not back from the lab. What steps should you take? Divide into discussion groups and report at least three solutions to the problem.

4. A new patient calls for an initial exam but tells you that she will not let the practice take x-rays. Describe in detail how to handle a scenario like this one. Write out the dialog between the patient and yourself.

Challenge Your Understanding

Select the response that best answers each of the following questions. Only one response is correct.

1. The complete patient file should contain the:
   a. First and last name of the patient
   b. Clinical record, financial, and informed consent forms
   c. Medical/dental history and necessary radiographs
   d. All of the above

2. Personal information or attributes about the patient should be included as part of the clinical or financial records.
   a. True
   b. False

3. Most practices conduct routine computer searches or manual audits of patient files to:
   a. Keep patients from becoming lost mid-treatment
   b. Locate the patients who may have cancelled appointments without rescheduling to complete treatment
   c. Ensure that patients are notified of their recall appointments when due
   d. All of the above

4. It is the _____ job to contact and reschedule those patients who have incomplete treatment or are past due for their recall appointment.
   a. dentist's
   b. sterilization assistant's
   c. office manager's
   d. dental hygienist's

5. Which of the following represents the correct alphabetical order?
   a. Hansen, P.; Hansen, Peter; Hansen, Peter Ralph
   b. Ward, John Henry; Ward, John H.; Mr. John Henry Ward
   c. McMullen, Kathryn; McMullen, C.; McMullen, Sarah
   d. Garcia, J.J.; Garcia, José J.; Garcia, Jerry J.

6. The instructions "qid" to the pharmacist mean:
   a. Four times a day
   b. Every hour
   c. Every four hours
   d. Daily

7. A complete financial responsibility form should include all of the following *except*:
   a. The name, address, and phone number(s) of the patient and the responsible party
   b. Specific insurance information such as the name of the carrier, the insured's group and/or policy number, and expiration date
   c. The patient's tax ID from the previous year
   d. The responsible party's social security number and place of employment

8. The purpose of the medical health history is to alert the dentist to:
   a. Prescribed drugs currently being taken by the patient
   b. Current medical conditions and any known allergies
   c. The name and telephone number of a responsible party to contact in case of an emergency
   d. All of the above

9. When transferring patient records, the office manager should send legible, high quality duplicates of the record never the originals.
   a. True
   b. False

10. When forming a diagnosis, the dentist may require adjunct diagnostic aids including:
    a. Dental radiographs (x-rays) or digital radiography
    b. Study models
    c. Intraoral camera images
    d. All of the above

11. Periapical x-rays record the clinical crowns and interproximal areas of teeth and are used primarily for detection of carious lesions (tooth decay) not visible to the naked eye.
    a. True
    b. False

12. Periapical films are used for all the following except:
    a. Diagnosis of periodontal disease
    b. Subgingival and interproximal calculus
    c. Sinus infections
    d. Changes in pulpal health and abscesses

13. All of the following are true about panoramic x-rays except:
    a. The panoramic film is helpful to the dentist in detection temporomandibular joint disorders and orthodontic conditions
    b. The panoramic film produces a somewhat enlarged image that is more diagnostically accurate than a full mouth series
    c. The panoramic film is most often used in conjunction with a minimum of one set of posterior bitewing films
    d. The panoramic film is helpful in detecting impactions, supernumerary, and unerupted teeth

14. Radiation is cumulative, which means its effects dissipate quite rapidly.
    a. True
    b. False

15. Sometimes it is necessary for the operator to stand in the direct path of the x-ray beam to hold a film in a patient's mouth during exposure.
    a. True
    b. False

16. Which of the following are steps required to protect the patient during radiographic exposure?
    a. Place a protective lead apron with a thyroid collar on all patients being exposed to radiation
    b. Take only the minimum number of films required by the dentist
    c. Use proper film positioning, exposure and processing
    d. All of the above

17. Benefits of digital radiography include:
    a. Reduced radiation exposure for patients and dental team members
    b. Reduced procedure exposure time and storage space
    c. Enhanced diagnostic capability and high resolution with enhanced image quality
    d. All of the above

18. The intraoral camera is used to detect periodontal disease and dental caries between the teeth.
    a. True
    b. False

19. The subscription is the portion of the prescription that contains the name of the drug, dosage form, and amount of the dose.
    a. True
    b. False

20. All of the following information should appear on the outgoing lab prescription *except*:
    a. The shade (tooth color) required to match the patient's original or existing dentition
    b. The type of material required
    c. A copy of the patient's financial history form
    d. The date the prosthesis is required back in the office

CHAPTER 12

Scheduling to Optimize Practice Efficiency

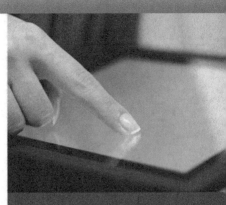

CHAPTER OUTLINES

KEY TERMS

block
call list
double booking
palliative
production scheduling
unit

LEARNING OBJECTIVES

1. List the priorities and considerations in scheduling appointments.
2. Describe the importance of time blocks/units in maintaining an efficient appointment system.
3. List the screening priorities of the office manager for handling and appointing emergency patients.
4. Describe scheduling considerations of special needs patients.
5. Describe duties of the office manager when handling late patients and no-shows.
6. Describe the procedure for recording/scheduling appointments, completing appointment cards, and sequential appointment scheduling.
7. Describe the office manager's role in appointment confirmation and technology available to make confirmations.
8. Describe the importance of maintaining a patient call list.
9. List the office manager's duties in posting the daily schedule, maintaining the recall system, and scheduling the hygienist who works with an assistant.

Appointment Scheduling

Scheduling is an essential business function of every successful dental practice. Some large practices employ staff that only schedule appointments, because of the importance of the role it plays. Scheduling determines

- the profitability of the practice;
- the quality of the care provided by the practice;
- the emotional and physical well-being of the clinical team; and
- the convenience and health of the patients.

Whether scheduling is completed manually in an appointment book or with a computer, the same basic principles of scheduling apply. Each treatment room has a designated column and it is necessary to view multiple days at a glance.

Scheduling for the Dentist's Preference

The first consideration in appointment scheduling is the dentist's energy level. Most practitioners prefer to perform more demanding procedures, such as difficult extractions, implants, or crown and bridge cases early in the day when they are most rested and alert. Oral surgery cases performed in the office with IV (intravenous) anesthesia are scheduled early in the morning because they require the patient have nothing by mouth for eight hours preceding surgery.

Every dentist has preferences for scheduling, making each schedule unique.

Scheduling to Maximize Production

A second consideration in appointment scheduling is a practice's requirement to meet production goals in the form of cash flow. **Production scheduling** decisions must follow the practice's strategies to generate adequate daily revenues to cover the overhead costs involved in running the practice, as well as optimize profitability.

The office manager can meet these goals by scheduling more productive procedures first, and at times most convenient for patients, second. Thus, the dental office manager schedules for higher production figures first and then schedules shorter or less productive visits in a manner as not to rush or overburden the dental staff. Often, less complicated procedures can be staggered in between lengthier procedures to allow the patient several rest breaks throughout the procedure. For example, the dentist may leave the room to conduct an oral exam on the hygiene patient or to give anesthetic to the next patient scheduled for restorative treatment. In this way every patient receives courteous, attentive care and the practice has the necessary staff available to offer the patient excellent care soon after being seated.

A common example of scheduling that keeps profitability high yet allows the clinical team to provide outstanding care is multitreatment room scheduling. This scheduling method permits the dentist to see patients in several different treatment rooms during the same period of time. The dentist begins a restorative appointment by giving Patient A anesthetic, after which the patient is monitored by the chairside assistant to ensure there is no reaction. During the waiting time, the dentist can see Patient B for five or ten minutes and then return to Patient A. When the dentist finishes the restorative care for Patient A, he or she can move on to give anesthetic to Patient C in the next treatment room or check any hygiene patients needing an exam. The clinical assistant stays with the Patient A and completes any treatment as directed by the dentist, accompanies Patient A to the front desk so the next appointment can be scheduled, then returns to the treatment area, cleans the treatment room, and sets up for Patient D. By using multiple rooms there is no "down time" when the room is cleaned and disinfected between patients but it is most effective with two or more clinical chairside dental assistants.

> **Note:** The general rule with scheduling is to keep the doctor busy and productive and at the same time utilize the chairside dental assistants in an efficient manner.

Blocking Out the Appointment Schedule

Whether using the computer or a manual appointment book system, the office manager must plan ahead and block out specific times in which not to schedule patients. These times include lunch, before and after business hours, and time away from the office (e.g., vacation or continuing education classes). Some offices also block out time for emergencies and staff meetings. The sample computerized schedule displays all the necessary components of electronic scheduling (Figure 12-1).

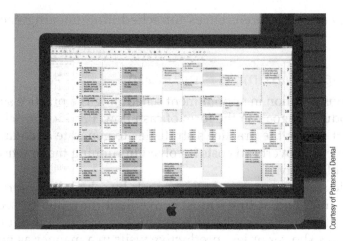

FIGURE 12-1 Sample of a computerized scheduling system.

Appointment Columns

Dental appointments are scheduled in blocks or units of time; most often a unit equals 10 or 15 minutes. This helps keep the staff on time and optimizes production. Once an office decides on the amount of time they will use for a unit, it is not easy to change so the decision is important when setting up the appointment book.

If the dentist works on 15-minute time units and requests one hour to treat a patient, the office manager would reserve four units. In an office that uses 10-minute units, this same appointment would require six units. If a procedure takes four units, the equivalent time is 40 minutes on 10 minutes per unit schedule verses an hour on a 15-minute per unit schedule. Generally office staff talks in units, not actual time, so no conversion is necessary.

To schedule efficiently, allowing neither too much nor too little time to complete procedures, the office manager must obtain from the dentist the desired number of appointment units for the most routinely performed procedures. These times can be added to dental management software such as Dentrix to facilitate appointment scheduling. Other considerations of determining the number of units each procedure will need include the following:

- How much appointment time does the dentist need and how much time is needed by the assistant?
- Has clean-up/setup time been included in the time requirement or must it be added separately?
- Does the scheduler have the ability to override the system when patients require more time?

Reevaluation of procedure times is something the office manager is responsible for monitoring. If your office is continually behind schedule or you seem to have staff standing around, you'll need to look at the procedure requirements and determine if they are accurate.

Multiple Appointments/Double Booking

Secondary appointments or double bookings may be scheduled throughout the day, such as postoperative checks for surgical patients, dental hygiene checks, and denture adjustments. The office manager may also schedule additional restorative patients and book them to arrive and be seated at staggered times. This takes practice and an excellent understanding of how the dentist works and uses clinical staff. With practice, multitreatment room schedules using a staggered schedule can be an excellent way to increase office production.

Sample of Appointment Book with Staggered Scheduling

Using the sample schedule in Figure 12-2, all three patients scheduled for 8 A.M. would be seated in their respective treatment rooms. The dentist would see Mary Brown to determine what x-rays the assistant needs to take to make a diagnosis. As the dentist is doing that, the assistant in treatment room 2 is reviewing health history and taking the panoramic radiographs as scheduled and when the dentist finishes in treatment room 1, Sally Hayes in treatment room 2 is ready for exam and consult. After the dentist finishes the consult, the office manager will go over treatment plan and finances either in the same treatment room or preferably in a consultation room so the assistant can set up for the next patient. The dentist then returns to treatment room 1 and completes Mary Brown's appointment and then he has time to check Patricia Abbott in treatment room 3 who is now finished with her hygiene appointment; however, notice that Patricia also has an appointment with the dentist after her hygiene appointment so efficiency will be improved for the dentist to do his exam during her restoration appointment. Meanwhile after Sallys treatment is complete in room 2 and she goes to the front desk to make her next appointment, the assistant will seat Elizabeth Reeves and take the FMX for her so when the dentist is done treating Mary, Elizabeth will be ready for her exam.

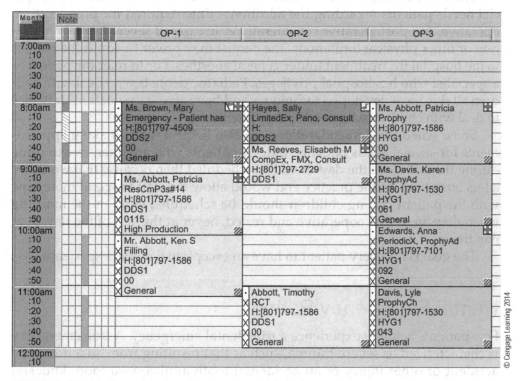

FIGURE 12-2 Sample of a staggered schedule.

It is important for the entire office staff to understand the schedule to make it work. Morning meetings can help with this by visualizing the flow of the day before beginning the schedule. If you are curious what the assistant who was working in treatment room 2 is doing from 9:20 A.M. to 11 A.M., that would be time when instruments are sterilized, supplies ordered, rooms restocked, and so on. She is also available to assistant in hygiene or as an extra pair of hands in treatment room 1.

Treatment Codes

Because many practices accept some form of third-party coverage toward payment for services, the office manager not only needs to understand what procedure is being done for each patient but also its procedure code so it can be billed accurately. These standardized codes known as Current Dental Terminology (CDT) codes, were mandated as part of HIPAA and are established by the American Dental Association. Everything done in the office has a code and some offices will also use those codes as part of their schedule.

Scheduling Special Needs Patient

Patients having special needs may require additional units added to their appointment time. Special needs patients include, but are not limited to, patients with known dental phobias, children, patients with bleeding disorders, physically or mentally challenged individuals, elderly patients requiring assistance, patients with heart conditions, patients requiring premedication for management of anxiety, or patients with special anesthesia needs. Patients covered by the Americans with Disabilities Act may have special needs requiring additional treatment time.

The office manager should check with the dentist before scheduling special needs patients regarding the additional time required for preoperative, operative, and postoperative considerations. In cases of severe mental retardation or other physical limitations, the dentist may prefer to admit the patient to the hospital for treatment under general anesthesia or to refer the patient to a specialist who has hospital privileges. Pediatric dentists who deal with children all day have developed techniques and have access to sedation strategies to deal with children who need special attention.

Some scheduling considerations are also helpful when making appointments for special needs patients. Elderly patients who are often free to come during the middle of the day should be scheduled then because that would be a less busy time for the practice and would allow the staff to spend more time with the patient. Young children should be scheduled early in the morning when they are most cooperative and rested, never at the end of the day, or at nap time.

The goal is for every patient to have an exceptional dental experience.

Dental Emergency Patients

Few patients actually experience a true dental emergency. A true emergency is characterized as severe trauma, such as that resulting from an automobile accident or other injury or an accidental tooth avulsion—a tooth knocked out of the socket, or jaw fracture. In most true dental emergency situations, patients are taken to the emergency room for treatment and/or referred to an oral surgeon or other specialists. Occasionally, however, individuals call the office requiring immediate treatment related to pain, swelling, or a lost or broken prosthesis or restoration. These are often referred to as emergencies in the dental practice.

Most practices are committed to treating all emergency patients promptly, regardless of the inconvenience to the dentist and staff.

In most practices, emergency visits are palliative only, which means the dentist treats only the immediate source of the pain or nature of the problem (such as cementing a crown back in place) and then reappoints the patient, if necessary, at another time to complete the treatment. The goal is to make the patient comfortable. The patient should be made aware of this when the appointment is made so the expectation for treatment is met. For example, the office manager might say, "Mrs. Smith at this appointment our goal is to make you comfortable. Depending on what is causing your discomfort, you may need to make another longer appointment to repair the problem. As you know, Dr. Crawford is an excellent dentist and he will take very good care of you."

If the patient is new to the practice, he or she will need to complete a new patient history form including a medical history. Even if the emergency patient is visiting from out of town and will be returning to their own dentist, a complete health history and treatment records are required.

Screening and Scheduling Emergency Patients

Emergency patients must be screened by the office manager to determine the following: (1) whether the caller is a patient of record; (2) the extent, onset, and severity of symptoms; and (3) other related circumstances. The office manager may use the following questions to obtain additional information and screen emergency callers:

- Have you seen Dr. Jones before? Ask this only if unfamiliar with the patient's name.
- Can you describe what kind of symptoms you are having? Which tooth is it? Try to get as complete a description as possible.
- When did the problem start? Is it constant?
- Rank the discomfort from mild to severe. Does it keep you up at night? Are there times when it is worse?
- Does it bother you if you eat or drink something hot or cold? Sweets? Pressure?
- Are you presently under the care of a physician for any other medical conditions or taking prescription medications? Have you been premedicated for dental treatment in the past?
- Do you have any known drug allergies or sensitivities?

The more complete the information obtained by the office manager is, the more efficient the clinical staff can be when treating the patient.

Some practices have specific times reserved in the daily schedule to accommodate emergencies. These times are often just before or after the lunch hour. Other practices prefer to handle dental emergency calls as needed.

Screening Telephone Requests for Prescription Drugs

In some instances, known or suspected drug abusers may call the office in pain, requesting prescriptions for narcotics. The office manager should alert the dentist to possible drug abusers who might be "shopping" for pain medication. The conscientious dentist is very careful not to provide prescription drugs to individuals that might abuse or resell controlled substances.

At the decision of the dentist and after examination, an emergency patient may be given a prescription for an antibiotic if an infection must be brought under control prior to initiating corrective treatment and, if needed, medication for pain management.

Recording Appointments

Upon request to schedule an appointment and with the knowledge of the necessary procedure and number of units required, the office manager works with the patients preferences to schedule an appointment. A significant key to practice building is availability of appointment times for patients.

Rather than just assigning an appointment time, the patient is usually asked if there are days or times that work better and are offered a couple of appointment times that would match that request as closely as possible. Patients like to be given choices, where possible, rather than being assigned one specific time only. If possible offer the patient two appointment options to choose from, this gives the patient some choice regarding the appointment without overwhelming the patient with options.

If you have lots of appointment times available, it is to your advantage not to share that with the patient. Patients want to go to a doctor that other patients are happy seeing; after all who wants to go to an unpopular dentist. When making an appointment and providing too many choices, patients may be more likely to cancel because they assume it won't be a problem rescheduling because, after all, you had so many appointment times available.

The office manager needs to accommodate the patient at the same time maintaining control of the appointment book. Overbooking is stressful for the entire dental staff and giant gaps in the schedule cut into the profitability of the practice.

Regardless of when the appointment is scheduled or whether it was done in an appointment book or on a computer, care must be taken to record it correctly on the schedule. The patient's name, the procedure being done, and the time requirements are needed but it is also helpful to note medical alerts including premedication or any other treatment needed such as x-rays. Accurately recording patient appointments as soon as you make them will help you avoid the embarrassment of having a patient arrive at the office who is not on your schedule. Writing it on a sticky note is not good enough when making an appointment.

Sequential Appointment Scheduling

When a series or sequence of planned treatments is indicated, some dentists prefer that the patient be scheduled for all appointments at the beginning of treatment. This keeps the planned treatment on schedule and prevents patients from becoming lost in the system during treatment. In such cases, the dentist should indicate the number of appointments needed, the number of units to schedule for each, and the anticipated treatment to take place during each appointment.

The office manager should note when outside laboratory work is required with the case, and allow sufficient time for the case to be sent out, fabricated, and returned in time for the patient's next scheduled visit.

When patients are scheduled for multiple appointments, some offices also set up payment schedules to correspond to the planned treatment visits for patients to pay as they go. This helps the patient schedule appointments according to his or her other financial obligations and also informs him or her of all anticipated treatment costs prior to the appointment. This pre-estimation helps avoid financial surprises and gives the patient a clear idea of planned treatment and his or her financial responsibility.

Issuing the Patient's Appointment Card

If the patient is present during the appointment scheduling, the office manager provides an appointment card containing the date of the scheduled appointment, as well as the date, including the year, time, and day of the week. The appointment card should have the practice's phone number, making it convenient for patients to call with any questions regarding the appointment. A notice usually appears at the bottom of the appointment card requesting that any change in the appointment be requested 24 hours in advance. For further information on completing appointment cards, see Chapter 7 (Printed Communications).

Appointment Confirmation

Once an appointment or series of appointments has been established, it is important that the office manager contact patients to confirm their scheduled appointments. This most often occurs the day before the appointment via a telephone call. Office managers find early mornings and late afternoon or evenings the most effective time to reach patients at home to confirm their appointments.

The office manager creates a list of scheduled appointments on the daily schedule. From the daily schedule the patient charts are pulled, if the office still uses them, and from the schedule calls patients to confirm their appointments. As patients are reached and their appointments confirmed, the office manager indicates that the patient has been reached and or that the message has been left. If a message is left, noting whether it was left on an answering machine with left message machine (LMM) or left message person (LMP) when an actual person received the message can be helpful.

If a patient lists a daytime telephone number other than their home, usually their work or cell phone they may also be contacted during the workday to confirm appointments unless they have indicated otherwise in their patient record. The confirmation call is brief and to the point and may be as follows, "Hello, Mr. Daniels, this is Mary calling from Dr. Edward's office. I'm calling to confirm your 9:30 A.M. appointment for tomorrow, April 10." The patient is given the opportunity to respond. To avoid confusion, use the actual date of the appointment rather than only tomorrow or Friday.

Some patients are difficult to reach and the office manager may leave a message on their voice mail or personal answering machine. You may leave only that there is an appointment with your office and the day and time. Because of privacy concerns no other details of treatment should be included.

Computerized Appointment Confirmation

Some offices use computerized or automatic appointment confirmation. The office computer dials numbers of the appointed patients and plays a recorded message such as, "This is Shannon at Dr. Olson's office, calling to confirm Courtney's appointment for tomorrow April 10 at 2 P.M. If you would like to hear this message again press 1, to confirm your appointment press 2. If you have questions regarding your appointment, please call our office at 512-555-1212." The automated confirmation system can be set to call during the hours that patients are most likely to be home and it will print out the results of its calls. For example, with Courtney it can indicate that someone answered the phone listened to the entire message but did not respond or that it called three times between 6 and 8 P.M. but there was no answer. Rarely are patients given the opportunity to cancel an appointment on an automated system because the practice wants the opportunity to reschedule the appointment at the time of cancellation. Remember you are not asking the patient if they want to keep the appointment; you are confirming an appointment that they made and should already have on their calendar. This is a courtesy call.

Using practice management software, many offices also have the option of confirming appointments using email or text messages.

Technological timesavers help free the office managers time to focus on face-to-face relationships with patients regarding treatment. Successful communication has always been and will always be interpersonal skills.

Handling Late Patients

Occasionally, patients cannot help being detained and arrive late for their appointment. Unfortunately, it may be necessary to reschedule the patient, provide less than the planned treatment for that day to keep on schedule, or make patients who arrived on time for their appointments wait when the latecomer is seen.

Every office has patients who are chronically late for appointments. First you need to ask yourself if you have trained patients to be late by never being on time yourself. If so, fix your problem before attempting to help the patient. If not, the office manager needs to talk to the patient in private about the necessity of being on time and let them know that if they come to appointments late they will need to reschedule. It is difficult to follow through with this and occasionally a patient will never return; however, is it worth losing good patients that come to appointments on time and expect to be seen on time for one that doesn't? Keeping chronically late patients in the practice increases the amount of stress for everyone.

It is very tempting to give the late patient an appointment card with an earlier time but lying to a patient even about something this small is still lying. When you get caught and you eventually will, the patient will wonder what else you lied to them about. It just isn't worth it. If the patient comes at the time written on the appointment card and has to wait, it isn't motivation for them to be on time in the future. Be honest in all aspects of your career.

It is important for the office manager to note in the chart late arrivals and any discussion that may have taken place about the problem.

"No-Show" Patients

Patients who fail to keep confirmed appointments are commonly referred to as "no-shows." Failing to keep an appointment is sometimes called a disappointment or failure. Practices that experience a high rate of "no-shows" should evaluate their appointment making and confirmation process.

Not scheduling "no-shows" quickly is sometimes helpful; if patients are able to reschedule right away they tend to reschedule more frequently. Imagine if you had waited several weeks or months for an appointment, you'd think twice about rescheduling. Some offices charge a fee if appointments are not rescheduled at least 24 hours in advance giving the staff an opportunity to call other patients to fill the schedule. Unfortunately, this is often not collectable and for many people is not a deterrent. At a certain point, suggesting a patient seek treatment from another office will actually be more profitable for your practice than to continue to schedule the "no-show" patient.

It is important for the office manager to determine if the patient is a "no-show" for a specific reason such as concerns about finances or fear of dental treatment. If that is the case, financing options can be worked out or the dentist may be willing to assist the patient with medication to relieve anxiety.

Maintaining a Call List

A call list is a handy reference for the office manager to fill a cancellation in the appointment schedule on short notice. Some especially busy practices have a long waiting period for appointments even providing a space on their new patient registration form to ask patients if they are available on short notice or would like to be placed on a call list to be contacted should another patient need to reschedule and an appointment becomes available on short notice. A great call list may be even more critical for a small practice with a smaller patient base from which to draw.

The call list may be a manually written list or notebook of patients that have asked to be contacted on short notice for required treatment; it can also be maintained on the office computer. The following information should be included on the call list: the date the patient was added to the call list, the name of the patient, the type of procedure needed, the required number of appointment units and the daytime telephone number. Note that once a patient has been contacted and appointed earlier in the schedule, his or her name should be: (1) removed from the call list to avoid the future embarrassment of calling to schedule treatment already completed; and (2) moved from the original space in the appointment book or computer scheduling program.

When using the call list, watch carefully for appointments that are part of a sequence and must stay in order or appointments requiring lab work that might not be available at the earlier date.

When a cancellation occurs in the schedule with short notice, the office manager should always start with the top of the call list, reviewing patients in the chronological order of their placement on the list. This avoids the potential for favoritism and treats all patients on the call list fairly.

The Daily Schedule

The office manager maintains a daily schedule based on the appointment book or computerized program. It is the office manager's responsibility to see that scheduling is carried out according to the dentist's preference, to meet production goals, and to accommodate patient schedules.

Each day a copy of the next day's schedule is provided to the clinical staff for review. This brings them up to date on which patients are scheduled, which patient appointments were confirmed, and alerts them to medical concerns or special needs of patients. Staff members are expected to review the schedule for the day prior to the morning meeting. Schedules should not be hung where patients could see them but kept in a secure area to comply with HIPAA.

Occasionally, changes in the daily schedule occur. It is the office manager's job to note changes on the daily schedule and to alert the clinical staff to those changes.

Scheduling Recall Appointments

Recall appointments are addressed in several areas throughout this text. A competent office manager knows that recall appointments are a vital lifeline in sustaining the growth and productivity of the practice. Many practices set specific recall goals for scheduling returning patients. Most dental management experts agree that 85 percent return rate of recall patients is successful.

Recall Appointment Confirmation

The office manager handles and confirms recall (also called recare) appointments for the hygienist in the same manner as the doctor's appointments. Charts are pulled the day prior, using the appointment schedule or computer program; a day sheet is compiled listing the names and appointed times patients are scheduled, and the type of procedure anticipated. The office manager calls to confirm the patients or uses an auto confirmation system.

Once the hygienist has completed the patient's recall appointment, the office manager either reschedules the patient for the next due recall appointment or enters the date for the next recall notification into the computer or manual recall filing system. If the patient requires restorative treatment, the office manager sets up the required series of appointments for the patient to return to be treated by the dentist.

Scheduling the Hygienist Who Works with an Assistant

In some practices the hygienist works with an assistant who provides chairside services not specifically delegated by the State Dental Practice Act to the hygienist. This helps the hygienist work more efficiently and makes the practice more productive.

The office manager schedules the hygienist's time for the procedures he or she is responsible for such as prophylaxis, subgingival scaling, curettage, administration of local anesthesia, and suture removal. The office manager may schedule the hygienist's assistant to provide such services as completion or updating of necessary forms, treatment room clean-up and setup, instrument preparation and sterilization, taking required x-rays, coronal polishing, pit and fissure sealants, topical fluoride application, and oral hygiene instruction. *Please note that all of these expanded duties are not available to assistants in all states and the office manager is responsible for knowing the laws in the state where the practice is located.*

In practices using assisted hygiene, the hygienist and assistant usually work between two treatment rooms alternating patients. Typical assisted hygiene flow may be as follows:

8:00 A.M. Hygiene assistant seats the patient in treatment room 1 and updates the medical history; opens sterile instrument pack in front of the patient; takes any required x-rays. The assistant would develop traditional x-rays or make sure digital x-rays are on the computer monitor. Then, the assistant moves to treatment room 2 to repeat the process with patient 2.

8:15 A.M. Hygienist enters treatment room 1 and performs an oral hygiene evaluation and oral screening exam, does periodontal charting, and any necessary scaling.

8:45 A.M. Hygiene assistant returns to treatment room 1 and does the coronal polishing for the patient then makes sure everything is ready for the dentist to do his or her exam. As this is being done the hygienist is seeing the patient in treatment room 2.

At the conclusion of the hygiene appointment, the hygiene assistant accompanies the patient to the front desk, informs the office manager of the patient's subsequent scheduling needs, and returns to the treatment room for clean-up, removal of contaminated instruments, room disinfection, replacing of protective barriers, and other procedures required to ready the treatment room for the next patient.

Scheduling for efficiency and productivity is a key responsibility of the office manager. Possessing skills in appointment schedule management are essential in assuming an office management position.

 ## Skill Building

These optional activities and exercises are designed to help the student put into practice information learned in the chapter.

1. You are the new office manager in a large urban practice. A caller with whom you are unfamiliar says he has been in pain with a terrible toothache for 24 hours. What actions should you take? What questions should you ask? Make a list of steps you would take and share with the class.

2. You arrive at 8:30 A.M. on Monday as the new office manager to discover that two patients have been inadvertently scheduled for the same appointment time with the dentist. What should you do? Make a list of possible solutions and share with the class.

3. Your patient, Kathy Peterson, is late again. She is one of your favorite patients but her habitual lateness is causing your clinical staff to see other patients later than scheduled. Role play how you would handle this situation.

4. Your patient, Bruce Smith, cancels an hour before his appointment. Not only will this affect today's appointment but it was number one in a series of three appointments. What might you do to convince Bruce to keep his appointment? Make a list of suggestions to share.

Challenge Your Understanding

Select the response that best answers each of the following questions. Only one response is correct.

1. What consideration must be taken into account when scheduling for productivity?
   a. The time of day preferred by the dentist to perform the procedure
   b. The daily cash flow requirements of the practice
   c. The impact of scheduling decisions on patient flow
   d. All of the above

2. Palliative treatment involves diagnosis and restoration of the emergency problem.
   a. True
   b. False

3. Which of the following information should be included on the call list?
   a. The date the patient was added to the call list
   b. The type of procedure needed, day and hours available
   c. The required number of appointment units
   d. All of the above

4. Times blocked out of the appointment schedule usually include all of the following *except*:
   a. Lunch hours
   b. Holidays
   c. Visits from dental supply representatives
   d. Time for emergencies and staff meetings

5. Appointment blocks or units of time are most often in _____ increments:
   a. 1–2 hour
   b. 10–15 minute
   c. 15–30 minute
   d. Varies

6. Multitreatment room scheduling is a technique used to:
   a. Manage habitually late or no-show patients
   b. Maximize the doctor's time efficiently
   c. Save space in the appointment book
   d. a and b only

7. Treatment codes are assigned to each procedure to facilitate third-party payment.
   a. True
   b. False

8. Special needs patients who may require adjustments in the number of units needed when scheduling include:
   a. Those covered under the Americans with Disabilities Act
   b. Patients who require premedication for management of anxiety
   c. Patients who require additional anesthesia
   d. All of the above

9. Few patients actually experience true dental emergencies.
   a. True
   b. False

10. What is the proper sequence for scheduling and confirming an appointment?
    a. Make out the appointment card, call the day before to confirm the appointment, record the appointment in the book or computer database
    b. Call the day before to confirm the appointment, make out the appointment card, record the appointment in the book or computer database
    c. Record the appointment in the book or computer, make out the appointment card, call the day before to confirm the appointment
    d. There is no set way to schedule and confirm appointments

11. Early mornings and later afternoon and evenings are the most effective time to reach patients at home to confirm their appointments.
    a. True
    b. False

12. An auto-dialer allows practice personnel to make important calls to patients and replaces sound patient relations skills.
    a. True
    b. False

13. The daily schedule:
    a. Is posted in each treatment room, usually late the prior afternoon
    b. Brings all clinical personnel up to date on which patients are scheduled and confirmed for the next day
    c. Alerts staff to raise concerns or ask questions at the next monthly staff meeting
    d. All of the above

14. Young children should be scheduled for late appointments when they are at a lowered activity level and are generally more cooperative.
    a. True
    b. False

15. Some practices have a specific time reserved in their daily schedules to accommodate routine emergencies. These times are often:
    a. Just before or after lunch
    b. At the end of the day
    c. Whenever the patient can come into the office
    d. a or b only

16. Having an assistant helps the hygienist work more efficiently and makes the practice more productive.
    a. True
    b. False

17. The office manager should:
    a. Accommodate a late patient
    b. Dismiss a late patient from the practice
    c. Reschedule a late patient
    d. Discuss the problem first in private with the patient

18. As a general rule, scheduling to maximize profits:
    a. Reduces quality for the patient
    b. Keeps the doctor busy through the day
    c. Relies on a trained dental assistant
    d. Both b and c

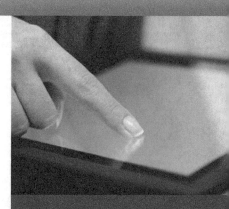

CHAPTER 13

Managing Accounts Receivable

CHAPTER OUTLINES

- **Managed Care Programs**
  Health Maintenance Organizations
  Preferred Provider Organizations
  Exclusive Provider Organizations
  Point-of-Service Plans
- **Insurance and Third-Party Claims Processing**
- **Terminology and Procedures**
- **The ADA Insurance Claim Form**
  ADA Procedure Codes
  ICD Diagnostic Codes
- **Predetermination and Preauthorization**
- **Signature on File**
- **Use of Digital Radiographs and Intraoral Photographs**
- **Electronic Claims Processing**
- **Claims Tracking and Rejection**
- **The One-Write System**
- **Methods of Payment**
  Cash
  Personal Check
  Dental Care Cards
  Health Care Savings Plans
  Credit Cards and Debit Cards
  Direct Reimbursement
  Series of Payments
  Finance Plans

KEY TERMS

assignment of benefits
beneficiaries
benefit
birthday rule
capitation
carrier
coordination of benefits
copayment
credit check
deductible
diagnostic codes
direct reimbursement
dual insurance coverage
electronic claims processing
exclusion
explanation of benefits (EOB)
fee-for-service
International Classification
  of Diseases (ICD)
indemnity
managed care
one-write system
pegboard system
predetermination
provider
release
signature on file
subscriber
Table of Allowance
usual, customary, and
  reasonable fee (UCR)
walk-out statement

LEARNING OBJECTIVES

Upon completion of this chapter, the reader should be able to:

1. Define managed care and describe alternative payment plans with regard to the dental practice.

2. Describe and define insurance and other third-party payment claims processing and related terminology; complete a standard insurance claim form accurately.

3. Describe the use and components of a one-write system.

4. Describe the benefits of electronic claims processing.

5. Describe methods of patient payment for dental treatment.

6. Describe the procedures for entering payments.

7. Explain the procedure and rationale for performing a credit check.

8. Describe the procedure for collection of past-due accounts.

Managed Care Programs

Managed care involves any third party's participation in the management of health care delivery with regard to finance. It includes predetermination of benefits and claims reviews, as well as fully managed capitation programs. Patients who enroll in managed care choose a specific participating office according to a list of dentists who enroll and agree to the managed care company's terms. The office is then responsible for all of the general, and in some cases specialty, dental services required. Billing and reimbursement varies widely based on the plan.

Managed care is a cost-containment system that directs the utilization of health benefits by limiting the type, level, and frequency of treatment; limiting access to care; and controlling the level of reimbursement.

The primary advantage for a dentist to sign up for a managed care program is a guaranteed flow of new patients. This is especially appealing to a new dentist just starting out in practice or trying to build a practice.

The main types of managed care organizations are Health Maintenance Organizations (HMOs), Preferred Provider Organizations (PPOs), Exclusive Provider Organizations (EPOs), and Point-of-Service Plans (POSs).

Health Maintenance Organizations

HMOs are broken down into four types: staff models, group models, Individual Practice Associations (IPAs), and network models.

The classic HMO is the staff model, in which the health care plan owns the facility and pays providers (dentists) to work in them. In this type of plan patients are restricted to the HMO providers (doctors and hospitals) and must seek treatment from primary caregivers before being referred to specialists. About 10 percent of all HMOs are staff model.

The group model is a variation on the staff model. In the group model, the HMO contracts with an individual provider group to care for its patients. The provider group is managed independently and reimbursed on a capitated basis. Capitation refers to a method of payment for services where the insurer pays providers a fixed amount for each patient treated, regardless of type, complexity, or number of services required. About 10 percent of all HMOs are group model.

Individual Practice Associations (IPAs) are the most common type of HMO, comprising 65 percent of all plans. IPAs contract either with individual providers or with networks of providers who practice in their own offices. Some providers and networks are paid a discounted fee-for-service; however, many are capitated.

The fourth type of HMO is the network model, which comprises approximately 15 percent of dental managed care plans. It is similar to the IPA model because it forms a network of independent providers, which may be single or multi-specialty. Providers in the network model may be paid by either discounted fee-for-service or capitation and may continue to provide services to their own private patients.

Preferred Provider Organizations

Under a PPO, a third party (an insurer, an employer, administrator, or other sponsoring group) negotiates discounted rates for dental services directly with selected provider dentists. Subscribers, also known as beneficiaries (those eligible or enrolled patients in the plan), covered by the PPO may use providers outside the PPO network, although financial incentives encourage patients to use preferred providers. Providers in a PPO are selected based upon their professional qualifications and performance; they benefit through increased patient volume and prompt payment. In return, providers agree to a fee schedule and agree, if requested, to have their performance reviewed.

Exclusive Provider Organizations

EPOs evolved from PPOs. The EPO is an indemnity arrangement where a group of providers contracts with an insurer, third-party administrator, employer, or other sponsor. The provider agrees to accept the negotiated level of reimbursement, to follow utilization review procedures (audits), to refer patients to other EPO-contracted providers, and to use only contracted hospitals if a patient requires extensive work under anesthesia.

In contrast with a PPO, the EPO provider can be prohibited from treating patients not enrolled in the organization. Patients must seek services only from participating providers. In an EPO any dental services provided by unaffiliated providers are not reimbursed.

Point-of-Service Plans

Members of a POS receive care from participating providers designated by the network, but have the option of obtaining care outside the network. Both HMOs and PPOs may offer a POS plan as a method of expanding members' options of providers. These agreements are called "open-ended." If a member receives treatment from a provider who is not part of the network, the care is covered, although it will likely include a high copayment. The copayment is the amount the patient pays at the time of service for treatment.

Insurance and Third-Party Claims Processing

Dental practice payment options often include insurance participation. In fact, the majority of dental practices accepts and/or participates in some form of insurance or third-party coverage for their patients who have coverage. Third party means that someone other than the dentist or patient is involved in financial responsibility for treatment.

It is the dental office manager's responsibility to complete and submit insurance claim forms. Some practices, especially large groups, employ staff members who deal exclusively with insurance claims processing and tracking.

Many patients who have obtained dental insurance have the misconception that their dental care is covered completely by insurance. To avoid misunderstandings, before treatment begins, it is the office manager's duty to explain that usually only a certain percentage of the total fee is allowable and covered by the insurance company. Ultimately it is the patient's responsibility to pay the remaining portion in those cases. It is important to stress to the patient that coverage is based on a contract between themselves or their employer and the insurance company. Fees and percentages are determined by that contract and not by the dentist.

> **Note:** Medical insurance rarely covers anything related to general dentistry; the patient must have a specific dental policy or coverage. Oral surgeons would have procedures, relating to accident or disease, covered under medical policies.

Here is an example of insurance payments: A patient needs a crown at an estimated fee of $650, which is the reduced fee the dentist negotiated with the insurance company; his fee for service is $800. The patient's contract with the insurance company states that the company will pay 50 percent of this restorative procedure; so the insurance pays $325 and the patient is responsible for $325 and the dentist receives $650.

Terminology and Procedures

An important step to successful completion of insurance claim forms is obtaining all of the necessary information including all the third-party details and all of the patient and subscriber details. It is better to have too much information than not enough, so make sure acquaintance forms are entirely completed.

Some insurance companies allow for coordination of benefits when the patient is covered by more than one carrier or policy, as in the case of working spouses, both of whom carry insurance and they or their children are covered under both plans. In this circumstance, the dentist practice bills the primary insurance provider first and then after receiving payment submits the unpaid balance to the secondary company. Usually the secondary claim must be accompanied by an explanation of benefits, also called an EOB, giving the secondary provider details regarding what has already been paid.

When both insurance providers/carriers participate, this is termed dual insurance coverage. It requires further research by the office manager to ensure that coordination of benefits is permitted and the extent to which both carriers provide coverage.

Dependent children of dual coverage parents are covered as "primary" by the plan of the respective parent whose birthday falls earlier in the calendar year. This is called the birthday rule. Dependent children with divorced or legally separated parents are covered according to the court decree or to the following guidelines if the decree does not mention health/dental care for the children:

1. The biological parent who has custody
2. The spouse of the biological parent with custody
3. The noncustodial biological parent
4. The spouse of the noncustodial parent.

Before starting any extensive treatment, the dental office manager would be wise to clarify who is the financially responsible party for fees not covered by insurance and to make sure that individual understands the fees involved. Working with divorced or separated parents can be challenging, and determining financial responsibility before treating the patient can save time and potential collection problems later.

If the dentist participates in a program with usual, customary, and reasonable fees (UCR), he or she files the UCR fees with the carrier. Payment is based upon the percentage covered by the group.

If the dentist participates in a fixed fee program, this means a fixed fee has been predetermined for every allowable procedure. Dentists who participate in fixed fee programs must accept the fees established and are not legally allowed to charge the patient an additional amount for any difference between the fees normally charged by the practice and the fixed fee that the dentist has agreed to accept.

Each insurance carrier provides a table of allowance, which establishes a fixed dollar amount for each patient's dental services. In this case the patient is not financially responsible for any difference between the fee charged by the dentist and the table amount.

Benefit refers to the amount the insurance company pays toward services covered under a contractual plan. Carrier refers to the insurance company that sells or carries the insurance. *Coverage* refers to the extent of the insurance policy or the benefits included. **Deductible** refers to the amount the patient or responsible party must pay toward services before the carrier will begin paying on insurance claims. **Exclusion** refers to services not covered under the terms of the policy.

The ADA Insurance Claim Form

The following information is required when completing a third-party insurance claim form. Missing or incomplete information may cause a delay in payment or trigger the claim to be rejected. The office manager must ensure the following information is completed and reported on every insurance claim form.

The insurance claim form is divided into three parts:

1. The top section of the claim contains information about the carrier, subscriber, and the patient.

2. The middle section is information regarding treatment including a description of treatment, its ADA procedure code, and the fee charged by the dentist.

3. The last part of the claim is the details about the dentist.

Completing an ADA claim form will require the following information in the numbered fields on the claim (Figure 13-1):

- (1) On the ADA form this will be the type of claim you are filing. If the work has been done, this is an actual claim; if you are getting an estimate of coverage for a procedure, it is a predetermination.

- (2) If this claim was already predetermined and is now being submitted for payment, enter that information.

- (3) Insurance Company/Dental Benefit Plan Information: This is the company that you are sending the claim to and expecting payment from; they are also referred to as the carrier.

- (4–11) If more than one person has dental insurance the name and information for the secondary carrier goes here.

- (12–17) The details regarding the policyholder/subscriber, who is the primary person on the insurance coverage.

  Note: This person is not necessarily a patient in the practice.

- (18–23) Patient: The patient is the person having the dental work done and is covered by the dental insurance policy.

- (24–32) This is the record of services provided and includes the date of the procedure, area of the oral cavity, tooth charting system, tooth numbers or letters, procedure code, description, and fee. 29a and 29b are new to the 2012 claim form and relate to the diagnosis codes.

- (33) This area is to chart any teeth that the patient is missing.

- (34, 34a) These fields are new on the 2012 ADA claim form and are for diagnosis codes.

- (35) This area is for comments or remarks regarding treatment.

ADA American Dental Association® **Dental Claim Form**

HEADER INFORMATION

1. Type of Transaction (Mark all applicable boxes)

☐ Statement of Actual Services ☐ Request for Predetermination/Preauthorization

☐ EPSDT / Title XIX

2. Predetermination/Preauthorization Number

INSURANCE COMPANY/DENTAL BENEFIT PLAN INFORMATION

3. Company/Plan Name, Address, City, State, Zip Code

OTHER COVERAGE (Mark applicable box and complete items 5-11. If none, leave blank.)

4. Dental? ☐   Medical? ☐   (If both, complete 5-11 for dental only.)

5. Name of Policyholder/Subscriber in #4 (Last, First, Middle Initial, Suffix)

6. Date of Birth (MM/DD/CCYY)

7. Gender ☐ M ☐ F

8. Policyholder/Subscriber ID (SSN or ID#)

9. Plan/Group Number

10. Patient's Relationship to Person named in #5 ☐ Self ☐ Spouse ☐ Dependent ☐ Other

11. Other Insurance Company/Dental Benefit Plan Name, Address, City, State, Zip Code

POLICYHOLDER/SUBSCRIBER INFORMATION (For Insurance Company Named in #3)

12. Policyholder/Subscriber Name (Last, First, Middle Initial, Suffix), Address, City, State, Zip Code

13. Date of Birth (MM/DD/CCYY)

14. Gender ☐ M ☐ F

15. Policyholder/Subscriber ID (SSN or ID#)

16. Plan/Group Number

17. Employer Name

PATIENT INFORMATION

18. Relationship to Policyholder/Subscriber in #12 Above ☐ Self ☐ Spouse ☐ Dependent Child ☐ Other

19. Reserved For Future Use

20. Name (Last, First, Middle Initial, Suffix), Address, City, State, Zip Code

21. Date of Birth (MM/DD/CCYY)

22. Gender ☐ M ☐ F

23. Patient ID/Account # (Assigned by Dentist)

RECORD OF SERVICES PROVIDED

	24. Procedure Date (MM/DD/CCYY)	25. Area of Oral Cavity	26. Tooth System	27. Tooth Number(s) or Letter(s)	28. Tooth Surface	29. Procedure Code	29a. Diag. Pointer	29b. Qty.	30. Description	31. Fee
1										
2										
3										
4										
5										
6										
7										
8										
9										
10										

33. Missing Teeth Information (Place an "X" on each missing tooth.)

1 2 3 4 5 6 7 8 9 10 11 12 13 14 15 16

32 31 30 29 28 27 26 25 24 23 22 21 20 19 18 17

34. Diagnosis Code List Qualifier ☐   (ICD-9 = B; ICD-10 = AB)

34a. Diagnosis Code(s)   A _____   C _____

(Primary diagnosis in "A")   B _____   D _____

31a. Other Fee(s)

32. Total Fee

35. Remarks

AUTHORIZATIONS

36. I have been informed of the treatment plan and associated fees. I agree to be responsible for all charges for dental services and materials not paid by my dental benefit plan, unless prohibited by law, or the treating dentist or dental practice has a contractual agreement with my plan prohibiting all or a portion of such charges. To the extent permitted by law, I consent to your use and disclosure of my protected health information to carry out payment activities in connection with this claim.

X _____

Patient/Guardian Signature   Date

37. I hereby authorize and direct payment of the dental benefits otherwise payable to me, directly to the below named dentist or dental entity.

X _____

Subscriber Signature   Date

BILLING DENTIST OR DENTAL ENTITY (Leave blank if dentist or dental entity is not submitting claim on behalf of the patient or insured/subscriber.)

48. Name, Address, City, State, Zip Code

49. NPI

50. License Number

51. SSN or TIN

52. Phone Number ( ) -

52a. Additional Provider ID

ANCILLARY CLAIM/TREATMENT INFORMATION

38. Place of Treatment ☐ (e.g. 11=office; 22=O/P Hospital)

(Use "Place of Service Codes for Professional Claims")

39. Enclosures (Y or N) ☐

40. Is Treatment for Orthodontics? ☐ No (Skip 41-42) ☐ Yes (Complete 41-42)

41. Date Appliance Placed (MM/DD/CCYY)

42. Months of Treatment Remaining

43. Replacement of Prosthesis ☐ No ☐ Yes (Complete 44)

44. Date of Prior Placement (MM/DD/CCYY)

45. Treatment Resulting from ☐ Occupational illness/injury ☐ Auto accident ☐ Other accident

46. Date of Accident (MM/DD/CCYY)

47. Auto Accident State

TREATING DENTIST AND TREATMENT LOCATION INFORMATION

53. I hereby certify that the procedures as indicated by date are in progress (for procedures that require multiple visits) or have been completed.

X _____

Signed (Treating Dentist)   Date

54. NPI

55. License Number

56. Address, City, State, Zip Code

56a. Provider Specialty Code

57. Phone Number ( ) -

58. Additional Provider ID

FIGURE 13-1a Sample of the ADA Dental Claim Form.

ADA American Dental Association®

America's leading advocate for oral health

The following information highlights certain form completion instructions. Comprehensive ADA Dental Claim Form completion instructions are printed in the CDT manual. Any updates to these instructions will be posted on the ADA's web site (ADA.org).

GENERAL INSTRUCTIONS

A. The form is designed so that the name and address (Item 3) of the third-party payer receiving the claim (insurance company/dental benefit plan) is visible in a standard #9 window envelope (window to the left). Please fold the form using the 'tick-marks' printed in the margin.

B. Complete all items unless noted otherwise on the form or in the CDT manual's instructions.

C. Enter the full name of an individual or a full business name, address and zip code when a name and address field is required.

D. All dates must include the four-digit year.

E. If the number of procedures reported exceeds the number of lines available on one claim form, list the remaining procedures on a separate, fully completed claim form.

COORDINATION OF BENEFITS (COB)

When a claim is being submitted to the secondary payer, complete the entire form and attach the primary payer's Explanation of Benefits (EOB) showing the amount paid by the primary payer. You may also note the primary carrier paid amount in the "Remarks" field (Item 35). There are additional detailed completion instructions in the CDT manual.

DIAGNOSIS CODING

The form supports reporting up to four diagnosis codes per dental procedure. This information is required when the diagnosis may affect claim adjudication when specific dental procedures may minimize the risks associated with the connection between the patient's oral and systemic health conditions. Diagnosis codes are linked to procedures using the following fields:

Item 29a – Diagnosis Code Pointer ("A" through "D" as applicable from Item 34a)

Item 34 – Diagnosis Code List Qualifier (B for ICD-9-CM; AB for ICD-10-CM)

Item 34a – Diagnosis Code(s) / A, B, C, D (up to four, with the primary adjacent to the letter "A")

PLACE OF TREATMENT

Enter the 2-digit Place of Service Code for Professional Claims, a HIPAA standard maintained by the Centers for Medicare and Medicaid Services. Frequently used codes are:

11 = Office; 12 = Home; 21 = Inpatient Hospital; 22 = Outpatient Hospital; 31 = Skilled Nursing Facility; 32 = Nursing Facility

The full list is available online at "www.cms.gov/PhysicianFeeSched/Downloads/Website_POS_database.pdf"

PROVIDER SPECIALTY

This code is entered in Item 56a and indicates the type of dental professional who delivered the treatment. The general code listed as "Dentist" may be used instead of any of the other codes.

Category / Description Code	Code
Dentist A dentist is a person qualified by a doctorate in dental surgery (D.D.S.) or dental medicine (D.M.D.) licensed by the state to practice dentistry, and practicing within the scope of that license.	122300000X
General Practice	1223G0001X
Dental Specialty (see following list)	Various
Dental Public Health	1223D0001X
Endodontics	1223E0200X
Orthodontics	1223X0400X
Pediatric Dentistry	1223P0221X
Periodontics	1223P0300X
Prosthodontics	1223P0700X
Oral & Maxillofacial Pathology	1223P0106X
Oral & Maxillofacial Radiology	1223D0008X
Oral & Maxillofacial Surgery	1223S0112X

Provider taxonomy codes listed above are a subset of the full code set that is posted at "www.wpc-edi.com/codes/taxonomy"

FIGURE 13-1b (*continued*)

- (36, 37) Authorization or signatures are in this area. The number 36 field is the contract for service between the dentist and patient and 37 allows the insurance payment to go directly to the dentist. If no signature appears in the number 37 field, payment for services will be sent to the patient.

- (38–47) This part of the claim shows ancillary claim and treatment information. It contains information regarding where the treatment took place and if it involved orthodontics, prosthetics, or was the result of an accident.

- (48–58) These areas are reserved for information about the dentist including address, license number, and tax ID or social security number, where the patient was treated, and additional information about the treatment by the dentist.

ADA Procedure Codes

Third-party reimbursement processing requires the use of treatment codes when claims are submitted for payment. This is to ensure that each procedure is properly billed and that the correct amount is paid to the provider. Procedures for which no code is provided are not reimbursed.

The American Dental Association publishes a book called *CDT* (*Current Dental Terminology*) that contains codes by category. The book is updated regularly and can be purchased and kept at the front desk for reference; codes are also embedded into practice management software.

Some office managers prefer to make up a short list of the codes most commonly used in the practice to save time.

ADA codes are divided into groups or categories. Each code begins with D designating it as a dental code followed by a number indicating its category and the last four digits of the code specify the procedure (Table 13-1).

ICD Diagnostic Codes

Beginning in 2014, International Classification of Diseases (ICD) codes will be implemented for the first time in dentistry. These codes are related to the CDT codes and explain why the procedure was done.

The 2012 ADA insurance claim form (Figure 13-1) has included an area for diagnosis coding. The actual diagnosis is made by the dentist but the dental office manager is responsible for adding correct codes to insurance forms. Office managers will initially be using ICD-10 codes, but like procedure codes, diagnosis codes are updated periodically. The number 34 field on the insurance claim form should be completed with AB to specify when ICD-10 codes are used. ICD-10 codes for dentistry are found under Diseases of the Digestive System, K00–K95, with K00–K14 being diseases of the oral cavity and salivary glands. Books can be purchased that contain all ICD codes, and both medical and dental or the specific dental codes can also be found online.

Here is an example of how a diagnostic code helps clarify a procedure code to improve patient care and insurance reimbursement for the dentist. Let's examine one of the most common dental procedures billed to insurance: Dental Caries. The procedure code we're using, for our example, is D2150, which indicates a two-surface amalgam restoration. By using a diagnostic code, the disease that existed creating the need for the restoration can be

TABLE 13-1 Current Dental Terminology (CDT) Codes

Diagnostic	D0100–D0999	Diagnostic codes would include exams, radiographs, and tools needed for the dentist to determine treatment necessary and create a treatment plan.
Preventive	D1000–D1999	Preventive codes would include procedures used to prevent dental disease such as prophylaxis, fluoride, pit and fissure sealants, and patient education. These codes would include many procedures performed by the hygienist.
Restorative	D2000–D2999	Restorative codes are used for procedures involving reconstruction of teeth damaged by decay or injury such as fillings using a variety of materials.
Endodontic	D3000–D3999	Endodontic codes are used for root canal therapy and diseases of the tooth's pulp.
Periodontics	D4000–D4999	Periodontal codes are used to designate treatment to the supporting structures surrounding the tooth both hard and soft tissue.
Prosthodontics — Removable	D5000–D5899	Removable prosthodontics codes are used for dentures or partial bridges
Maxillofacial prosthetics	D5900–D5999	Maxillofacial prosthetic codes are used for restoration of facial structures as a result of birth defect, injury, or disease
Implants	D6000–D6199	Implant codes cover the surgical insertion of implants into the jaw to anchor prosthesis
Prosthodontics — Fixed	D6200–D6999	Fixed prosthodontics involves artificial teeth that are not intended for removal once they are cemented in place
Oral and maxillofacial surgery	D7000–D7999	Oral surgery codes include all extractions involving impacted teeth, and repair of injuries, and reshaping bone because of trauma or disease
Orthodontics	D8000–D8999	Orthodontic codes are used for braces and appliances to control growth
Adjunctive general services	D9000–D9999	These codes are for anything that is not included under another category.

coded as caries limited to enamel (K02.51), as caries penetration into dentin (K02.52), or caries penetrating into the pulp (K02.53).

With diagnostic codes the dental practice can describe the disease more precisely. The area on the 2012 insurance claim form dealing with the diagnosis code(s) is 34a. For the example above, let's designate the appropriate code as K02.52. That would be entered in the "A" space. The "record of services provided" section of the claim form has a diagnosis pointer (29a) and quantity (29b) to allow the person completing the claim form to reference the diagnosis code, A through D, that is appropriate. For our example, the dental office manager would enter A in space 29a and 1 in space 29b on the line with the procedure D2150. Many claims contain multiple services provided, so this simplifies the diagnostic coding process.

> **Note:** ICD codes are used to designate only diseases, and procedures relating to dental health and prevention presently have no codes.

Predetermination and Preauthorization

Many insurance companies request that a predetermination is filed in advance of performing some extensive procedures. Predetermination means the amount or percentage the insurance company estimates it will pay toward the total fee for treatment but it is not a guarantee of payment. Preauthorization indicates if the insurance will or will not cover a specific procedure as diagnosed by the dentist.

Signature on File

Most dental insurance companies accept a Signature on File status on all claims for the current benefits year. The office manager should be aware of the insurance company policy regarding Signature on File and the Release and Assignment of Benefit Forms and be certain they are updated as required by the policy.

The release applies to dental records and authorizes the insurance claims examiners to review the diagnosis and treatment. Many procedures require dental radiographs to verify the need for treatment and subsequent claim for payment.

The assignment of benefit refers to the benefit paid by the insurance company and authorizes the company to send payment directly to the dentist, rather than to the patient.

Most practices have a signature on file box on their new patient registration forms. When the patient first enrolls in the practice, the patient or responsible party signs this box in lieu of having to sign an insurance claim form each time dental care is provided. The signature on file is also essential in practices when using electronic claims processing because there is no place to sign a form that is electronically submitted. Because the claim form is usually done after the patient leaves the office, the signature on file saves the practice from having the patient return for a signature.

Use of Digital Radiographs and Intraoral Photographs

Most third-party carriers require preoperative and occasionally postoperative radiographs or intraoral photos supporting treatment submitted for payment. When insurance claims were submitted traditionally through the mail, copies of the original radiographs were often included in the envelope with the claim requesting payment. This consumed the office manager's time, postage, processing costs, and often delayed payment for six to eight weeks.

Today, most plans accept computer-generated images either scanned or attached from the patient file and submitted with the electronic claim. The average cost per claim is low and it takes only minutes to process. The cost of submitting an electronic claim is offset by the fact that it requires no paper or mailing cost.

Electronic Claims Processing

Electronic claims processing is one of the technologies available to assist dental practices in filing insurance claims for payment. Electronic claims processing uses the practices computer to store, generate, and submit third-party claims to respective insurance company's computers via a clearinghouse. The change to electronic filing is part of the HIPAA Administrative Simplification Rule. It was initiated to reduce administrative costs for health care providers by making it easier and faster to file claims electronically.

Dental practices that utilize electronic claims processing find many advantages in this type of paperless claims submission:

- The predetermination cycle is often eliminated, saving valuable treatment time and paperwork
- Preoperative x-rays and photos are also sent electronically
- Electronic filing saves on filing space, postage, and paper processing costs
- Quicker filing time
- Faster payment
- Security of direct deposit into the dentist-designated bank account instead of processing and mailing paper checks
- Fewer clerical errors
- HIPAA compliance.

Claims Tracking and Rejection

Occasionally, the claim may be lost, misplaced, or never received by the insurer. Whether using a manual or electronic method of claims processing, the office manager should keep a record of claims submitted by date, patient/responsible parties' name, group number, insurer, and amount. If the payment is not received within the customary timeframe anticipated, the office manager should contact the third party to track the status of the claim.

The claim may also be rejected by the insurance carrier, most often because a vital piece of information has been omitted from the claim. This often is the responsible party's identification number or group number. Missing codes or completed treatment records may also cause a claim to be rejected. Sometimes a claim may be rejected because the insurance company does not cover the particular procedure. In such cases, predetermination and preauthorization would probably have caught this rejection. It is the office manager's responsibility to make financial arrangements with the patient before treatment commences based on the most accurate information available. The office manager then closely monitors the activity of all third-party claims. This is most efficiently conducted by printing out computer reports that supply a breakdown of payment on outstanding third-party payments to obtain the following information:

- All claims that have been submitted for predetermination
- All outstanding claims submitted for payment

- Charges for claims generated but not yet submitted
- Claims that have been returned or rejected that have not been resubmitted.

Many states have mandated timelines during which an insurance company must respond to a claim that has been submitted. Response does not automatically mean payment; it can be a response requesting additional information.

The One-Write System

Although the majority of dental offices use computers for accounts receivable, some practices still use the **one-write or pegboard** manual system (Figure 13-2). The components of the system include a plastic or metal writing surface onto which pre-punched preprinted forms fit using a system of raised pegs on the left side. Forms are designed to fit over each, using a carbonless transfer system. This eliminates the need to make duplicate bookkeeping entries, thus saving time and reducing mathematical errors.

The Daily Journal sheet or day sheet provides a listing of activities for each patient seen during the business day. It also serves as a method of recording payments received on accounts during the day.

The office manager manually enters the dates, the patient's account number, the patient's name, and the service code. The office manager also enters in the necessary information under the columns designated for the fee charged, the payment received, the balance, and the previous balance.

The pegboard or one-write system also provides receipts, fees slips, and ledger cards, onto which the information is automatically transferred using carbonless forms. The one-write ledger is stored in a ledger file tray and provides the office manager with an instant billing system. A photocopy of the ledger becomes the patient's statement.

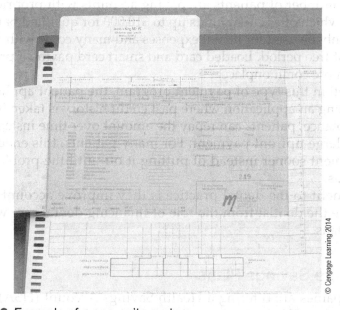

FIGURE 13-2 Example of a one-write system.

Methods of Payment

In addition to third-party payments, received either as paper checks or transferred electronically into the doctor's bank account, other methods of accepting payment for dental services are also utilized in the dental office. Although monthly statements are the most commonly used method of requesting payment of an account, the following are ways the dental office may receive that payment.

Cash

Cash is one method of payment though becoming less and less common; many practices offer a discount to patients using cash for payment of services in full. Discounts for payment in full at the time of treatment are offered because paid-in-full patients do not require statements saving the practice time, billing costs, and improving cash flow in the practice. The office manager must issue a receipt to the patient or responsible party for all cash sums paid. Discounts for accounts paid in full are tracked separately as part of the accounts receivable system; they are not just subtracted from the treatment fee.

Personal Check

Many patients prefer to pay their balance due by personal check. Paying by check has many advantages, including proof of payment through the canceled check; also, writing a check is safer than carrying large sums of cash. Most offices will offer a discount for payment of services in full to patients paying by check. Tracking this discount would be the same as with a cash payment. Payment in full by cash or check discounts are popular with patients who do not have dental insurance.

Dental Care Cards

A growing number of patients are paying accounts with proprietary dental care cards, which offer credit limits up to $10,000 for qualified patients. These cards can only be used for dental expenses and many come with an introductory interest-free period. Loaded card and smart card payment processing are becoming more commonplace.

To enroll in this type of payment program, the patient applies for credit by completing an application where past credit history is taken into account. After acceptance, patients can repay the amount over time instead of having to make a large upfront payment. For many patients, this enables them to have treatment sooner instead of putting it off until the problem becomes more serious.

The benefit to the dental practice is they improve accounts receivable and remove the dentist from the role of financing dental care with lengthy payment plans.

Health Care Savings Plans

More companies are offering a Health Savings Account (HSA) or Flexible Savings Account (FSA) to their employees and are doing so with a smart card. These cards look and work like debit cards against the amount the employee has designated to be withdrawn from their paycheck. This enables the employee to use pretax dollars to pay for health care, including dentistry.

The benefit to the dental practice to participate in payment by these cards is that the payment is guaranteed and paperwork and processing times are reduced.

Credit Cards and Debit Cards

Acceptance of any type of credit card costs the practice a fee, usually a percentage of the payment. Terms regarding the installation of a card reader and the fees associated with using it can vary among companies. Fees may be different if the office swipes a card or manually enters the numbers. The advantage of accepting major credit cards for payment is that payment is virtually guaranteed, and paperwork, billing, and collection times are reduced. If the credit card fees to the practice are 2 to 6 percent of the purchase, this amount is more than offset by the fact that no further collection or billing charges need to be incurred and the patient can schedule treatment right away. Any finance charges are assumed by the patient.

If the practice accepts credit cards, the office manager can display signage of the credit associations such as Visa, MasterCard, American Express, and/or Discover card. This payment option should also appear on all statements sent out by the practice. For patients who want the option of credit card financing this can attract them to the practice and encourage them to pursue treatment.

In some cases, patients do not have available limits on their personal credit cards or want to pay for treatment over several months rather than in a lump sum. In these cases the patients may agree to preauthorize the office manager to initiate a monthly charge to their credit cards of a predetermined amount over several months to make treatment affordable. Credit card payments over the period of treatment are very popular with orthodontic offices where treatment extends a year or more.

Modern "point-of-sale" technology validates credit availability electronically, eliminating the risk of accepting an over the limit or expired credit card as payment; this method of processing is not free. Electronic credit account processors are being compensated for this type of data access at a percentage of the fee. The cost is only a few cents on the dollar; however, processing fees should be considered before making the decision to install the reader.

Direct Reimbursement

Direct reimbursement is a popular method of payment with dentists. The reason is that the patient may choose whomever he or she wishes as a provider of dental care. The patient pays the dentist at the time of service and submits a copy of the paid receipt to his or her employer's benefit administrator. The administrator then generates a reimbursement check to the employee/patient, usually within 30 days.

Direct reimbursement plans usually have a ceiling amount of reimbursement for an employee or their family members per year or they reimburse a percentage of the total fee. For example, the employer may cover 80 percent of all routine preventive treatments, 50 percent of all restorative treatment, and a flat, one-time benefit of $2,500 for orthodontic treatment.

In cases where the patient requires extensive dental treatment, the appointments may be planned in sequential phases through several benefit periods until the treatment is completed. This maximizes the patient's return on direct reimbursement.

Series of Payments

Many patients prefer to take advantage of in-office financing, if it is available, making a series of payments to the dental practice during the time treatment is being rendered. A series of payments is made per a written financial agreement between the practice and patient. Some offices add a small finance charge for offering this option to patients, especially if the payments extend beyond the treatment.

Once the dentist has completed a diagnosis and the treatment plan and the charges are explained to the patient with a written copy of the treatment plan provided to the patient or responsible party, it is the office manager's responsibility to make financial arrangements.

An example of an agreement for a series of treatments is as follows. The total treatment fee for Mr. Green's treatment is estimated at $1,800 and the treatment will take from three to six months to complete. Mr. Green states he would like to begin treatment and make monthly payments of $100 each for 18 months with no interest charges. The office manager explains that the doctor would like to be able to offer these terms to him; however, it is the doctor's policy that at least half of the treatment is paid for when treatment is initiated and payment in full by the final appointment.

The office manager then suggests to Mr. Green that he make a down payment of $1,000 at the initial appointment, with the additional sum of $200 due the 15th of each month for the next four months, at which time the treatment will be completed. With Mr. Green's acceptance, the office manager completes a financial agreement statement, which is dated, signed by both parties, and so noted on Mr. Green's financial record either manually or in the computer. One copy of the completed financial record goes into Mr. Green's file and the other is given to Mr. Green. The office manager then sets up the necessary appointments for Mr. Green, being sure to allow sufficient time for lab work to be returned between appointments. It should be noted that if more time is required by Mr. Green to make payments or if finance charges are to be added, this information must be included in the financial agreement. Terms should also address the consequences should the patient not complete all planned treatment, fail or "no-show" for scheduled appointments, or fail to meet the terms of the agreement. Obviously practices want to use good judgment when extending credit as repossessing treatment is not possible. In-office financing is an unsecured loan.

Performing a Credit Check
Some offices use credit checking services prior to beginning extensive cases. A credit check is legal, provided the patient is aware of the credit check and gives consent.

Credit checks may be performed using local credit agencies, either via telephone or electronically. The office is charged a fee for this service and the patient must be informed and consent to having it done.

Finance Plans

Some practices prefer not to carry patients for any type of financing program and instead refer them to financing institutions such as local banks or programs sponsored in cooperation with the local dental association.

> **Note:** Making sure the financial responsibility form is completed for all patients is the office manager's responsibility.

Under a financing program, the office manager may assist the patient or responsible party in completing a standard finance application and then fax or phone the information to the participating bank, credit union, or lending institution. Approval or denial is usually confirmed within 30 minutes.

If approved, the bank or lending institution provides payment in advance to the patient, made out in the dentist's name. The patient makes a monthly payment to the bank similar to a mortgage or auto loan payment. Fulfillment of the loan, including interest charges, is the responsibility of the patient or responsible party.

Cycle Billing

Cycle billing means statements are sent out on a regular, 30-day cycle. Some practices send out all statements on the same day of the month, and many indicate a due date to encourage patients to pay promptly. Payments can be made in any of the previously discussed methods of payment.

Other practices stagger the 30-day cycle billing, usually by dividing patients alphabetically by last names and billing a segment of the alphabet (A–D, E–K, L–P, and Q–Z) each week. Staggering of statements makes processing easier in practices that send a large amount of statements to private pay patients. This also evens out the cash flow throughout the month. Although all practices vary somewhat in their receivables management, the following is an example of a typical lifecycle of an account.

The Typical Billing/Collection Cycle

- Cycle 1–30 days: The statement is mailed, usually at the end of the month, within 30 days or at completion of treatment.
- Cycle 2–60 days: A second statement follows, usually with a sticker or other notation or a personally handwritten reminder from the office manager that payment is due.
- Cycle 3–75 days: At this time, the office manager should make the first formal telephone collection contact.
- Cycle 4–90 days: If payment still has not been received, the office manager usually sends an ultimatum letter stating something to the effect of, "If payment is not received within 10 days, or if we have not heard from the financially responsible party in 10 days, this account will be turned over to a collection agency."

Many offices collect the patients' estimated portion of the treatment fee at the appointment, minimizing the need for statements and collections strategies. The cycle billing shown is just one example and some practices may choose to call patients who have not made a payment more quickly.

Walk-Out Statement

At the conclusion of each treatment visit, many offices issue a walk-out statement to the patient or responsible party. The walk-out statement provides documentation regarding the appointment, the fee for the service provided, the amount paid and the balance on the account. The walk-out statement may be used by the responsible party to pay the statement personally, submitting the information to the employer's benefit administrator to receive direct reimbursement, or to retain as a personal financial record.

Procedure for Entering a Payment

Regardless of whether payment is made on a patient's account from a third party, from the patient, or another financially responsible party, and whether using a manual, pegboard, or computerized accounts receivable system, the procedure for entering a payment is the same.

If payment is made by check, the office manager endorses the check with the doctor's bank stamp. If payment is made in person by cash, the office manager provides the patient with an official receipt.

The office manager enters the amount of the payment on the patient's financial record and then the remaining amount due, if any. The payment is recorded on the bank deposit slip, which is totaled at the end of the day and deposited. Note that some dentists like to review the total payments received for the day prior to making the bank deposit.

Collection of Past-Due Accounts

It is most often the office manager's responsibility to collect overdue or delinquent accounts. The following general rules should be followed when collecting overdue balances.

Collection Telephone Calls

The office manager must follow certain rules or guidelines when making telephone collection calls. He or she must make every effort to communicate in a firm, businesslike manner in a way that conveys, "Let's work together to resolve this issue." The office manager should never make threats, which only intimidate or alienate patients. Following are general guidelines from the Fair Debt and Collection Act, *the* practice may also be governed by laws that vary from state to state.

In general, the office manager should do the following:

1. Make collection calls at a reasonable time; not before 8 A.M. or after 9 P.M.
2. Identify himself/herself as collecting a debt only to the financially responsible party. No message regarding the debt should be left at the person's home or place of business. It is permissible to leave a message requesting the person return the call.
3. When the responsible party is reached, the office manager should identify himself or herself and the employer, as well as the nature of the call.
4. During the week, the office manager may make only a maximum of two calls to the delinquent party at his or her home; or a maximum of two calls

to his or her place of employment during one month; a total of 10 calls is the maximum allowed.

> **Note:** Calls to the responsible party's workplace are not allowed if forbidden by the employer.

5. In placing collection calls, the office manager must keep in mind that she or he is a trained professional, and as such, may not harass, oppress, or abuse the financially responsible party. This behavior is not only unethical, but illegal, as well; it could possibly damage the professional reputation of the practice.

6. The office manager must not threaten further action if there is no intent of following through. Nor may she or he state that the patient's debt will influence his or her credit rating.

7. The office manager should thoroughly review the responsible parties' account ledger or computer screen data and have specific amounts and dates readily available. If the responsible party makes specific statements about when he or she will pay any amount, the office manager records this information. The office manager then summarizes what the responsible party agreed to do.

8. Sometimes the amount of the balance or overdue debt is disputed by the patient. In this case, the office manager is prohibited from taking further action or contacting the debtor until sufficient verification can be provided. In this instance the office manager must send the responsible party written notice of his or her right to dispute the debt within five days of the initial communication. The responsible party then has 30 days from the receipt of notification to take action.

> **Note:** Verification may be a copy of the statement of the overdue account or a copy of the agreement creating the debt.

9. If the responsible party sends the office a letter requesting that he or she may not be contacted, the office must cease communication, except to notify the person of pending legal action.

> **Note:** The office is entitled to add interest and other charges to past-due accounts only if the agreement stating that the debt allows it or if it is permitted by individual state law.

Small Claims Court and Collection Agencies

If after all traditional collection attempts are made and payment is not received, the office has a final option of small claims court or turning the account over to a collection agency, which usually claims at least one-third of the monies retrieved. Small claims court usually handles sums not in excess of $1,500. Before making such a drastic decision, always consult with the doctor as the final decision rests with him or her.

Skill Building

These optional activities and exercises are designed to help the student put into practice information learned in the chapter.

1. Obtain a blank insurance form to complete. Review the information required for completing an insurance form provided in the chapter. Using information provided by your instructor, complete the insurance form.

2. Mr. Alexander's account of $460 is 60 days past due and no payment has been received, despite two statements being sent to his home. You bring this to the attention of the dentist, who instructs you to place a collection call to Mr. Alexander. Divide into pairs and take turns role-playing the office manager and Mr. Alexander. Be persistent. Do not back down. Ask probing questions of Mr. Alexander. Invite feedback and coaching strategies from your classmates. Have you stayed within the collection guidelines provided?

3. Mrs. Garcia calls the office and is very angry. She tells you she has paid her account in full but just received a bill, which does not reflect her final payment. Divide into pairs and role-play the scenario. Ask your classmates for feedback. Could this scenario have been prevented? What steps could have been taken?

Challenge Your Understanding

Select the response that best answers the following questions. Only one response is correct.

1. Advantages to the dentist of signing onto a managed care program include:
   a. A guaranteed flow of new patients
   b. Minimal administration cost
   c. A guarantee cash flow and patient base
   d. All of the above

2. In a group model HMO, the HMO contracts with the individual provider group to care for its patients. The provider group is managed independently and reimbursed on a capitation basis.
   a. True
   b. False

3. In an EPO plan, all dental services provided by unaffiliated providers are automatically reimbursed.
   a. True
   b. False

4. Having a claim rejected by the insurance carrier might be eliminated by which of the following:
   a. Having a treatment plan
   b. Filing a preauthorization
   c. Signing assignment of benefits
   d. Making sure a release is on file

5. All of the following are true of PPO providers *except*:
   a. They are selected based on their professional qualifications and performance
   b. They benefit through decreased patient volume
   c. They must agree to a fee schedule and review of their performance
   d. They receive prompt payment for services rendered to patients enrolled in the plan

6. The term *third party* means someone other than the dentist or the patient is involved in financial responsibility for treatment.
   a. True
   b. False

7. Information required on claims submissions for payment includes:
   a. The name of the insured party, the responsible party, the spouse, or parent or guardian of the insured party
   b. The name of the employer, employer code, or group number
   c. The address and telephone number for submitting claims and the acceptable method(s) for claims submission(s)
   d. All the above may be required

8. The term *deductible* refers to:
   a. The amount the insurance company pays toward services covered under the contractual plan
   b. The company that sells or carries the insurance
   c. The amount the patient or responsible party must pay toward services before the carrier will begin paying on insurance claims
   d. The extent of the benefits provided by the insurance policy

9. Treatment codes are necessary when filing for third-party reimbursement to:
   a. Ensure that each procedure is properly billed
   b. Ensure that the correct amount is paid to the provider
   c. Ensure dual coverage benefits
   d. a and b only

10. Predetermination indicates whether the insurance will or will not cover specific procedures diagnosed by the dentist as necessary.
    a. True
    b. False

11. Procedures for which no code is provided are generally reimbursed when the patient has proof of insurance coverage.
    a. True
    b. False

12. The term *release* applies to dental records and authorizes the insurance claims examiners to review the diagnosis and treatment. Many procedures require dental radiographs to verify the need for treatment and subsequent claim for payment.
    a. True
    b. False

13. The term *assignment* refers to the benefit paid by the insurance company and authorizes the company to send payment directly to the patient, rather than the provider.
    a. True
    b. False

14. The walk-out statement provides handwritten or computer-generated information including all of the following *except*:
    a. The patient's name and date
    b. The patient's social security number
    c. The type of service provided
    d. The insurance code, the fee, the amount paid, and the balance, if any

15. The walk-out statement may be used by the financially responsible party to:
    a. Pay the statement personally
    b. Submit the information to his or her employer's benefits administrator to receive direct reimbursement
    c. Personally submit to a third-party payer
    d. All of the above

16. Electronic claims processing uses the practice's computer to store, generate, and submit third-party claims to respective insurance companies' computers via a clearinghouse.
    a. True
    b. False

17. Advantages of electronic claim processing may include:
    a. Compliance with HIPAA
    b. Saving on file space, postage, and paper processing costs
    c. The security of direct deposit into the dentist's designated bank account
    d. All of the above

18. Each insurance company has its own set of codes to identify treatment procedures.
    a. True
    b. False

19. The office manager should issue a receipt to the patient or responsible party for all cash sums paid.
    a. True
    b. False

20. According to the guidelines set forth by the *Fair Debt Collection Act*, the office manager should:
    a. Identify herself or himself as collecting a debt only to the financially responsible party
    b. Not leave a message at the person's home or place of employment that contains personal information
    c. Not make calls to the responsible party's workplace if not allowed or forbidden by the employer
    d. All of the above

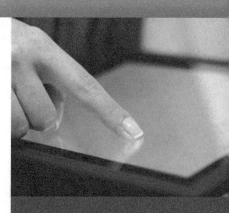

CHAPTER 14

Managing Accounts Payable

CHAPTER OUTLINES

- **Understanding Accounts Payable**
- **When an Invoice Arrives**
- **Embezzlement**
- **Understanding Overhead**
  Fixed Expenses
  Variable Expenses
  Controlling Practice Overhead through Budget Goals
  Categories of Practice Expenses
- **The Office Checking Account**
  Components of a Check
  Bank Deposits
  Understanding the Bank Statement
  Reconciling the Bank Statement
  Electronic Funds Transfer and Automatic Payment Systems
  Other Forms of Payment
- **Payroll Records and Reporting Procedures**
  Employer Identification Number
  Employee's Withholding Allowance Certificate
  Employee Earnings Record
  Payroll Deductions
  Federal Insurance Contributions Act (Social Security and Medicare Taxes)
  Income Tax Withholding: Federal and State
  Depositing Withheld Income Tax and Social Security (FICA) Taxes
  Federal Unemployment Tax
  Wage and Tax Statement
  Report of Withheld Income Tax
  Retaining Payroll and Tax Records

KEY TERMS

accounts payable
audit
automatic payment systems
cash on delivery (COD)
electronic funds transfer
embezzlement
fixed expenses
overhead
petty cash voucher
restrictive endorsement
variable expenses

Upon completion of this chapter, the reader should be able to:

1. Define the term overhead as it pertains to the dental practice.
2. Define and differentiate between fixed and variable overhead expenses associated with the dental practice.
3. Be familiar with the most commonly used forms of accounts payable, including check writing systems used by the office manager; also the seriousness and consequences of embezzlement.
4. Be familiar with common categories of overhead and types of expenditures associated with dental practice including handling COD payments, automatic deposits, and monthly expenditures.
5. Describe standard taxes withheld from employee paychecks and the importance of sound record keeping for all payroll procedures.
6. Describe and list the purposes of common tax forms and required payments, including quarterly filing and annual employee withholding statements.

Understanding Accounts Payable

Chapter 13 (Managing Accounts Receivable) addressed payments owed to the office. This chapter addresses accounts payable, the system of distributing money owed by the practice. It is the office manager's job to ensure that the accounts payable duties are conducted efficiently, accurately, honestly, ethically, and in a timely manner.

Often, the office manager is responsible for the distribution of large sums of money owed by the practice to a variety of suppliers, government tax agencies, and other vendors. Accurate accounting methods are essential to maintain an efficient system of bookkeeping, including accounts payable.

The office manager may be expected to perform the following tasks associated with maintaining accounts: writing checks, endorsing checks and making bank (or electronic) deposits, keeping accurate account balances, and reconciling bank statements.

When an Invoice Arrives

When an invoice, either a bill or statement, arrives, the office manager should check the vendor's invoice number against the original packing slip or invoice enclosed to ensure they are for the same amount and that all goods or services ordered were indeed delivered. Invoices should be filed alphabetically by vendor, paid monthly, and retained for a minimum for three years.

Embezzlement

The office manager should understand the responsibility for ensuring that all bookkeeping functions of the practice are accurate and balanced. Any discrepancies are the responsibility of the office manager. Further, the claim of embezzlement, the fraudulent appropriation of money entrusted into one's care, is a serious allegation that if proven, may result in immediate termination, denial of unemployment benefits, failure to find future employment, and possible indictment, imprisonment, and/or fines.

Understanding Overhead

The term overhead means the operating expenses associated with running the dental practice. Expenses included in overhead include such items as the rent or mortgage payment; property taxes (if applicable); payroll and independent contractor expenses; outside consultants, including legal and accounting services; supplies, dental laboratory bills, utility bills, marketing costs, insurance premiums; other services not included with payroll such as cleaning and housekeeping, laundry and dry cleaning; outdoor maintenance such as landscaping; equipment warranty/service contracts; front office and stationery supplies; professional and reception area publications; entertainment; professional licensing, incorporation fees; and more.

When faced with such an enormous list of overhead expenses, the office manager may feel overwhelmed at keeping them organized, let alone paid in a timely manner. In many dental practices today, overhead runs 70 percent or higher.

Fixed Expenses

The term fixed expenses include those office expenses that remain fairly constant from month to month. These are generally the larger bills, such as rent or mortgage, payroll, utilities, and lease payments on equipment.

Variable Expenses

The term variable expenses include the office expenses that vary from month to month, or are received only on occasion. These may include dental supplies and lab fees, new equipment purchases, and new services.

Controlling Practice Overhead through Budget Goals

Many dental practices set annual budgeting goals as a cost-containment strategy. Just as they establish production goals to achieve maximum practice revenues, budget goals help contain costs incurred by the practice. Some practices reward the office manager for keeping practice overhead revenues within an established percentage of production.

Categories of Practice Expenses

The following categories and percentages of practice overhead may be used as a guide in determining anticipated office expenses at annual budget review time. They are based upon gross collections of a solo practitioner office.

Personnel Expenses

The highest category in overhead is associated with payroll, including salaries and taxes, which average between 18 and 25 percent. Another 2 to 4 percent of personnel expenses go toward employee benefits.

Occupancy Expenses

The cost of physical occupancy of the practice may run from 5 to 9 percent. This includes the lease or mortgage payment plus interest, depreciation, insurance on the building and contents, cleaning and maintenance services, and utilities.

Administrative Expenses

The cost of administering the practice may run from 6 to 9 percent and includes accounting and legal services, collection costs and bank charges, related computer expenses, continuing education, dues and subscriptions, insurance (including disability, malpractice, and business overhead), laundry and dry cleaning, licenses and permits, front office and printing supplies, postage, repairs and maintenance to equipment, taxes, telephone, and other miscellaneous administrative expenses.

Equipment and Furnishings

The cost of equipment and furnishings may run from 4 to 6 percent and includes lease payments and interest on equipment and/or cash purchases of equipment. The cost may be as high as 25 percent in new practices.

Clinical/Dental Supplies

The cost of dental supplies associated with patient care may run from 4 to 7 percent. However, the inclusion of additional infection control and barrier protection costs associated with compliance with government regulations may raise this cost as high as 10 to 12 percent.

Lab Fees

The cost of dental lab fees varies greatly, depending upon the type of practice and its volume of prosthetic or orthodontic cases. Generally, lab fees range from 2 to 4 percent.

Marketing Costs

The cost for marketing expenses also varies from practice to practice. Marketing costs may include giveaways, gifts and donations, telephone directory space advertisements, practice newsletters, holiday cards, mailings, and media costs. Experts currently establish marketing costs at about 5 percent of the practice's overhead.

The Office Checking Account

The office checking account is the primary means by which bills (accounts payable) are paid. Most bills are paid on a monthly basis. Payroll is paid weekly, biweekly, or monthly. In most practices, only the dentist/owner of the practice has the authority to sign checks. In some offices two signatures are required as a system of checks and balances for checks to be payable. These signatures may be of the dentist/owner and the office manager. A few practices authorize the office manager to sign checks. The signature of the person authorized to sign checks must be on file with the bank where the account is held.

It is the office manager's duty to ensure that all bills and payroll are paid promptly and correctly. Ensuring that bills are paid on time establishes a good credit rating for the practice and eliminates additional interest or other finance charges assessed for a late payment. This saves the practice money in the long run.

Regardless of whether the office uses a manual check writing system, a One-Write check writing system, computerized software check writing system, or electronic bill pay, the following components of check writing apply.

Components of a Check

A check is a written order to the dentist's bank to pay a specified amount of money to a designated person. Writing a check requires entering or displaying the following minimal information.

The Magnetic Ink Character Recognition (MICR) numbers are included along the bottom of the check to facilitate high-speed machine processing. The first part of this number is the bank's ABA (American Bankers Association) identification number; the second part is the dentist's checking account number. The name of the bank also appears on the check. Each check is sequentially numbered at the top of the check for easy tracking.

The name and related information about the practice is printed at the top of the check, usually at the left side, including the practice's address. The date the check is written must be filled in, as well as the name of the person to whom the funds are being paid, for example: ABC Dental Supply, Inc.

The amount of the check must be entered in two different ways. This is required to reduce the incidence of error and for clarification by the bank, should a question arise about the exact amount. The numerical amount of the check is entered first, such as $233.86. It is then entered in longhand or typed into the computer as two hundred thirty-three and 86/100 _____ dollars on the next line.

Note the long dash or wavy line following the amount; this is used to prevent the alteration of the original amount for which the check was written.

Many checks also feature a memo line to make note of the reason or purpose for writing the check, for example, dental supplies. Finally, there is the signature line where the authorized person signs. Figure 14-1 provides an example of a sample check.

Note that it is imperative that this identical information be recorded in the checkbook stub area, which corresponds to the number of the check written. The office should complete the stub portion first, to avoid confusion as to the amount of the check, the date written, or the name of the party to whom the check was written. This saves embarrassment, confusion, and valuable time later.

Bank Deposits

Another important role in maintaining the practices checking account is preparing the nightly deposit for the bank. Most often it is the responsibility of the office manager to prepare the daily bank deposit slip in preparation for the deposit. In some practices, the office manager is also personally

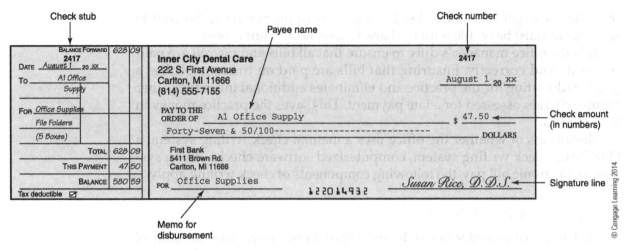

FIGURE 14-1   Sample of a properly written check.

responsible for making the deposit. In other practices, the dentist completes this task. Note that deposits may be made in person at the bank, by mail, by night deposit, or by automatic teller machine (ATM).

When the dentist opens a checking account, deposit slips are printed with the dentist's or practice's name and account number. Spaces are provided to enter the date and the total amount of checks and cash to be deposited. Whether using the manual check deposit system, a One-Write system, or a computer software banking program, the process for making bank deposits is the same.

Prior to depositing checks into the account, each check must be endorsed by the dentist/practice to which the check is written. Endorsement may be made by signing the back of the check or using an ink stamp **restrictive endorsement**. Note that if the check is signed, for example, "Dr. Ralph Jones," anyone finding that check may attempt to redeem it for cash at a bank. This is called blank or open endorsement and is not recommended for security purposes.

The restrictive endorsement contains special conditions or restrictions limiting the receiver of the check concerning use that may be made of the check. Most often ink stamp endorsement reads for deposit only on the first line and features the doctor's name or the name of the practice on the second line. This significantly reduces the potential for bank fraud.

When making a manual deposit, the office manager lists the name of each patient next to the amount of the check. When making cash deposits, the office manager makes a list of patients and the corresponding amount paid and clips it to the duplicate deposit slip.

The deposit slip is made out manually or computer generated from the day sheet. Note that creating a computer-generated deposit slip from the day sheet significantly reduces the likelihood of an error, omission, or embezzlement, as it provides a detailed accounting of all patients scheduled for the day including those for whom no charge or payment was received or entered.

Many offices make a photocopy of each production day's deposit slip as a method of tracking daily deposit amounts.

Understanding the Bank Statement

The bank provides a monthly bank statement containing all checks by chronological order cleared and all deposits made by amount and date the transaction occurred. Other items that appear on a monthly bank statement may include overdrafts, interest accrued, bank service and ATM charges, printed check charges, and electronic payments such as federal withholding tax, as well as, starting and ending balances.

The office manager should review the bank statement upon receipt carefully, to ensure that no errors have occurred and that all deposits were duly noted. Banks do make mistakes. The office manager should then reconcile the bank statement. Some banks return the physical checks, whereas others retain them and send only the bank statement and other banks include a photocopy record of the checks. Because not all checks written on the office account clear immediately, it is necessary to reconcile the statement to determine the exact amount in the account. Many banks are providing statements online eliminating the paper and mailing costs.

Reconciling the Bank Statement

To maintain an accurate checking account record and statement balance, the office manager is responsible for reconciling the bank statement. The following steps are necessary:

1. Compare and verify the amount of the canceled checks with the amounts indicated on the bank statement. The office manager will note that the canceled checks, or the check numbers printed on the statement, will be arranged or reported sequentially.

2. Arrange the canceled checks in chronological order if they are enclosed in the statement.

3. Compare the amounts reported on the canceled checks and the deposits to the amounts entered into the checkbook register at the time the check and deposits were made. Indicate with a check mark or other visual symbol checks and deposits in your checkbook register to determine which items do not correspond.

4. List any outstanding checks with the corresponding check number and the amount of each. An outstanding check is one that has not yet been returned to the bank for payment. Total the amounts of the outstanding checks.

5. If a deposit was made but does not appear anywhere on the bank statement, add the amount to the bank statement balance. Likewise, if the bank account earns interest add that amount. Subtract and total the amount of the outstanding checks.

6. Review other charges listed on the bank statement such as service charges, debit memos, ATM privilege charges, automatic withdrawals, or overdraft fees; subtract them from the checkbook register.

Bank statements and canceled checks (if returned from the bank) should be retained for 7 years, in case they are required for an **audit**. During an audit the accuracy of dental accounts including income and expenses are checked by a third party.

Electronic Funds Transfer and Automatic Payment Systems

Some practices prefer to save time by using **electronic funds transfer** and/or **automatic payment systems** to pay routine bills.

THINK Green

Using paperless banking systems is one more step toward a greener practice.

Electronic transfer of funds may be conducted easily through the computer. Automatic payment systems deduct the amount of a specific payment, for example a utility payment and transfer that amount directly into the account of the party the practice owes money. This saves time, paper, and postage costs of writing and mailing a check. It is important to note when automatic payments are withdrawn you should debit them from your bank account so you don't find yourself overdrawn.

Other Forms of Payment

Although check writing is the most common type of payment system used by dental practices in accounts payable management, other forms of payment are also used, including petty cash, cash on delivery (COD), and charge cards.

Petty Cash

While the office manager is strongly advised against storing large sums of money in the office, out-of-pocket expenses sometimes arise. Occasionally, a small amount of cash is needed to make some change for cash paying patients or for lunches, tips for delivery personnel, and so on. Petty cash in an office rarely exceeds $50.

When such expenditures are required, often on short notice, the office manager is responsible for completing a **petty cash voucher** as a receipt of proof of outlay of cash. Preprinted petty cash vouchers or forms may be purchased from a stationary supply company, or the office may elect to create a handwritten petty cash voucher for minimal expense.

Information contained on the petty cash voucher should include the date, the person or party to whom the cash was paid, the reason for the payment, and the name or initials of the person who distributed the money.

Cash on Delivery

Occasionally, suppliers or vendors require payment at the time of delivery (**cash on delivery [COD]**), rather than through a monthly billing procedure. This is called cash on delivery, abbreviated COD. Such a delivery may be paid from the petty cash fund.

Some COD orders exceed $50 and vendors will accept a check upon delivery. In this instance the office manager may draft a check for the total and obtain the doctor's signature at the time of delivery. Before doing so, however, contents of the package should be checked to ensure the goods are intact and are what was ordered.

Charge Cards

It has become increasingly popular for practices to make purchases using charge cards, especially when the dentist is away from the practice attending continuing education seminars, for airfare, hotel accommodations, and meals. When a charge card is used for payment, the office manager must keep a file of charge card receipts, the reason for the expenditure, and the amount due. These receipts are compared with a monthly charge card statement for accuracy.

At the direction of the dentist, the office manager writes a check for the entire amount due, a portion of the amount due, or the minimum amount due. Note that late payment or partial payment on a charge account accrues interest charges.

Payroll Records and Reporting Procedures

Depending upon the size of the staff and amount of the payroll, some practices prefer to handle payroll in-house, either manually or electronically on a computer software system; others prefer to have an outside payroll administration company administer payroll.

Whether preparing the payroll information for in-house administration or for an outside agency, it is most often the office manager's responsibility to maintain accurate payroll records and other accounting procedures.

Federal and state laws require records to be kept on information regarding wages paid and for the preparation of required tax reports. The dentist/employer must obtain a copy of the Internal Revenue Service's (IRS's) *Employer's Tax Guide*, which summarizes the employer's responsibility for computing, depositing, paying, and reporting all taxes. The office manager should be aware that laws change frequently and that a current copy of this table should be kept on file for the latest withholding and reporting information.

Employer Identification Number

As an employer, the dentist must have an employer identification number. This nine-digit number assigned to either sole proprietors or corporations for the purpose of filing and reporting payroll information is required by the federal government. This may be applied for through the IRS.

Employee's Withholding Allowance Certificate

Each employee of the practice must complete an *Employee's Withholding Allowance Certificate, Form W-4*. The withholding certificate determines the status of each member for income tax deductions from earned wages. The following information is required on this form: the employee's full name, Social Security Number, home address, marital status, total number of allowances/exemptions claimed, and any additional amount desired to be withheld. The employee must sign and date the form. If the employee changes the number of exemptions claimed, a new *Form W-4* must be completed.

Employee Earnings Record

By law, the dentist as employer must maintain all employees' earnings records, including a summary of individual staff members' earnings. This information is important because it provides the employer with information required for quarterly and annual tax reporting. The employee's earnings record should provide the following general information:

1. The employee's name, address, Social Security Number (SSN), rate of pay (hourly or salary), the number of withholding exemptions claimed, marital status, and any other special deductions, including garnishments for child support, automatic savings programs, or health insurance or retirement plan contributions.

2. The number of pay periods in the reporting quarter and the date when each pay period ends.

3. Regular earnings, overtime earnings, and total earnings.

4. A column for each type of deduction and total deductions.

5. The net amount paid to the employee or net pay. Net refers to the amount paid after deductions are taken from the gross pay.

6. Accumulative taxable earnings, which gives the employer information for taxable earnings, FICA, and taxable wages for contributions to unemployment taxes.

7. Amounts for quarterly and annual totals. This information is used when the employer submits quarterly and annual tax payments and reports.

Payroll Deductions

At the time of employment, a specific wage is agreed upon by the employer and employee. This may be paid as an hourly or salaried amount and paid weekly, biweekly or bimonthly, or monthly depending on the terms of their agreement. Often, the office manager is responsible for calculating deductions and determining net wages reflected in the paychecks.

> **Note:** Confidentiality regarding payroll is a must. The office manager may not discuss payroll with any other staff members as this constitutes a breach of confidentiality and may be grounds for dismissal.

Federal Insurance Contributions Act (Social Security and Medicare Taxes)

These deduction amounts vary from year to year and differ with the amount of income earned. It is the dentist/employer's and office manager's responsibility to seek out the latest information in payroll tax deductions.

The Social Security portion is a flat percentage based on the amount earned. The ceiling on this tax varies. The Medicare tax a flat percentage on all earnings with no ceiling amount.

Tax tables are available free of charge from the IRS. *An Employer's Tax Guide* with a sliding scale can be obtained from the IRS and used for easy reference.

Income Tax Withholding: Federal and State

The amount of withholding tax varies depending upon the number of exemptions the employee claims on *Form W-4, Employee's Federal Withholding Certificate.* The more exemptions claimed the less tax withheld. Thus, two employees earning the same amount may have a differing net or take-home pay, depending upon the number of exemptions claimed and marital status.

State income tax may be deducted by states that have personal income taxes. Other withholding amounts may include automatic savings to a bank or credit union, child support, and others.

After computing the individual employee's net pay, checks are written or the information is sent to a payroll processing company outside the office who will use the information submitted and automatically print out checks or automatically deposit funds into the employee's designated bank account.

The information is then recorded on each staff member's individual earning record. If a One-Write or pegboard accounting system is used, the information on the employee's earnings is recorded directly onto the earnings record, as well as the monthly expense disbursement sheets when the check stubs are recorded. This reduces the amount of time required and also helps eliminate human computing errors.

Depositing Withheld Income Tax and Social Security (FICA) Taxes

The IRS automatically sends the dentist/employer a federal tax deposit coupon book with coupons to deposit all types of taxes. Additional forms may be obtained or ordered using the *reorder form*.

For clarification, the dentist/employer owes taxes when wages are paid, not when the payroll period ends. Instructions provided in completing Form 941 provide further information. Returns and tax payments are due as outlined in Table 14-1.

Note: It is now possible for the IRS to do electronic transfers.

Federal Unemployment Tax

The employee or dentist must also pay federal unemployment tax on each employee at the rate of 6 percent of the first $7,000 in earned income. Note that employees do not contribute to unemployment benefit funds—only employers do.

The dentist must determine federal unemployment taxes quarterly and deposit the amount on or before the last day of the first month after the close of the corresponding quarter, reporting with Form 941.

Wage and Tax Statement

Each year the dentist/employer must supply for each employee a copy of *Form W-2, Wage and Tax Statement*, no later than January 31. This information is crucial because the employee must supply this when filing his or her personal federal and state income tax return. A total of six copies of the *Form W-2* are provided. One copy is for the IRS, one for the state, city, or local tax department, three copies to the employee (one for the federal tax return filing, one for state or local filing, and one for the employee's permanent files); a final copy is retained by the dentist/employer.

TABLE 14.1 Deadline for Tax Returns and Payments

Quarter	Quarter Ends	Date Payment Due
#1: January–March	March 31	April 30
#2: April–June	June 30	July 31
#3: July–September	September 30	October 31
#4: October–December	December 31	January 31

© Cengage Learning 2014

The *Form W-2, Wage and Tax Statement* contains the following important information:

1. The employer's identification number, name, and address
2. The employee's social security number, name, and address
3. The amount of federal income tax withheld
4. The total sum of wages paid the employee
5. The total FICA employee tax withheld
6. The total wages paid subject to FICA
7. All state and local taxes withheld, where applicable

Report of Withheld Income Tax

The dentist/employer must also submit, on or before February 28 of each year, all *W-2* forms issued for the previous year and *Form W-3, Transmittal of Wage and Tax Statement*, to the IRS.

Retaining Payroll and Tax Records

It is the responsibility of the dentist/employer to retain all records regarding employment taxes, for at least four years following the date of taxes they pertain to, should the IRS order an audit. The following information is the minimum that should be retained by the employer regarding employee payroll and tax records:

1. The amounts and dates of all wages paid to employees
2. The names, addresses, occupations, and Social Security number of all employees
3. The dates of all staff members' employment
4. Any periods in which employees were paid when absent because of illness or occupational injury
5. All employees' income tax withholding allowance certificates
6. The employer's identification number
7. Copies of returns filed with dates and amounts of required deposits made

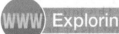 Exploring the Web

Detailed instructions regarding withholding wages and filing taxes
    www.irs.gov/pub/irs-pdf/p15.pdf

A collection of current articles regarding office overhead and management
    www.dentistryiq.com/index/Practice_Management/financial/overhead.html

 Skill Building

These optional activities and exercises are designed to help the student put into practice information learned in this chapter.

1. Using the IRS.gov website obtain a copy of *An Employer's Tax Guide—Circular E*. Using the charts provided by the IRS, determine the net pay for dental assistant earning $600 per week, who is married and claims two exemptions.

2. Invite a payroll administration company representative to visit your class to provide a demonstration of how payroll is administered for a small business, such as a dental office.

3. Bring in a copy of your personal checking account monthly statement. Using the steps provided in the chapter, reconcile your checking account.

4. Using the percentages for specific types of budgeting of office overhead provided in the chapter, set up a hypothetical budget for a practice having a $300,000 production budget.

> **Note:** approximately 30 percent should be applied to the dentist income. Compare your figures to those of your classmates.

 ## Challenge Your Understanding

Select the response that best answers each of the following questions. Only one response is correct.

1. Accounts Payable is a system of/for:
   a. Distributing money owed by the practice
   b. Collecting money owed to the practice
   c. Making collection calls to patients who have overdue bills with the practice
   d. Receiving direct reimbursement from insurance companies

2. Which of the following procedures would the office manager be expected to perform related to managing accounts?
   a. Writing checks
   b. Making bank deposits
   c. Reconciling bank statements
   d. All of the above

3. The term overhead pertains to the operating expenses associated with running the dental practice.
   a. True
   b. False

4. Overhead, which, includes those office expenses that remain fairly constant from month to month is:
   a. Variable
   b. Income
   c. Fixed
   d. Reconciled

5. Embezzlement is a serious charge that may result in
   a. Immediate termination
   b. Denial of unemployment benefits
   c. Possible arrest, imprisonment, and/or fines
   d. Any or all of the above

6. In many dental practices today the average overhead runs at _____ percent or higher.
   a. 50
   b. 60
   c. 70
   d. 90

7. The cost of administering the practice includes all of the following except:
   a. Accounting and legal services
   b. Collection cost and bank charges
   c. Payroll
   d. Continuing education, dues, and subscriptions

8. The signature of the person authorized to sign checks must be on file with the bank where the account is held.
   a. True
   b. False

9. Ensuring that bills are paid on time:
   a. Establishes a good credit rating for the practice
   b. Eliminates additional interest or caring/finance charges assessed for a late payment
   c. Saves the practice money
   d. All of the above

10. The Magnetic Ink Character Recognition (MICR) numbers are encoded along the bottom of the check
    a. Facilitate high-speed machine processing
    b. Include the banks ABA (American Bankers Association) identification number
    c. Include the customer's checking account number
    d. All of the above

11. When writing a check, the office manager should complete the checks tab portion after completely filling out the check.
    a. True
    b. False

12. A/An _____ endorsement contains special conditions or restrictions limiting the recipient of the check concerning how the check can be used.
    a. Blank or open
    b. Closed
    c. Restricted
    d. Implied

13. The monthly bank statement lists:
    a. All deposits made by amount and date the transaction occurred
    b. Overdrafts, interest accrued, and bank service charges
    c. Starting and ending balances
    d. All of the above

14. When reconciling the office checking account the office manager should:
    a. List any outstanding checks with the corresponding check number and the amount of each
    b. Total the amount of the outstanding checks
    c. Indicate with a check mark or other visual symbol all canceled checks and deposits in the check register
    d. All of the above

15. Automatic payment systems automatically deduct the amount of a specific payment from the payers checking account every month by prearrangement and deposit the amount into the account of the party owed.
    a. True
    b. False

16. A petty cash voucher is a receipt of cash withdrawal and documentation.
    a. True
    b. False

17. The employer identification number:
    a. Is a nine-digit number assigned for the purpose of filing and reporting payroll information as required by the federal government
    b. May be applied for through the Internal Revenue Service
    c. Replaces the dentist's Social Security Number
    d. a and b only

18. An employee's withholding allowance certificate, *Form W-4*:
    a. Remains the same throughout the duration of employment
    b. Requires the employee's full name, Social Security number, home address, marital status, total number of allowances/exceptions claimed, and any additional amount desired to be withheld
    c. Determines the status of each staff member for income tax deduction from earned wages
    d. Both b and c

19. The employee's earnings record provides the following information:
    a. The employee's name, address, Social Security number, rate of pay, the number of withholding exemptions claimed, marital status, and other special deductions, including garnishments for child support, automatic savings programs, or health insurance or retirement plan contributions
    b. The number of pay periods in a reporting quarter, the date when each pay period ended, regular earnings, overtime earnings, and total earnings
    c. The total deductions, the net amount paid to the employee, accumulated taxable earnings, amounts for quarterly and annual totals for the employer to use when submitting quarterly, and annual tax payments and reports
    d. All of the above

20. The *W-2 Wage and Tax Statement Form* contains the following except:
    a. The employer's identification number, name, and address
    b. The total sum of wages paid the employee
    c. The employees spouses Social Security number
    d. The total FICA employee tax withheld

CHAPTER 15

Supply Ordering and Inventory

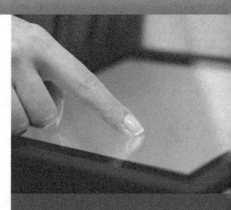

CHAPTER OUTLINES

- **The Importance of Managing Supply Inventory**
- **Types of Supplies**
  Consumable Supplies
  Disposable Supplies
  Expendable Supplies
  Equipment
- **Managing Supply Quantity Needs of the Practice**
  Shelf Life
  Rotating Stock
  Storage Considerations
  Rate of Use, Reorder Point, and Flagging System
  Storage of Controlled Substances
  Computerized Ordering and Inventory Control
  Quantity Discounts
  Buying in Bulk
  Automatic Shipments
  Bids and Contract Buying
  Supply Order Tracking
  Order Form
  Purchase Order
  Packing Slip
  Invoice
  Back Order
  Credit Invoice
  Warranties and Repairs

KEY TERMS

automatic shipments
 back order
consumable supplies
credit invoice
disposable supplies
equipment
expendable supplies
flagging system
inventory
invoice
packing slip
purchase order
purchase order number
quantity discounts
rate of use
reorder point
shelf life
supplier
vendor
warranty

LEARNING OBJECTIVES

Upon completion of this chapter, the reader should be able to:

1. Describe the office manager's role in managing dental office supply inventory.
2. Describe the necessary steps in tracking and managing supply quantity needs of the office.
3. Define supply inventory terms, such as shelf life, rotating stock, and storage considerations.
4. Describe the necessity of security precautions for in office drug inventory and dispensing.
5. List the steps, manual or electronic, in ordering supplies and inventory control.
6. Be familiar with the methods of saving the office money on supplies, including bulk quantity purchases, automatic shipments, and contract purchases.
7. Understand the terms associated with the dental supply ordering and receipt, such as packing slip, back order, and credit invoice.
8. Describe the office manager's role in maintaining equipment warranties and service repairs.

The Importance of Managing Supply Inventory

The inventory in a dental office includes supplies the practice keeps on hand, for example, gloves, patient napkins, prophy paste, and toothbrushes. An important part of the office manager's job is maintaining a sufficient amount of dental supply inventory and purchasing those items at the lowest price. Because most dental practices spend upward of 10 percent of their total overhead on dental supplies, the supply budget represents a significant expenditure by the office and must be managed accordingly.

Types of Supplies

Supplies may be broken down into four categories: consumable, disposable, expendable, and equipment.

Consumable Supplies

Consumable supplies are those that are completely used up or consumed with use. These include pit and fissure sealant material, cements, impression materials, and gypsum products for making dental models.

Disposable Supplies

Disposable supplies are single-use items that are discarded immediately after the procedure for which they are used. These include paper cups, exam gloves, dental dam, cotton rolls, anesthetic needles and carpules.

Expendable Supplies

Expendable supplies are those items that are relatively low in cost and are replaced frequently. This includes burs, matrix bands, plastic impression trays, and small office supplies like paper clips, pens, and rubber bands.

Equipment

Equipment items are those major purchases that are used for five or more years and may be depreciated by the office over a number of years. These include such items as computers, chairs, dental units, sterilizers, lasers, hand pieces, and intraoral cameras.

Managing Supply Quantity Needs of the Practice

In purchasing and recording supplies it is important to note that a sufficient quantity must be ordered so as not to run out of the necessary item, at the same time taking care not to order too many units only to have insufficient storage space or determine that the shelf life may expire before the item can be used.

Shelf Life

The shelf life is the amount of time a product is guaranteed fresh. The product should be used before it reaches the expiration date marked on the label and discarded after the expiration date. Examples of items with a shelf life include medications, cements, impression materials, and dental radiography film. Some suppliers will exchange or discount the next order when supplies expire to encourage the practice to continue using them as a supplier.

Rotating Stock

The office manager must ensure that when new supply items are received in the office the oldest items are used first; new items are placed farthest back in the storage area and brought forward as the older items are removed from the front. This ensures product freshness and also keeps products and supplies from becoming lost in storage.

To ensure an organized supply storage area, the office manager should label shelves, cupboards, and bins appropriately with the product name or type of product for easy retrieval. Examples of labels include "patient napkins," "cements," "HVE tips," "burs," "alginate," "dental dam," and "restorative materials".

The following are some guidelines for storing supplies[1]:

- Store supplies in one central area. Keeping them together helps make maintenance and inventory easy.

- Keep a minimum amount of product on hand. Maintaining too many supplies costs the practice money and many products have a shelf life.

- Be alert to products that are light- or heat-sensitive. Read all bottles and package labels to check for expiration dates and storage instructions. This includes items such as gloves, cements, and anesthetics.

- Use storage bins to organize supplies. Plastic or cardboard bins that are high in back and low in front help facilitate rotation and avoid expiration of shelf life. They also keep hard to stack items neat and organized.

- Plan to spend a minimum of one hour each week to check supplies, determine reorder points, and throw away outdated supplies.

Storage Considerations

Consideration must be given to special storage requirements on product labels, such as light and heat sensitivity, refrigeration, storing in a cool dark area, or keeping certain hazardous materials apart from each other. For example, as referenced in Chapter 4 (Hazard Communication and Regulatory Agency Mandates), ammonia and bleach should not be stored next to each other, as they may cause an explosion; also, the resulting fumes may be fatal, if inhaled.

> **Note:** Some items for use in the treatment areas may require special storage. For example, dental film must be stored at no less than 50°F nor more than 70°F (10°C to 20°C) and between 30 percent and 50 percent relative humidity. Items requiring refrigeration must be stored separately from edible items, such as staff lunches and beverages.

Rate of Use, Reorder Point, and Flagging System

Offices vary widely in the quantity of supplies used and the rate at which they use them. Many office managers determine a rate of use on commonly used items to establish a routine reorder point for each. Rate of use refers to the rate of consumption of items and supplies commonly used in the office. The reorder point is predetermined minimum quantity of a specific supply left in inventory. When the item reaches the minimum quantity, additional units are to be ordered to avoid running out, especially if the item is frequently back ordered by the supplier.

If using a manual system for supply inventory and reordering, a flagging system may be used to signal the predetermined reorder point. If a computerized system is used, the computer will automatically alert the office manager to the appropriate reorder time when the item is taken out of inventory at the reorder point.

Storage of Controlled Substances

With an increase in sedation dentistry, more offices stock and dispense controlled substances to patients. To prevent abuse of a controlled substance,

---

[1] Adapted from Jill L. Sherer, *Taking Stock: How to Order, Store, and Maintain Dental Supplies.*

unauthorized disbursement, or theft, an office that uses these prescription medications should consider a double-locked storage system.

A double-lock system requires two separate keys to open the storage box. Two different people in the office must each maintain one key, independent of the other.

Dispensing of prescription drugs also requires that known drug allergies and sensitivities be entered into the computer database for each patient, as well as other known medications taken by the patient. This is to prevent the likelihood of overdosing or double dosing patients, as well as dispensing two or more drugs that may cause an adverse reaction or serious drug side effect if taken simultaneously by the patient.

Computerized Ordering and Inventory Control

Many practices take advantage of computerized supply ordering and inventory control. Having the capability to order supplies by computer also facilitates printing out a list of supplies by name, manufacturer, usage rate, and reorder time required.

The office manager may use a computer wand across the barcode on the product label or package at reorder time, or may use specific software provided by the individual supplier/vendor. The advantages of ordering supplies via computer electronically are time savings in order processing and receipt and avoidance of duplication of orders.

Quantity Discounts

Because offices spend a significant amount of money on supplies annually, they often take advantage of supplier's quantity discounts. Quantity discounts are extended to offices for buying large numbers or units of a single item to receive a discount per item.

Buying in Bulk

In an effort to save the office money on supplier specials and large order quantity discounts, the office manager may be tempted to order excessive amounts of products. Careful planning must take into consideration the rate at which consumables, disposables, and expendables are used, the amount of available storage space, and the need for special storage.

For example, a case of cotton rolls normally sells for $29.95 and the quantity discount rate is three cases at $26.95 each or 12 cases for $23.95 each. The office would save $3 per case by buying three (a $9 saving) or it would save $6 per case by buying 12 cases (a $72 saving).

If the office has sufficient space to store 12 cases of cotton rolls and uses them quickly, this inventory may represent a significant savings to the doctor. Because cotton rolls have no special storage requirements, such as refrigeration, the cost saving may be justified. If, however, few cotton rolls are used, storage space is minimal, it may be wiser to order a smaller amount.

Automatic Shipments

Many offices take advantage of quantity discounts on bulk purchases and save valuable storage at the same time. When storage considerations, product freshness, or rate of use are of concern, they may still take advantage of these savings through automatic shipments arranged with an individual supplier.

For example, if an office uses two cases of gloves monthly, 24 cases per year, the office manager may wish to take advantage of a supplier's quantity special on gloves but they have no way to store such a large order. Using an automatic shipment plan, the office manager may order the gloves at the lowest price per case and arrange with the supplier to have two cases shipped automatically per month. With this shipping option, the office benefits by always having a fresh supply of gloves available, without bulky storage requirements.

Bids and Contract Buying

Many large group practices and clinics prefer to send their supply needs out on bid and enter into an annual contract with the supplier who bids the lowest on the total supply budget for the year.

This system relies on one supplier for the majority of dental supplies purchased for the year and helps the office maintain a sound inventory supply system. The inventory is a written or computer printed list that includes all supplies on hand, the amount ordered, the manufacturer/supplier, the reorder frequency (approximately how often to place another order), and the per unit price.

Supply Order Tracking

Part of the office manager's job is to order supplies and track all paperwork and records for accuracy and to ensure proper payment for invoices.

Order Form

An initial order for a product or supply is placed with the vendor, also known as the supplier. This is the person working for a dental supply sales company or a manufacturer's representative who sells dental products over the telephone, by mail, or via computer websites. Regardless of how the order is placed, information is necessary to complete the order.

Information necessary to place an order includes the name of the vendor/ supplier, the appropriate address, telephone, fax and email, the quantity, the item number, the description of the product, and any other important information, such as size, shade, unit pricing, and so on.

The vendor/supplier will need to know from the office manager the doctor's name and full mailing address, telephone number, and account number. If there are special shipping considerations, such as days the practice will be open to receive a package, or that an item is to be held until a specific date, the vendor/supplier will also need this information.

Purchase Order

Large practices and clinics sometimes place their orders, either on paper or electronically, using a purchase order. A purchase order contains the practice, clinic or institution's name, customer number, and all other pertinent order information.

An additional significant piece of information required on every purchase order is a purchase order number. The purchase order appears usually using a sequentially ordered numbering system in the same location on each purchase order. When placing an initial order or referring to an existing purchase or repair requisitioned, the purchase order number is vital and it should be used on all correspondence and communications with the vendor.

Packing Slip

After the order has been placed the merchandise will arrive at the office. It is the office manager's duty to sign for the package received if delivered by a vendor and to review the contents of the package for accuracy.

Inside the package or outer envelope is a packing slip, which lists the contents of the package. This information should be identical to the order form and the subsequent invoice, which is the bill requesting payment for merchandise. The office manager should review the information contained on the packing slip and compare it to the original order and the final invoice for payment. She or he should note any errors, omissions, discontinued items, or back ordered items. If there are discrepancies the office manager should contact the vendor immediately.

Invoice

After the order has been received and marked off against the original order, the items must be put away in the appropriate storage areas of the office. Within 30 days the office will receive an invoice requesting payment for the items.

The office manager must once again check the items and prices listed on the original order against the packing slip and invoice to ensure accuracy of billing. The invoice will also note a date the payment is due.

Back Order

Occasionally, items ordered are not in stock with the vendor/supplier and are not shipped with other items on the original order. In this instance, the item is placed on back order. This means that when the vendor/supplier receives the product it will be shipped separately to the dentist's office as part of the original order.

The office manager should take care not to place a duplicate order when checking on back ordered items and, likewise, that the office is not charged twice for one order.

Credit Invoice

Occasionally, the office will cancel an order or return an item for a refund. In this instance, the vendor/supplier may issue a credit invoice for the items canceled or returned. A credit invoice works exactly opposite of an invoice or statement and may be deducted from the bill or may be credited to the dentists account toward future purchases.

Warranties and Repairs

Part of the job of maintaining control of inventory is that of overseeing repairs and warranties on purchases and equipment of the practice.

Occasionally, a service representative must be contacted to repair existing equipment or install replacement parts. Similar to invoices for supplies, equipment repairs must also be tracked for accuracy.

Warranties on large pieces of equipment should be filed or stored in a designated place in the office for easy access and reference. When equipment is still under warranty for repairs or parts, the warranty information must be readily accessible when arranging for repairs or replacement.

Exploring the Web

The following are just a few dental suppliers, to find more try searching on dental suppliers online or in your area.

www.sullivanschein.com
www.patersondental.com
www.smartpractice.com
www.plaksmaker.com

Skill Building

These optional activities and exercises are designed to help the student put into practice information learned in the chapter.

1. The dentist asks you to place an order for one case of Caulk Fast Set, one bottle of Durelon cement, and three # 11R Buffalo Dental spatulas from ABC Dental Supply. Using the information provided, role-play placing a telephone order for the items requested; make-up the doctor's name, address, and telephone number. The office will be closed for vacation next week and would like the items delivered after Tuesday, the 20th of the month.

2. Break into small groups or teams to solve the following problem. A salesperson calls or stops in your office with an excellent buy on personalized toothbrushes (only $0.35 each). The offer is good only for today and you must order 5,000 units to take advantage of this special offer. The doctor is out of the office attending a continuing education seminar in another state. The office is running low on toothbrushes. What should you do? Discuss in your group or team and share your resolution and your rationale with the class.

3. You open an order from XYZ dental supply only to find that you have been billed twice for one item and that two other items are missing; however, your bill reflects you have received the items. What should you do?

4. Using the Internet, investigate three dental supply companies and compare prices for similar items.

5. List three advantages and disadvantages of doing business with one or two suppliers; list three advantages and disadvantages of using multiple suppliers.

Challenge Your Understanding

Select the response that best answers each of the following questions. Only one response is correct.

1. Which of the following is not an important part of the office manager's job in inventory control and management?
   a. Maintaining a sufficient amount of dental supplies
   b. Purchasing supplies at the lowest price
   c. Depleting inventory to the last unit before reordering
   d. Working with suppliers

2. Consumable supplies are single use items that are discarded immediately after the procedure for which they are used.
   a. True
   b. False

3. Because most dental practices spend upward of 10 percent of their total overhead on dental supplies, the supply budget represents an insignificant expenditure.
   a. True
   b. False

4. Which of the following is not considered an equipment item?
   a. Plants in the reception area supplied and maintained by an outside florist
   b. An intraoral camera
   c. Items that may be depreciated by the office over a number of years
   d. Major purchases that are used for five years or more

5. If the shelf life of a product has expired, the office manager should:
   a. Tell the chairside assistant to use it anyway
   b. Discard the item
   c. Call the supplier for an exchange or refund
   d. Place the item on back order

6. In supplying and storing supplies, the office manager should:
   a. Store supplies in one central area
   b. Spend a minimum of one hour each week to check supplies and determine reorder points and throw away outdated supplies
   c. Be alert to products that are light or heat sensitive
   d. All of the above

7. To ensure product freshness, the office manager should arrange supplies with the newest farthest back on the shelf and the oldest brought forward to be used first.
   a. True
   b. False

8. Special storage considerations for products the office manager must consider include:
   a. Storage requirement information on product labels
   b. Heat sensitivity
   c. Light sensitivity
   d. All of the above

9. A double locked storage system:
   a. Prevents abuse of controlled substances
   b. Controls and unauthorized disbursement or theft
   c. Requires two separate keys held by two different people to open the storage box
   d. All of the above

10. Some supplies for use in the treatment area that require refrigeration may be stored in the same refrigerator with items for personal consumption, such as lunches and beverages.
    a. True
    b. False

11. Which of the following is a benefit of entering an order via the computer?
    a. Time-saving in order processing and receipt time
    b. Increased order accuracy
    c. Automatic shipment
    d. Guaranteed lowest pricing

12. With careful planning the office manager may save the practice money on the supply budget using:
    a. Bulk purchasing
    b. Automatic shipments
    c. Annual purchasing contracts
    d. All of the above

13. The packing slip:
    a. Lists the contents of the package
    b. Should be identical to the original order form and to the subsequent invoice
    c. Notes back ordered items
    d. All of the above

14. A back order means that when the supplier receives the product it will be shipped separately to the dentist's office as part of the original order.
    a. True
    b. False

15. If the office manager notes a discrepancy on the packing slip he or she should:
    a. Refuse to accept the delivery for partial shipment
    b. Wait until the order is completed before checking off the contents
    c. Contact the supplier immediately
    d. Place an order for the missing items with another supply

16. A credit invoice may be deducted from the bill or may be credited to the dentist's account for a future purchase.
    a. True
    b. False

17. The office manager should keep a separate file of equipment warranties in the event of the repair or replacement problem.
    a. True
    b. False

18. The supply inventory is a written or computer printed list that contains:
    a. All supplies on hand
    b. The usual amount ordered
    c. The manufacturers/supplier
    d. All of the above

19. A case of patient napkins normally sells for $24.95 the office manager has the opportunity to save money by ordering 12 cases at $21.45 per case. If he or she places the order for 12 cases at the quantity discount rate, how much will the practice save on this order?
    a. $2.50 per case for a total savings of $30
    b. $3.50 per case for a total saving of $42
    c. $4.50 per case for a total savings of $54
    d. $5.50 per case for a total savings of $60

20. Careful planning of supply ordering and inventory control must take into consideration:
    a. The rate at which consumables, disposables, and expendables are used
    b. The amount of available storage space in the office
    c. Special storage requirements
    d. All of the above

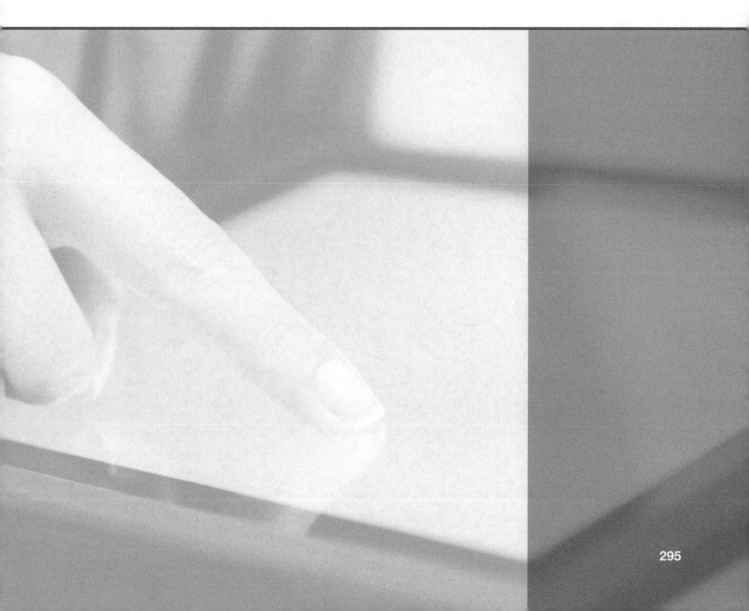

SECTION V

Dental Office Employment

CHAPTER 16

Employment Opportunities

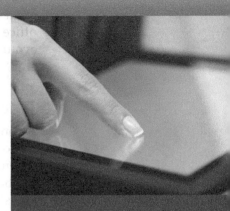

CHAPTER OUTLINES

- **Employment Opportunities**
  Type of Employment Desired
  Employment Opportunity Sources
- **Preparing for Employment**
  Preparing a Resume
  Preparing a Cover Letter
  Preparing for the Interview
  Terms of Employment
  Other Career Opportunities in Dentistry

LEARNING OBJECTIVES

Upon completion of this chapter, the reader should be able to:

1. Describe the types of practices where a dental office manager might seek employment.

2. Describe the steps in preparing for employment.

3. List the key parts of a resume for employment.

4. Describe the steps in preparing for an interview.
   Be familiar with the terms relating to employment.

5. Describe other dental employment opportunities outside of the traditional private practice.

KEY TERMS

cover letter
group practice
interview
reference
resume
solo practice
specialty practice

Employment Opportunities

Whether starting out in a career, reentering the job market, or as an experienced team member, an office manager will probably seek out a number of employment opportunities before finding the best possible job option. The dental office manager should plan a strategy to access as many leads as possible, evaluate those leads, and then pursue the ones that best fit the individual's employment goals.

Type of Employment Desired

At one time, the majority of dental office management positions were in fee-for-service, small, private, solo practices. Today, there are numerous options for employment. An office manager may want to examine a number of opportunities prior to making a decision and accepting a position. The following are types of employment options a dental office manager might want to consider.

Solo Practice

Today, about two-thirds of all dental practices are privately owned by one dentist (solo practice), offering fee-for-service procedures. The trend is fast-changing, however, because of a variety of factors including the increase in group practices to share overhead expenses, the increase in managed care practices, and the growing number of specialty practices.

Solo practices tend to be slower paced and the office manager may participate in variety of activities throughout the day from making appointments to filing insurance claims and everything in between. For office managers looking to build relationships with patients in a family atmosphere, a solo practice is a good choice.

Group Practice

The group practice (an office owned or operated by two or more dentists or other shareholders*) may represent a greater challenge for the dental manager who enjoys a busy environment but who may also enjoy a variety of activities such as scheduling, supervising, and managing the dental staff members.

The growing number of group practices is because of increasing overhead costs including the cost of complying with government regulations and infection control requirements. Decreasing revenues for procedures paid for by third-party payers, insurance companies, and managed-care companies have forced dentists to find more efficient ways to run a dental business. A group practice allows dentists to offer extended hours by working a varied schedule and sharing an office and staff.

Managed-Care Facility

Many managed care facilities operate identically to privately owned practices; however, the dentist and other providers of care, such as hygienists and assistants, may have a contract with a managed care company. The office manager may find it rewarding to work in this type of practice. Large managed care facilities may offer an opportunity for career development within the organization, as well as compensation and other benefits provided by managed-care

---

* Some states allow only dentists to own a dental practice so all shareholders in that case would be dentists.

corporations. The possibility for career advancement should be investigated prior to accepting a position.

Specialty Practice

A specialty practice provides a unique opportunity to serve dental patients requiring a narrower, more specialized field of dental treatment. In Chapter 2 (Introduction to the Dental Team), there was a complete listing and description of the nine recognized dental specialties. Many of those specialties operate practices similar to solo or group practices with the exception that they provide only one facet of dental care.

Specialty practices can provide unique challenges to the dental office manager because instead of developing long-term relationships with patients you are building relationships with family dentists that trust you to care for their patients. With a few exceptions, specialty offices have rapid patient turn over because once the patient receives treatment they return to the care of their family dentist. For example, a patient is referred to an oral surgeon for extraction of wisdom teeth. Once those teeth are extracted the relationship with the oral surgeon is over.

Employment Opportunity Sources

The office manager should contact a variety of sources to explore employment opportunities. Consideration must be given not only to the type of practice, but the geographic location and commuting distance. The following describes a variety of employment sources.

Newspapers

Traditionally the classified sections of the newspaper have contained a selection of employment opportunities generally located under health care opportunities; the ads are listed alphabetically as "dental assistant," "dental office manager," and other designations. Occasionally, specialty practices will appear alphabetically farther down in the health care column. Some classified advertisements are run as a blind ad, which means the identity of the employer is not disclosed to the applicant. This is to ensure confidentiality of the dentist/employer. It also reduces the number of telephone inquiries that may flood the office the day after an advertisement appears or masks the fact that an employee is being terminated from the practice. Some classified advertisements request that candidates send a resume to a PO box, office, home fax machine, or to an email address not easily identified with the practice. Sending a resume to an unidentified recipient is done to ensure confidentiality of the employer.

Several sources of employment opportunities have rapidly replaced newspaper classified ads.

Electronic Sources: The Internet and Websites

Many employers now offer the prospective employee the option of sending a resume or job inquiry via the Internet using an email address from their website. The advantages of job searching using electronic sources to the employment candidate are speed of inquiry and saving some postage and paper. An added value is the ability to save resumes into a database for instant retrieval.

Several dental employment sites, which are free to job seekers, have become part of the Internet over the last few years. With computer knowledge being a valuable asset for a new employee, more employers are looking for future dental team members on the Internet. There are sites that list jobs and sites for employees to post resumes. A few Internet sites will give a prospective employee the ability to enter job requirements and will automatically send an update email when a position that meets that description is posted.

Dental Associations

Some state or local dental associations have an employment referral service to match their dentist members with potential employment candidates. Of the associations that provide this service, many offer it at no cost as a benefit to their members.

A dental office manager moving out of state may wish to consider the city or geographic area of desired employment and contact the dental association in that area to see if they have an employee/employer matching service.

Campus Placement Programs

Many postsecondary campuses have a placement office that posts ongoing job openings for students and graduates of their programs. This service is offered free of charge and is updated frequently. The goal of campus placement programs is to match students with employers in the area. Dentists in the area may call a local school that trains dental auxiliary when they are looking for new employees particularly if they have been happy with the quality of past program graduates.

Telephone Directories

When seeking employment, the office manager may wish to consult telephone directory yellow page listings for dental offices in the area. The advertisement may give you an idea regarding the type of practice and how they view themselves. Ads that focus on "catering to cowards" indicate a different type of practice from one that advertises "beautiful smiles and cosmetic dentistry."

> **Note:** Don't make the mistake of organizing a "mass mailing" to whom it may concern from phone book listings. If you contact an office take the time to personalize the contact.

Dental Supply Sales Representatives

Dental supply sales representatives cover a specific geographical or regional area and are often aware of open dental office positions within their sales territory. The office manager may contact local dental supply houses to speak with a sales representative who covers the territory within their desired area of employment.

The benefit to the sales representative to assist the dental practice in finding an employee is it maintains the practice as one of the sales "reps" happy customers.

Employment Agencies

Employment agencies are privately owned or franchised companies who prescreen and pretest applicants for employers. They work on a flat fee or commission basis to place ads, evaluate applicants, and conduct preliminary employment interviews before sending applicants to interview with the perspective dentist/employer.

Some dentists prefer to work through employment agencies, paying a percentage based on the employee's salary to save screening time and administrative costs. If the dental office uses a consultant or practice management company, that company also may be aware of available job candidates and will charge a finder's fee similar to the employment agency to match the dental practice and job candidate.

When the dental office manager is looking for employment, the ad that is posted may not be from the dentist at all but from an employment agency representing the practice. Rarely is any fee charged to the prospective employee but asking for clarification of the arrangement is always a good idea.

Employee Leasing Organizations

For office managers moving to a new area where they are unfamiliar with dental practices, working for an employee leasing organization can be a good start. Many employees love this type of arrangement for its variety and flexibility. Some employers, especially owners of large clinics, find it efficient to lease employees, rather than hire them out right. This saves the practice a significant amount of time and money spent in advertising, screening, interviewing, and hiring. These companies have traditionally been referred to as "temp agencies" because they are also useful in finding employees for a limited duration to cover vacations and maternity or sick leave. In addition to short-term jobs, these agencies have expanded their services to include long-term employees as well.

Employee leasing companies also handle payroll, administration of benefits, and other human resource services for the employee and bill the dentist an agreed upon rate.

Preparing for Employment

Once the geographic area and type of employment desired have been determined, it is time to prepare for employment. This includes developing a resume or multiple resumes, a cover letter, getting ready for actual interviews, and being prepared for follow-up.

Preparing a Resume

A **resume** is a review of the candidate's credentials that states his or her qualifications for employment (Figure 16-1). It contains the candidates' biographical information such as name, address, current phone number, and email. The resume indicates the type of employment sought, education, and previous work experience relevant to desired employment. Relevant is a very broad term and can include directly related employment but also jobs that show a strong work history in another field.

There are two types of resumes: chronological and functional. A chronological resume states the job objective, work history in reverse order so that the most recent is listed first including education, past employment, skills, and references. A functional resume states skills and experience related to the job. The functional resume is most often used by career reentry candidates where the candidate has held a variety of jobs and wishes to focus on one area of employment.

KAREN COPELAND

1033 First St.
Seaside, CA
831-555-1234
kcopeland@email.com

SUMMARY
Team player motivated by challenges that allow utilization of interpersonal, organizational, and creative skills that aid in profitability, productivity, and quality results. Detail oriented multi-tasker with customer service expertise and the ability to solve challenges.

SKILLS & ABILITIES

- Professional correspondence
- Scheduling to maximize production
- Filing insurance claims
- Working knowledge of Dentrix practice management software
- Knowledge of x-rays, infection control procedure, and sterilizing equipment

EXPERIENCE

Office Manager/Receptionist   **David Smith, DDS**

June 1998 to Present   **Seaside, CA**

Responsible for all incoming and outgoing calls; computer scheduling; insurance verification and filing of claims including electronic claims; professional correspondence; patient statements, and collection of delinquent accounts.

Chairside Assistant   **George Watkins, DDS**

December 1995 to May 1998   **Seaside, CA**

Performed chairside functions; OHSA compliance for infection control and hazard communication; ordered office supplies; x-ray certified.

EDUCATION

Dental Office Management – Certificate of Completion   **1998**

Pacific University   Seaside, CA

Dental Assisting Program – Graduate   **1994**

County Community College   Newburgh, NY

REFERENCES
References furnished upon request

FIGURE 16-1 Sample resume.

Preparing a solid resume is crucial to getting a good job. The following are some resume rules:

- Start out with a bang! The appearance of your resume should be professional and appealing. If yours is one of several resumes received it needs to be the one that the hiring manager wants to read.
- Always have at least one person proofread your resume.
- Use good grammar and avoid slang.
- Spell check and grammar check are for your benefit—use them but you still need to proofread.
- Choose one easy to read font and stay with it—multiple fonts can be confusing.
- Make sure your resume is for the job you want. It might be helpful to have several versions of your resume stored on your computer that correspond to different jobs such as one for a specialty office and one for a family practice, or one for a solo practice and one for a larger group practice.
- Translate your previous job skills into new job assets.
- Keep your points brief use short bulleted statements.
- If you had accomplishments in a previous job make sure to list them specifically; such as, increased collections 16 percent over a12-month period rather than increased collections.
- Double check how your resume looks when received by email by emailing to yourself or a friend. Does the formatting stay consistent?
- It's a good idea to take a copy of your resume to any interview. Make sure it is printed on high-quality paper.
- Try to keep your resume to one or two pages.
- Don't include irrelevant information such as your favorite foods or hobbies. If you volunteer with an organization or speak a second language, it's okay to mention that information.
- Be honest! You can be enthusiastic about your accomplishments but don't embellish them beyond recognition.
- And last but not least: if your personal email address is one that should stay personal, for example "partygurl@abc.com" or "hotchick@abc.com," get a professional email for job hunting.

Likewise, there is certain information that should not be included when preparing a resume:

- Never give reasons for termination or leaving a job on a resume.
- Never include your references, simply say references furnished upon request.
- Do not include your Social Security Number, marital status, or other personal information.
- Avoid using exact dates of employment or education; month and year are sufficient. If you were out of the workforce for a number of years, you may wish to prepare a functional resume, rather than a dated one.
- Never include your present employer's telephone number unless your employer is aware of your eminent departure.

- Avoid using professional jargon, unless it will be understood by the person interviewing you.
- Never include salary information on a resume. You may actually short-change your earning power in doing so.

Preparing a Cover Letter

A resume alone is an insufficient response to a classified advertisement or other notification of an available position. Although the well-prepared resume may accurately reflect all work experience, credentials, and the desired position, a letter of introduction should accompany the initial inquiry. This introduction is a **cover letter** and should accompany the original resume whether it is mailed, faxed, or emailed, in response to a job inquiry (Figure 16-2). A cover letter introduces the candidate and explains the reason for the inquiry, the job

---

Julie Newton

3724 Sunnyside Place Sommerville, CA 00234 | 831-555-6789 | jnewton@email.com

May 28, 20xx

John D. Molar, DMD
Family Dental Associates
123 Healthcare Circle
Sommerville, CA 00234

Dear Dr. Molar:

I was excited to see your posting for a Dental Office Manager on findadentaljob .com. Because of my training in Dental Management, I feel I am an excellent match for the job and a great fit for your practice. I would bring motivation, a commitment to dental excellence, and enthusiasm to your dental team at Family Dental Associates. My past employers will tell you I am prompt, trustworthy, and a team player.

At City College, I obtained specialized training in Dental Office Management; I have been educated on the dental basics, communication skills, written correspondence, information and inventory management, scheduling to maximize production, insurance, recall systems, financial arrangements, book keeping, dental practice software, office equipment, patient relations, and record keeping.

I would be happy to provide greater detail about my skills and experience during an interview. Thank you for your time and consideration.

Sincerely,

Julie Newton

Julie Newton

FIGURE 16-2 Sample cover letter.

desired, and where the candidate was informed of the job available. The cover letter should also state when the candidate is available for employment and how to be contacted to schedule an interview or for further information.

The cover letter is especially important when seeking employment as an office manager because professional correspondence is part of the job description. Make sure your cover letter represents your letter writing skills.

Preparing for the Interview

The interview takes place when the employer and prospective employee meet face-to-face to discuss the nature of the job and to obtain additional information from each other. Occasionally, the interview may involve not only the dentist and/or office manager but several of the dental team members. Group interviews provide an ideal environment to assess the ability of the candidate to function as a team member.

In some practices, part of the interview may include personality profile testing to determine traits and characteristics of the applicant.

In preparing for the interview it is important to make a good first impression. This includes wardrobe, professional demeanor, interviewing skills, and follow-up.

In an effort to interview only the most qualified candidates, some offices do a preliminary phone interview. After applying for a job the applicant needs to be ready to be called for a brief phone interview or to set up a face-to-face interview. There is nothing wrong with asking permission to return the call when it comes at an awkward time or if it is possible let it go to an answering machine or voice mail. If applying for multiple positions, the job candidate needs to keep track of those applications along with the office and date of application. If there are other people that could answer the phone number given in contact information, asking for their assistance can be helpful. Make sure the people who could answer the phone will best represent your interests and provide appropriate messaging and information to you for follow up with a future employer.

Appropriate Dress and Professional Demeanor

The candidate for employment should plan to dress conservatively and according to local conventional business dress codes. For women, this generally means conservative attire including closed toed shoes. The best guideline for how to dress for the interview is to dress like the practice business staff in the office you will be visiting.

> **Note:** the office manager should not wear scrubs or a uniform to the job interview! If the office manager is a male, he should wear a shirt and tie with conservative business slacks and shoes. Athletic shoes are not appropriate for men or women.

A conservative purse or briefcase is acceptable. Jewelry and other accessories should be kept to a minimum. A watch and wedding band are acceptable; conservative earrings include single pearls or small gold posts. Jewelry that makes a lot of noise with any body movement is not acceptable.

Nails should be short and clean, and may be polished with clear or a very neutral color. The free edge of the nail should be no more than 2 to 3 mm. Excessively long nails are unprofessional and artificial nails are not allowed in the clinical area.

The hairstyle should be professional and away from the eyes and face. Flamboyant hair accessories should be avoided and the applicant should not have to touch her hair during the interview.

Perfume, cologne, or aftershave should be minimal and the applicant should not chew gum, smoke, eat food, or drink during the interview. Children should be left at home with appropriate supervision.

Plan Ahead

The organized office management candidate plans to arrive early for the interview. If unsure of the exact location of the office or parking accommodations, it is acceptable to call the office to request this information, and/or take a trial drive ahead of time. By planning to arrive a few minutes early, many applicants will welcome having the time to freshen up at the office prior to meeting the interviewer/dentist.

Although sometimes unavoidable, car problems and traffic may delay the job candidate creating punctuality problems. It is advisable to make sure that reliable transportation is available and that sufficient travel time is planned.

In addition to having already sent a copy of the resume to the practice, the prospective employee should bring an extra copy or two, in the event the interviewer has misplaced the original. Having an extra copy allows the job candidate the opportunity to review the information included, as a refresher and to answer specific questions regarding information contained in the resume. Because the job candidate may be asked to complete an employment application prior to being interviewed, he or she should also bring a pen. Having a small notebook for notes regarding the practice or job is also a good idea.

During the Interview

Because first impressions are all important, the office management candidate should remember to walk, speak, and sit professionally. It is appropriate to introduce yourself and to extend your right hand to give a firm handshake upon arrival. Always smile, nod, and exude a positive attitude.

Maintaining good eye contact and composure ensures a competent professional appearance. The candidate should pay attention to the interviewer's questions and give only appropriate answers to them. Refrain from giving additional information or from asking probing questions until the end of the interview or until the interviewer asked, "Do you have any further questions?"

The office management candidate should also avoid nervous mannerisms such as finger drumming, nail biting, or repetitive movement of the feet or legs. Speak in a low, but direct voice, avoiding shrill noises and excessive laughter.

The job candidate should not bring up the manner of financial compensation and benefits; the interviewer should address this, as well as the starting date and other pieces of information critical to the nature of employment. However, the candidate should bring this up should the interviewer overlook it.

If the interview was with only one representative of the practice, there may be a second interview scheduled for the most qualified candidate or candidates. The job candidate(s) may also be invited back to undergo a working interview where the candidate actually participates in office management tasks, or at a minimum is asked, "How would you handle this?"

Information That May Not Be Discussed

Specific personal information may not be requested by an employer, such as marital status, number of children, racial origin, creed, spouse's employment, personal financial indebtedness, or lifestyle preference (see Chapter 3, Legal and Ethical Issues and Responsibilities for additional information regarding EEOC guidelines).

Authorization to Release References and Other Information

In some states it is illegal to release employment information without a person's consent. The interviewer may request information such as references from previous employers, college transcripts, and other information pertinent to past employment history or education.

To avoid confidentiality issues, the interviewer may ask the employment candidate to sign a waiver, granting release of this information or requesting permission to contact these parties.

> **Note:** *Personal information or information not relevant to the specific nature of employment may not be requested.*

Generally information that may be legally shared includes start and end dates of employment, name of direct supervisor, the job title, and the nature of job duties.

Drug Testing

The issue of drug testing as a pre-employment requirement is becoming more common. It is considered legal in most states and is designed to protect the practice, as well as the patients.

After the Interview

The employment candidate should let the interviewer conduct or lead the interview, and also close it. The candidate should not appear rushed, nor should she or he consume too much of the interviewer's valuable time.

Upon completion of the interview, the candidate should stand, extend their hand for a closing handshake, and thank the interviewer, using her or his name.

Regardless of the outcome of the interview, the job candidate should send the interviewer a personal thank you note for the opportunity to interview and be considered for the position. This should be done immediately after the interview and sent by mail.

Working Interviews

Being invited to do a working interview is becoming very common. The following are a few guidelines for a successful working interview:

- Think before you talk. Sharing too much personal information is not a good idea.
- Don't disparage your former employer.
- Arrive on time and ready to work.
- Be enthusiastic.

Terms of Employment

It is important for the prospective employee and employer to establish clear communication regarding all aspects of the position. This includes, but is not limited to, the nature of the job, including a detailed job description, the hours, compensation, benefits, and other office policies.

Before being asked to make a decision regarding the job, the candidate should understand the job description so that expectations can be met.

Letter of Employment

Some practices issue a letter of employment that serves as a written document outlining the terms of employment. A letter of employment clarifies the terms of the position for both employer and employee and serves as documentation of the employer's expectations. Putting the details of the job into a letter can eliminate misunderstandings and gives both parties something to refer back to for clarification.

Information may include duties and responsibilities, working/office hours, salary and benefits, uniform requirements and dress code, provisional employment, and continuing education guidelines.

Provisional Employment

Some employers establish provisional employment following a successful interview. Provisional employment, formerly referred to as a probationary period, provides a time for the prospective employee and employer to work together. The end result is that after a satisfactory probationary period an agreement is made for permanent employment. Provisional employment is further described in Chapter 3 (Legal and Ethical Issues and Responsibilities).

Salary Negotiations

Generally, the salary is determined by the dentist-employer as part of the job offer. However, in some instances, there may be specific needs or requests that may be negotiated once the job offer has been made to the prospective employee.

Other Career Opportunities in Dentistry

In addition to traditional employment in a dental office, there are many other employment opportunities. In recent years, the trend toward a variety of dental jobs has grown.

Teaching

The experienced office manager may have the desire to share her or his knowledge and skills with others by pursuing a teaching career. Most postsecondary dental teaching institutions require significant experience in the field and a degree from an accredited institution.

Sales: Retail Supply Houses, Dental Manufacturers, and Telemarketing Organizations

Some former dental assistants and office managers, who enjoy an especially fast-paced working environment, travel, and being with the public may secure employment in dental sales. Sales positions require attention to detail and working on a salary-plus-commission basis. However, the income opportunity for someone who is successful is very high.

Outside sales opportunities with retail dental supply houses and dental manufacturers who distribute through retail supply houses are another place to use dental skills out of the dental practice environment. Often, dental sales representatives exhibit a company's products at large dental trade shows and may also visit schools to give product demonstrations.

Inside sales positions may involve telemarketing promotions to dental offices.

Dental Consultant

Some dental office managers with significant experience may wish to join consulting companies or open their own dental consulting business. If considering opening a business, it is advisable to obtain additional information about the legal and financial considerations of self-employment.

Dental School Clinics

There are more than 60 dental schools in the United States that have positions for dental office managers, clinical dental assistants, clinical supervisors, supply and dispensing assistants, and instrument processing assistants. These jobs are especially advantageous for working parents with children at home during school vacations because dental schools have similar schedules.

Government Clinics, Public Health, and Correctional Facilities

Government-funded clinics serve a variety of the population's needs. They may be funded by county, state, or federal agencies and generally provide basic dental services or prepare statistical reports on dental health status and treatment needs for underserved populations.

Public health departments, usually funded by the state, may provide a source of alternative employment for the experienced office manager. Correctional facilities are owned privately or by the state or federal government and must provide dental care for the inmates. Working conditions in these facilities are rigid and the environment includes camera surveillance and security officers.

State Board of Dental Examiners

Occasionally, state dental boards have clerical, licensing, enforcement, investigative, and special service officer positions available. Former dental assistants/office managers may find these positions especially interesting, because of their dental background and familiarity with dental procedures. These positions are offered through state employment.

Insurance/Managed Care Corporate Offices

The rapid increase in third-party organizations and managed care has created a need for administrative staff, claims reviewers, and supervisors. Because of their familiarity with dental terminology procedures, dental office managers may find these positions of interest.

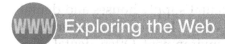

Exploring the Web

Resume and Cover Letter Templates
www.office.microsoft.com

Job Search Sites
www.dentalpost.net
www.indeed.com
www.mydentaljobs.com
www.craigslist.com

Skill Building

These optional activities and exercises are designed to help the student put into practice information learned in the chapter.

1. Prepare a resume for yourself using a chronological format. Assume this resume is going to a dental practice so be sure to highlight relevant skills.

2. Prepare a cover letter to send to David Good, DDS. His practice address is 3456 Santa Rita Ave.; Anywhere, CA 98070.

3. Take turns with classmates and role play a job interview. Make sure you are prepared to ask questions regarding the position, job description, starting date, and so on. Critique your interview; let your interviewer to critique your performance.

4. Prepare a thank you follow-up letter to Dr. Good.

Challenge Your Understanding

Select the response that best answers each of the following questions. Only one response is correct.

1. The trend towards solo, fee-for-service practices is increasing.
   a. True
   b. False

2. The office manager may find employment in:
   a. Private, general, solo, fee-for-service practices
   b. Group practices and managed care facilities
   c. Specialty practices
   d. Any/all of the above

3. Many classified advertisements are run as blind ads to ensure confidentiality of the employer/dentist
   a. True
   b. False

4. Electronic job searches:
   a. Increase speed of inquiry
   b. Save on postage and paper
   c. Allow employers to scan resumes into a database for instant retrieval
   d. All of the above

5. Campus placement offices do all of the following except:
   a. Charge a fee for applicant screening
   b. Post ongoing job openings for students and alumni
   c. Match students with employers in the area
   d. Include their fee within tuition charged

6. Employment agencies are privately owned or franchised companies that:
   a. Prescreen and pretest applicants
   b. Work on a flat fee or commission basis
   c. Save screening time and administrative costs for the dentist or employer
   d. All of the above

7. A resume contains all of the following except:
   a. A review of the candidate's credentials and qualifications for employment
   b. The candidates biographical information
   c. A follow-up thank you letter to the interviewer
   d. The educational and previous work experience pertinent to desired employment

8. The two types of resumes are:
   a. Provisional and organizational
   b. Organizational and chronological
   c. Provisional and functional
   d. Chronological and functional

9. A resume should always be printed out on bright color paper to catch the interviewer's attention.
   a. True
   b. False

10. A resume should be geared toward a specific job.
    a. True
    b. False

11. The prospective office manager should always include previous/present salary information on a resume:
    a. True
    b. False

12. A cover letter:
    a. Introduces the candidate
    b. Explains the reason for the inquiry
    c. States specific job desired and availability for employment
    d. All of the above

13. To make a professional impression, the office manager should wear a clinic jacket or scrubs to the interview.
    a. True
    b. False

14. To become an instructor, most post-secondary dental teaching institutions require which of the following:
    a. Certification as a Health Care Administrator
    b. A degree but experience working in a dental office is optional
    c. Registration as a dental hygienist
    d. Significant experience and a degree from an accredited institution.

15. The rapid increase in third-party organizations and managed care has created a need for administrative assistants, claims reviewers, and supervisors.
    a. True
    b. False

16. Employment in a dental school may be especially advantageous to working parents because most require evening employment.
    a. True
    b. False

17. A resume should always include:
    a. References
    b. Social Security number
    c. Spouse's occupation
    d. None of the above

18. A resume should always include specific contributions or improvements made in previous position.
    a. True
    b. False

19. A sales position in the dental field may include employment in the any of the following except:
    a. A retail dental supply house
    b. A dental manufacturing company
    c. A dental association
    d. A telemarketing organization

20. The present employer's telephone number should be included on a resume.
    a. True
    b. False

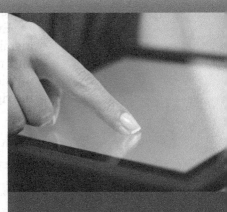

CHAPTER 17

Hiring a Dental Team

CHAPTER OUTLINES

- **Hiring the Right Person**
  Making an Employment Plan
  Terminating an Employee
  Writing an Employment Advertisement
- **Evaluating Resumes and Cover Letters**
  Initial Phone Contact
  Face-to-Face Interviews
  Working Interviews
  Offer Letters

LEARNING OBJECTIVES

Upon completion of this chapter, the reader should be able to:

1. List qualities for the ideal dental team member.
2. Describe the hiring process.
3. List five things that the hiring manager can't ask in an interview.
4. Discuss the importance of a working interview.
5. List the components of an employment ad.

KEY TERMS

employment ad
employment plan
offer letter
working interview

Hiring the Right Person

One of the key responsibilities of the dental office manager is to build a dental team that is highly productive in an atmosphere that attracts patients and makes them want to stay with the practice.

Every office is going to have different needs when hiring a new staff member. In Chapter 1 (Dental Office Management), the practice's philosophy and mission were discussed. When adding staff members, the practice's mission and philosophy play a key role in finding not just an employee but the right employee.

Making an Employment Plan

When considering a new employee, the first step is to establish an **employment plan**. What things would you "like" in a new employee and what things do you "need"? Depending on your practice these could be very different so it might be advantageous to use input from everyone in the office.

For example, two offices need to hire a dental assistant. Dr. Jones has a large staff that includes several highly trained expanded function assistants and is looking for someone in an entry level position. Dr. Smith works with two assistants and needs an experienced assistant who can be productive from day one. The perfect candidate for Dr. Jones's office is not a good match for the job available in Dr. Smith's office.

By involving your current staff you can also determine if you have a current team member who would like to change his or her role in the office that would also alter the job description for the new assistant. An example of this might be, the assistant leaving has been responsible for ordering supplies and one of your current assistants would like to take on that responsibility. By assuming that duty, the assistant may want to transfer one of her current duties to the new assistant. This would alter the job description for the new assistant.

Involving dental team members is tricky when the position that will be available is the result of the pending termination of an employee. If you have decided that an employee isn't working out and the employee needs to find employment elsewhere, this should be confidential until the employee is terminated and leaves the practice. It is never a good idea to start making plans with staff before the termination has actually occurred.

Things to consider in making an employment plan are the following:

1. What qualifications does the ideal candidate have?
2. Where are we willing to compromise to hire someone?
3. How long do we have to look for the perfect person?
4. Do we want to or are we able to train a new employee?
5. Does the job description reflect our mission statement or philosophy?

Terminating an Employee

Most dental office managers will need to remove someone from the staff at some point in their careers; it is often to your advantage to do it as soon as possible. Even when everyone else has to take on additional duties it may be preferable to having an unhappy or unproductive employee in your office.

Some terminations are obvious and with cause, such as theft, alcohol/drug use, or violations of patient privacy. Other terminations may need to occur to preserve office moral.

An employee may be technically proficient: however, their demeanor and attitude can have a detrimental impact on the dental team and the practice. These types of behaviors and attitudes include the following:

- *Excess baggage*: This employee can ruin the mood of the office the minute he or she walks in. They bring all of their personal problems to the office. If you have one of these employees, it is like having "one bad apple"; they are highly destructive. Patients pick up on the tone this employee sets on the "bad days." Dentistry can be stressful enough for many patients without adding this tension.

- *Helpless*: A helpless employee can never seem to catch on to anything but eventually it becomes obvious they are choosing to allow others to work for them. At first, these employees are fun because they make the helper feel good with praise but over time it becomes evident their motivation or lack thereof keeps other employees from their jobs and makes the office less efficient.

- *Undependable*: Often the undependable employee has a good excuse for frequent absences or habitual lateness but in a dental office the jobs are interdependent and everyone needs to pull their weight.

- *It's not my job*: This employee works hand in hand with "I only want the fun jobs." Not every job in the dental office is fun and certainly not glamorous. When one employee wants to only work with "easy patients" or "interesting procedures," it leaves everything else for the rest of the team. All jobs good and bad need to be spread evenly to create a happy productive office for the employees and patients.

- *Clicks and gossip*: These employees are especially damaging to office moral.

One of the problems with any unprofessional employee is the patients notice the added tension in the office. If one employee is snapping at another, it makes it more difficult for the patient to relax. A relaxed patient tends to imagine a good dental visit and positive outcome whereas an anxious patient imagines all the ways things could go wrong.

Writing an Employment Advertisement

Writing an ad for a new employee can be tricky. You want to find the best person you can without scaring away an excellent candidate in the process (Figure 17-1).

Things to include in an employment ad include the following:

- Dental jobs require different registration or licensure; make sure you are specific about what you want. If your dental assistant *must* be registered or have expanded duty certifications, include that in the ad. It will save you time and a potential candidate frustration. If you prefer registration but it is not an absolute requirement, word your ad to reflect it, such as "dental assistant registration preferred."

- Most offices prefer experience but keep in mind there are lots of great candidates looking for that first job.

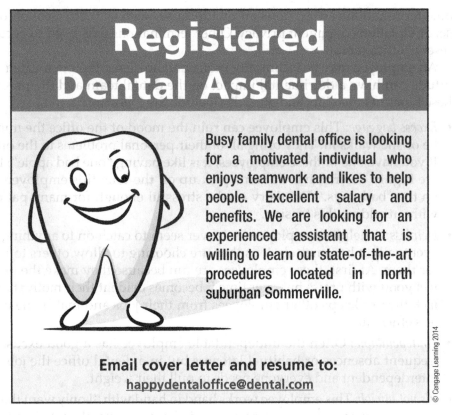

FIGURE 17-1 Sample dental employment ad.

- If your job is part-time or full-time make sure you are specific. Are you offering benefits? Include that to attract additional qualified candidates.
- Including an email address is an excellent way for potential employees to make an initial contact. As the office manager, having a resume in writing gives you the time to thoroughly evaluate the candidate's qualifications. Some offices will include a phone number but receiving numerous employment calls can be difficult in a busy office and distract the office manager from patient care.
- Giving a location can save time for everyone involved in the employment process.

Evaluating Resumes and Cover Letters

You've written an outstanding employment advertisement, posted it on several sites, and you are lucky to have multiple resumes arriving daily—now what? How do you choose the applicants who should be interviewed? Usually it is up to the dental office manager to make the decision regarding which resumes to bring to the dentist and dental team. Ideally you want to sort the resumes into groups based on your employment plan. If your employment plan put a high value on experience you would want to group the more experienced candidates together.

The easiest way to sort is electronically. Resumes arriving by email can be saved into groups making it easy for the dental team to look them over and comment. Resumes received as a hard copy can be scanned into the computer for easy retrieval. Resumes that are not a good fit for your office at this time can be moved into a low priority file.

Resumes in your high-priority group

- closely fit the employment plan; and
- show the candidates attention to detail, such as the letter was sent specifically to your practice not just sent "to whom it may concern," spelling and grammar are correct, and it has a polished appearance.

From your high-priority group, the dental team can choose the candidates for an initial phone interview.

Initial Phone Contact

The most common first contact with a prospective employee is by phone. As the office manager, contacting job candidates instead of having them contact you can have advantages. Having the office manager make the initial phone contact allows the dental office to maintain control of the phone interview. Making phone calls at the end of the work day or early evening eliminates having to interrupt the job candidate at the current place of employment. The initial call at an unexpected time can give the office manager insight into how well the potential employee handles phone calls and unexpected situations. When making phone calls after the work day, calls must be made early, not past 8 P.M. Although the job candidate might be taken by surprise when they answer the phone, anyone submitting a resume and asking to be called or contacted should understand that anytime the phone rings it could be regarding the job.

If you allow the job candidate to make the first contact by phone, it could be at a time that you are not able to devote your complete attention to the call.

Making a phone interview question list will help the office manager ask all the important questions in making the decision to interview the candidate in person. Even though some of these questions may have been answered in the resume, it can still give the office manager insight by having the job candidate review the information verbally.

Face-to-Face Interviews

After carefully reviewing resumes and records of the phone interviews, the list of potential employees can be narrowed once again to a group selected for a face-to-face interview. Usually this interview is scheduled with the office manager and dentist but may also include other staff members. Some offices like to have a group of questions ready to ask each candidate. Try to interview only your best candidates. It is difficult for some applicants to take time away from their current employment and demoralizing to not get a job they were hoping to be offered. Valuable staff time is also wasted interviewing too many applicants. Keep in mind if none of the candidates is acceptable after the interview, you still have all the resumes that were submitted.

Working Interviews

A **working interview** is an opportunity for the prospective employee to work as part of the team before being offered employment. After the face-to-face interview it is common to invite the top candidate(s) to work with the

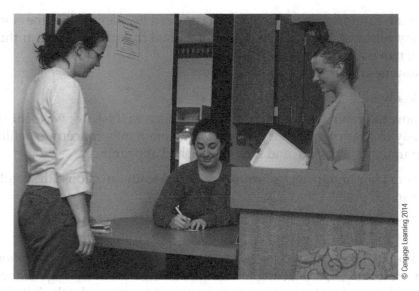

FIGURE 17-2 A working interview allows the dental team to evaluate the fit of the prospective employee with the practice.

dental team for a day or part of a day (Figure 17-2). This gives the current employees the opportunity to evaluate technical skills, the ability to learn new tasks quickly, how the prospective employee interacts with patients, and professionalism.

Generally because of the complications of bookkeeping a working interview is unpaid and considered part of the interview process. Some offices give candidates gift cards or other "thank you" for spending the day, especially if the candidate is doing the work a paid employee would be doing.

As the office manager, it is your responsibility to inform the candidate of exactly the expectation for the day such as arrival time, daily schedule, and appropriate attire. During the working interview, the job candidate is expected to be part of the dental team. Throughout the working interview, the office manager has the opportunity to evaluate if the job candidate would be an asset to the practice.

Before the working interview, it is a good idea to remind your dental team that there are some questions that they should not ask the job candidate and their recommendation for or against this candidate should be based entirely on skills both patient and technical.

Following the working interview the team should meet to share thoughts regarding if the candidate's technical skills are a good fit for the position available.

Offer Letters

Usually the job has already been verbally offered and accepted prior to sending the official offer letter. However, the offer letter protects both the employer and employee by putting the terms of their verbal agreement about the job into writing. The terms stated in the offer letter include:

- Salary and how the employee can expect to be paid
- Probationary period
- Expected start date

Exploring the Web

LinkedIn
www.linkedin.com

This professional networking site does require that you register your information but there is no fee to do so.

Skill Building

1. Role-play interviewing a job candidate. Critique things that went well and things that could be improved.

2. Put together an employment plan. Be specific.

3. Write several employment ads; one for an administrative assistant, one for a highly experienced clinical assistant, one for an entry level clinical assistant, and one for a multifunctional assistant.

4. Write an offer letter to a job candidate.

5. Discuss receiving a resume with some words spelled incorrectly and how that would affect your perception of the job candidate. Would this eliminate the candidate from consideration? Why or why not?

6. Your clinical dental assistant is extremely moody. What impact does this have on the team? Discuss an improvement plan including a solution.

Challenge Your Understanding

1. Employment advertisements should contain:
   a. Salary for the position
   b. Preference for gender of the candidate
   c. Location of the job
   d. Request for a photo of applicant

2. Resumes received from candidates not getting an interview should be discarded immediately.
   a. True
   b. False

3. The attention to _____ in a resume may predict the candidate's job performance in the dental office.
   a. Detail
   b. Accuracy
   c. Personalization
   d. All of the above

4. An employee with great technical skills should stay employed regardless of attitude.
   a. True
   b. False

5. The primary goal of adding dental team members is:
   a. Hiring a person with excellent education
   b. Hiring a person that fits the practice mission statement
   c. Hiring a person with exceptional experience
   d. Hiring a person that is willing to work for the least salary

6. An employment offer letter should include all of the following except:
   a. Salary being offered
   b. Expected hours of employment
   c. When to expect a raise in salary
   d. Benefits included with the job

7. The job of the dental office manager is to screen job candidates for the position.
   a. True
   b. False

8. The best time to conduct a phone interview is:
   a. After 8 P.M. to give a candidate with children a chance to put them to bed
   b. After work but before 8 P.M.
   c. First thing in the morning before the potential candidate goes to his or her current job
   d. During the day so the job candidate's current employer knows he or she is looking for another job

9. The most efficient way of managing resumes received for an available position is:
   a. Scan hard copy resumes into your computer system
   b. Print resumes out when they are received electronically
   c. Saving only the top candidates so the number of resumes is manageable
   d. Have both a hard and electronic copy

10. A phone interview is the last step before employment.
    a. True
    b. False

11. Which of these dental team members may ask only questions regarding the ability to do the job when interviewing a candidate?
    a. Dentist
    b. Hygienist
    c. Dental office manager
    d. All of the above

12. Before terminating an employee, the dental office manager should inform the rest of the team so they are not surprised.
    a. True
    b. False

13. When doing a working interview, should the job candidate be paid?
    a. There is no salary for an interview
    b. Minimum wage as according to state law
    c. A wage similar to the starting wage you'll be paying the employee
    d. Salary plus an appropriate bonus

14. A working interview is beneficial to:
    a. The dentist
    b. The job candidate
    c. The dental team
    d. All of the above

15. To make a phone interview more efficient:
    a. Set a time limit so the interview stays on track
    b. Have a written set of questions to use as a guide
    c. Use the phone interview to only give information about the job
    d. Call the job candidate at their current job when they are busy

16. Because the appearance of a job candidate's teeth is important for a job in a dental office, it is appropriate to request a dental health exam as part of the application.
    a. True
    b. False

17. Examples of employees that negatively affect the morale of the dental team include all of the following except:
    a. The employee that brings personal problems to work
    b. An employee that comes to the office but doesn't share in the work
    c. The employee who misses an extended amount of work because of pregnancy
    d. An employee who is chronically absent with little or no notice

18. When reviewing resumes, the dental office manager can consider a candidate that has been trained on the job for all of the following positions except:
    a. Administrative support staff
    b. Clinical dental assistant
    c. Dental lab technician
    d. Dental hygienist

19. Final selection of a new employee that will fit into the practice is most effective when done by:
    a. Dentist
    b. Dental office manager
    c. Employees working closely with the new hire
    d. A combination of those groups

20. After applying for a job, the candidate should be prepared to answer a phone interview call.
    a. True
    b. False

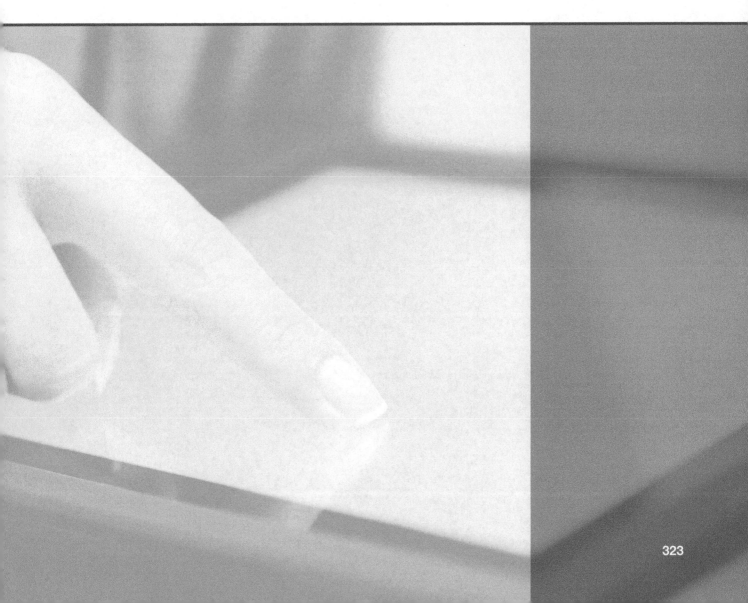

SECTION VI

The Use of Practice Management Software

CHAPTER 18

Dental Practice Management Software

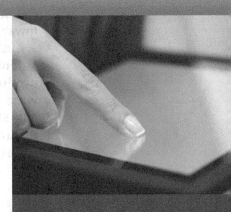

CHAPTER OUTLINES

- **Electronic Medical Records**
- **Dental Practice Management Software**
  Carestream Dental
  CurveDental
  Dentimax
  Dentrix
  EagleSoft
  EasyDental
  OCS Dental
  QSI
- **Use of the Dentrix Learning Edition CD**
  Installing the Dentrix G4 Learning CD
  User's Guide
  Registering Your Software
  Sample Practice
  Accessing Dentrix
  Web Sync Override
- **Summary**

LEARNING OBJECTIVES

Upon completion of this chapter, the reader should be able to:

1. Successfully install Dentrix Learning Software.
2. Register Dentrix Learning Software.
3. Access and navigate the Dentrix Learning Software.
4. List three dental management software programs in addition to Dentrix.

Electronic Medical Records

Making all medical records electronic by 2014 was a goal put into place in 2004 by former President Bush. Although the 2014 date is not mandated and did not specifically include dental records, many dental offices are moving toward paperless electronic charting and record keeping.

Integration of dental practice management software makes managing a dental practice more efficient and profitable; in addition, it increases productivity and also is user-friendly. Dental practice management software allows dental offices to organize patient information saving valuable staff time with activities such as accessing patient records, submitting insurance claims, sending appointment reminders, and handling patient correspondence.

Dental Practice Management Software

Dental offices have many excellent choices when it comes to choosing a dental software program. The Dentrix Learning software was chosen to be included in this text because of its popularity and ease of use. As a dental office manager, investigating other leaders in the dental software market will assist you in making an informed choice. The following is a short list of widely used dental practice management programs.

Carestream Dental

Carestream Dental offers several well-known multifunctional software programs to appeal to a large number of dental practices. Its products are server-based. Included are PracticeWorks and Softdent especially designed for family dental, periodontic, pedodontic, and prosthodontic offices; WinOMS for oral and maxillofacial surgeons; and OrthoTrac for orthodontists.

CurveDental

Software from CurveDental is cloud-based and doesn't need a server. Curve has very near 100 percent reliability because "crashes" are virtually eliminated. It is HIPAA-compliant even though data is stored outside of the dental office. Curve software offers a complete dental package including imaging.

Dentimax

Dentimax offers several simplified versions of full featured software on a server-based system. The software is marketed as easy to learn with training available on interactive CDs. Its dental imaging is compatible with 25 different digital radiography sensors.

Dentrix

Dentrix is available through well-known medical/dental supplier Henry Schein. It is a full-featured server-based software package with mobile capability for Apple iPad and voice activation. Dentrix offers training in dental offices and online.

EagleSoft

EagleSoft is a widely used market leader in dental practice management software. It is available through Patterson Technology and is a multifunctional server-based software package. EagleSoft offers easy access to staff training.

EasyDental

EasyDental's multifunctional software is marketed as easy to use and easy to own. It is server-based and uses Guru patient education that you will become familiar with through your Dentrix Learning CD.

OCS Dental

OCS has been publishing dental software since 1984. They provide full-featured front desk management programs on a server within the office.

QSI

QSI offers cloud-based multifunctional software that specializes in multioffice management. Because of the centralized data, it is easily accessed from multiple locations. It is HIPAA-compliant. Features include touch screen along with mouse and keyboard entry options, as well as, voice activated periodontal charting.

Use of the Dentrix Learning Edition CD

In the chapters throughout Section VI, the Dentrix Learning Edition CD will be used to provide an introduction to practice management software. This will provide a basic understanding of how software is used in a dental practice so students can be immediately productive in the office environment. Dental offices across the country use Dentrix for practice management so it is likely that the student will use it sometime during his or her career. Upon gaining confidence using Dentrix the student will be able to transfer these skills to dental software used in other dental offices as well.

When learning any new practice software system, there are several things that will improve your success:

- *Relax*: This is a learning environment so any mistakes made can be easily reversed so don't be hesitant to explore the system. Even in an office environment, errors can be edited easily as long as it is done before the end of the day.

- *Set a goal to improve keyboarding skills*: You will enjoy working with dental software more if you can add information quickly and accurately.

- *Practice, practice, practice*: Practicing with the software will build confidence and speed.

Installing the Dentrix G4 Learning CD

Before beginning to install the CD there are several important steps to follow. By following the instructions carefully, the installation will be successful and problems will be minimized.

1. Your computer system will need to meet the system requirements.
2. You will need adequate disk space available.
3. Make sure all other applications are closed when you install the CD.
4. Read the instructions for installation carefully.
5. Complete the entire installation process.

Insert the CD into the disk drive; the welcome screen should appear (Figure 18-1). There are several important items on this screen including instructions and prompt for installation of the G4 Learning CD. Review the Important Installation tips, which you will see at the top of your welcome screen, second from the left.

During the installation process, the Dentrix software will evaluate your computer system for compatibility. You will see the screen "Dentrix System Requirements Notice," showing you the system requirements along with your existing computer system. If all the check marks are green you are ready to proceed. Any component marked with a red "X" indicates a potential problem that could cause the installation to fail or cause the Dentrix software to run less efficiently. Correcting any issues appearing with a red "X" before proceeding will increase the potential for a successful installation and satisfaction with the software.

When installing the Dentrix Learning Edition, there are several times you will be prompted to continue the installation by selecting "Next" at the bottom of the screen. For example, Dentrix will confirm you have read the installation instructions and licensing agreements before continuing. For the easiest setup,

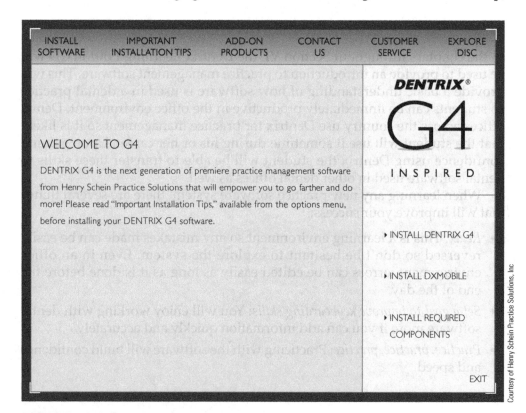

FIGURE 18-1 Dentrix welcome screen.

hit "Next" to continue with the recommended installation. You will also want to install the *Guru Limited Edition Server*; follow the instructions to do so. Last, you will need to allow access through your computers firewall; you can do this automatically by selecting yes or you can modify your firewall manually if you prefer.

> **HELPFUL HINT**
>
> Throughout this section we will be working with the Dentrix program; your instructions are shown in numbered bold text for easy identification. Read instructions carefully before attempting the task. Additional information is in regular text and hints will be provided throughout.

The installation process is fast but it does take a few minutes so make sure you allow yourself enough time to complete it.

1. Go to "Install Software" on the right side of the screen under the G4 logo and begin your installation.
2. Remember, let your software install completely!

User's Guide

When the Dentrix Learning Edition CD installation is complete, you will see some new icons or short cuts on your desktop that will make it easy to access patient records and information. Among those icons, you will see the User's Guide Icon (Figure 18-2). The User's Guide will answer questions you may have as you work through these exercises or questions you have in the future. Even daily Dentrix users refer to the User's Guide when doing tasks that occur only occasionally or making changes to their practice setup. The User's Guide is also available from the Start menu and from drop-down menus throughout the software.

FIGURE 18-2
Dentrix User's Guide Icon.
Courtesy of Henry Schein Practice Solutions, Inc

> **HELPFUL HINT**
>
> Sullivan Schein technical support does not assist users of the Dentrix Learning Software so if you have a problem you will need to consult the User's Guide for an answer.

1. **Double Click on the User's Guide Icon now.**

   The User's Guide has more than 1,000 pages so you'll want to refer to your computer copy instead of printing it. At this time, read through the table of contents to see the variety of things you can learn to do with Dentrix. There is a page counter to allow you to get to any topic you would like to read more about. Let's practice.

2. **Find page 6 in your User's Guide by typing 6 in the page count box and click on enter.**

   You will discover a guide to important to know icons that Dentrix uses to make navigation easy. The User's Guide will show you two examples of the icon. The icon on the left was used in earlier versions of Dentrix that are still used in many dental offices and the icon to the right is the newer version. Most of the icons are descriptive in their graphics but reading through these will help you as we proceed through the exercises.

3. **Continue exploring the User's Guide until you feel comfortable finding information quickly.**

Registering Your Software

During the setup process, you will be asked if you would like to register your Learning CD.

Registering your Dentrix Learning CD is optional. If you have Internet access and would like to use some of the online learning tools, you must register your Dentrix Learning CD. It is easy and will enable you to access the *On Demand Training* resources. To register the Learning CD you will need to enter an email address and a password of your choice. After you complete the registration information, a code will arrive via email using which you can login. Your email address is not used to send you advertising or spam.

If you choose not to register your CD, this textbook will still guide you through using the Dentrix practice management software.

FIGURE 18-3
Dentrix Toolbar Icon.
Courtesy of Henry Schein Practice Solutions, Inc

Sample Practice

The Dentrix Learning CD is preloaded with a complete staff and 71 patients. It is also possible to add patients up to a total of 100. Although you can't change the staff, you can work with the patient charts to practice and learn with the existing staff members already on the CD.

Accessing Dentrix

There are several easy ways to start the Dentrix software after you have installed the program.

1. You can use your start menu, go to programs, find Dentrix and then select the function you would like to use.

2. Dentrix has installed a quick start button on your tool bar (the lower right hand icons on your computer screen). This button shows a graphic of a white circle with a dark red tooth in the middle of it (Figure 18-3). Right clicking on the icon will allow you to select specific functions within the practice management system.

3. From your desktop you can also select the shortcut icon for the function you would like to use.

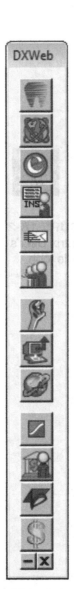

Web Sync Override

Dentrix uses an automatic Web sync that is set to run every day at the same time of day. Although this is great in an office, it makes more sense to run it only as required as you are learning the system.

1. **Go to Web Sync Reminder icon on your lower toolbar and right click. A tool bar will open (Figure 18-4).**

2. **Select the button for settings (a wrench icon) and then select Web Sync Wizard.**

3. **Set the Web Sync to run only when requested.**

FIGURE 18-4
Dentrix Web Sync Toolbar.
Courtesy of Henry Schein Practice Solutions, Inc

Summary

This section of the textbook is designed to help you become a confident Dentrix user by not only guiding you through common office tasks but also showing you how to accomplish tasks you will use only occasionally.

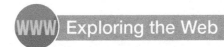

Exploring the Web

www.carestream.com

www.curvedental.com

www.dentimax.com

www.dentrix.com

www.patterson.eaglesoft.net

www.easydental.com

www.ocsdental

Challenge Your Understanding

1. All dental offices must be paperless by:
   a. 2015
   b. 2012
   c. There is no specific dental mandate
   d. 2014

2. Dental practice management software allows offices to:
   a. Eliminate staff
   b. Increase productivity
   c. Access patient records quickly
   d. Both b and c

3. Which of these will improve your dental software skills?
   a. Relax
   b. Improve your keyboarding
   c. Practice
   d. All of the above

4. Registering your learning software will:
   a. Give you access to tech support
   b. Allow you access to On Demand Training
   c. Allow you to add and delete staff members
   d. All of the above

5. To use On Demand Training you must:
   a. Have Internet access.
   b. Have Dentrix correctly installed
   c. Find the help drop down
   d. All of the above

CHAPTER 19

Entering, Updating, and Maintaining Patient Information

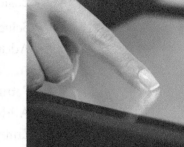

CHAPTER OUTLINES

- **Managing Patient Charts**
  Selecting a Patient
  Adding a New Patient
  Adding Patient Photos
  Adding Medical Alerts
  Adding a Patient Referral
  Insurance Information
- **Summary**

LEARNING OBJECTIVES

Upon completion of this chapter, the reader should be able to:

1. Demonstrate retrieving patient information using different search methods.
2. Demonstrate entering a family group into Dentrix.
3. Demonstrate entering a new patient including employment and insurance information.
4. Accurately add a patient referral source.
5. Successfully add a medical alert to a patient chart.
6. Demonstrate how to add patient insurance information for both primary and secondary carriers.
7. Organize new insurance companies in your established database.

KEY TERMS

head of household
medical alert
primary insurance
referral
secondary insurance
toolbar

Managing Patient Charts

One of the main functions of all practice management software is adding and retrieving patient information. With dental software, all the patient charts are easily accessed on the computer; however, it is still necessary to locate patient records and add or update information.

Basic patient management tasks include the following:

- Selecting a patient
- Adding a new patient
- Adding a patient photo
- Setting up a family file
- Adding medical alerts
- Entering referral sources for tracking
- Adding or updating patient insurance information

Selecting a Patient

1. **For this exercise start Dentrix by going to the start menu, select Programs, select Dentrix Learning Edition, and then select Family File. You can also click on the Family File shortcut icon or right click on the quick start button from the toolbar at the lower right of your screen and then click on Family File.** If you have completed the task correctly you should be looking at the screen pictured in Figure 19-1: Dentrix Family File.

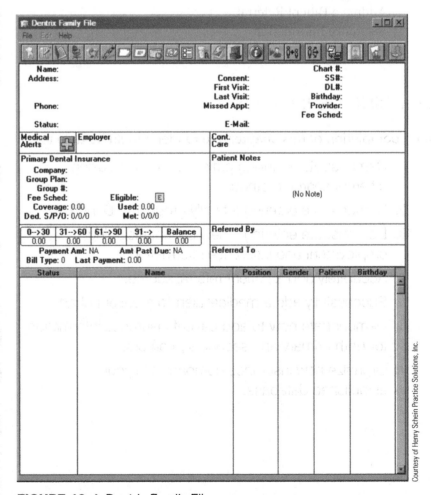

FIGURE 19-1 Dentrix Family File

At the top left you will see identification of this screen as the Dentrix Family File. Underneath you will see "File" and "Help." The option "File" will allow you to access several tasks that are indicated as instructions by the bold text in this book. The "Help" button gives an overview of the family file as well as additional information about services available through Dentrix. "Help" also allows you access to the user's manual information through specific tasks listed in contents. The next line is your toolbar; it has icons to allow you to move through the Dentrix program.

2. **Without clicking on the icons, move the cursor along the toolbar to learn the function of each one.**

Currently the information on the screen is blank so the next step is to "Select a Patient." The "Select a Patient" icon is found toward the right side of the toolbar (Figure 19-2). Locating patient information is a task that every member of the dental team does throughout the day so it is important that you should be able to do this quickly. You will see this icon throughout the program so you can select a patient from most Dentrix screens.

FIGURE 19-2
Select Patient button
Courtesy of Henry Schein Practice Solutions, Inc.

Dentrix allows you to search for a patient in six different ways:

- By name last/first
- By name first/last
- By preferred name such as a nickname
- By home phone number
- By chart number
- By social security number

Once you choose how you would like to search for a patient, Dentrix will continue to search using this method until you reset the selection method. When there are multiple computer users, generally an office will leave the system set to one search method but it's always nice to have an alternative.

> **HELPFUL HINT**
> If you reset the search criteria remember to change it back. If the criteria that the employees normally use are changed, it is frustrating for other employees to use the system.

Think about why you may need to search for a patient using a method other than the patient's name. If the primary search method (usually name) returns no result, and the patient has seen the doctor before, another search method needs to be used to locate the patient record. The most common reason why this would happen may be because of an error made in spelling the patient's name when it was originally entered into the system. By having an alternate search method, it is still possible to retrieve the patient's information.

3. **Using the toolbar, find the "Select Patient/New Family" icon and click on it bringing up the "Select a Patient" dialog box as seen in Figure 19-3: Select a Patient.**

In the upper right of the screen are the "Search By" choices, this is set to last name. To select a patient, simply start typing the last name; as you add letters the number of patients to choose from is reduced and the selection becomes easy.

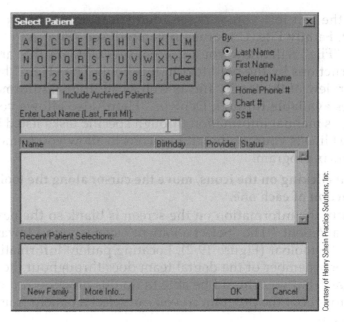

Courtesy of Henry Schein Practice Solutions, Inc.

FIGURE 19-3 Select a Patient dialogue box

HELPFUL HINT

This function is helpful if you aren't sure how to spell the name. In a small family practice, patients expect you to know who they are. If you can remember how the name begins, Dentrix can help you identify the patient with a small amount of information.

---

4. **The cursor is set automatically in the selection field. Begin using the patient "Henry Myers" from the Dentrix tutorial database for this exercise. Start typing his last name, do this slowly so you can see how it reduces the number of patients available for selection with each letter you type. Experiment with typing his name incorrectly to see what happens.**

5. **When you have identified Henry as the patient you are looking for, double click on the highlighted line or on OK and his information, along with anyone in his family group, will be displayed.**

6. **As you look at the family file note the information at the top including address and personal information; it will also have insurance information and a list of family members.**

7. **By double clicking on the patient's name from the list you can switch between family members.**

8. **By double clicking on one of the squares within the screen, for example "Patient Information," you can edit it.**

HELPFUL HINT

In practice, you will have patients updating their personal information and this is one point to make that change. It will change the information for everyone in that family file.

---

9. **Practice moving around the family file until you can do it easily and with confidence.**

Adding a New Patient

You can also add a new patient/new family from this screen.

1. **To add a new patient you do not have to move from the current family file screen. Just choose the icon for "Select a Patient" that was used in the previous exercise.**

2. **You will see the same dialog box you used to type in the patient's name to select a patient. At the lower edge of that box is a "New Family" button for patients not already in the database.**

> **HELPFUL HINT**
>
> Occasionally you will encounter a patient who is certain he or she saw the doctor a long time ago and can't recall if their information is in the computer system. Before entering this patient as a new patient and accidently creating a duplicate chart, try marking the archived patient box directly under the number/letter pad at the top right of the dialog box. This will allow you to see if their patient information is available and stored in your system. If you retrieve a patient from archive don't forget to update his or her information.

3. **Dentrix groups patients into family units so you will want to begin creating the family group with the head of household; usually this person is the person financially responsible for the account or the person who carries dental insurance for the family. After determining the patient or family is indeed new and who the head of household is, just enter their information in the fields provided. A non-patient can be the head of household, just choose the appropriate patient or non-patient status from the drop-down menu. Accuracy is important, so it is better to leave a field blank than to fill it with incorrect information. Add the following new patient information using Figure 19-4 as an example.**

   Robin Belinda Cooper
   Female
   Preferred name: Binky
   D.O.B. 12/10/1970
   Salutation: Robin
   2145 Wright Avenue
   Jacobs, Washington 91319
   Home: 101-555-0154
   Work: 101-555-5445
   Email: cooperfamily@email.com
   Driver's License WA522780
   Assign primary provider as Dennis Smith
   Assign secondary provider as Sally Hayes RDH
   Patient requests no phone calls
   Allergic to codeine
   Heart murmur

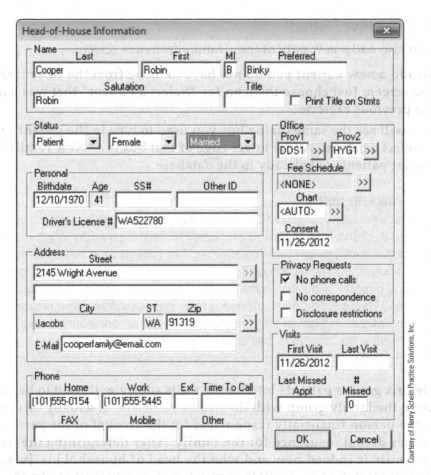

FIGURE 19-4 Entering a new patient

4. **You can increase your speed by entering patients using the tab key to jump to the next field. If the patient has a preferred name such as a nickname make sure you include it. By knowing what a patient likes being called you help create a more personal practice; however, you should use a formal/legal name in the name field so that insurance forms or future referrals will be accurate and more professional. The salutation field can be used to indicate a name you would like to use for written correspondence. At this point you can assign a status to the patient such as patient, inactive, or non-patient from the drop-down menu.**

> **HELPFUL HINT**
>
> Remember preferred name is also a patient search category so if a patient identifies himself or herself by a preferred name you can also search by that name.

5. **There is a field for email address. This is helpful if your office sends reminders, confirmations, or any correspondence electronically. Several fields are available for phone numbers. If you are using an auto-dialing system for confirmation calls, it will use the home number field as the**

number it calls. When entering a phone number you do not need to include dashes or hyphens.

6. At the right of the new patient information there are additional fields, such as provider, which is helpful in multiple doctor offices. There is also an area for privacy requests. If your office has multiple hygienists you can use provider 2 as a hygiene preference.

7. When you have completed the necessary information, click on OK and you have a new family file.

8. Entering the next family member is easy; on the toolbar next to the "Select a Patient" you will see a stick figure with a plus sign pointing to another stick figure to its right. When you click on the icon a window will open that allows you to add another patient as part of this family. Notice Dentrix has already completed the address and other details for you. Add the rest of Robin Cooper's family members to the group (Figure 19-5).

> Timothy Cooper, husband, D.O.B. 5/13/1969
>
> Male
>
> Timothy's preferred name is Tim
>
> Marianne Cooper, daughter, D.O.B. 7/22/2002
>
> Marianne's preferred name is Mari
>
> Female

9. Congratulations. You know how to enter a patient into Dentrix and create a new family group. With practice you will become faster and the process effortless.

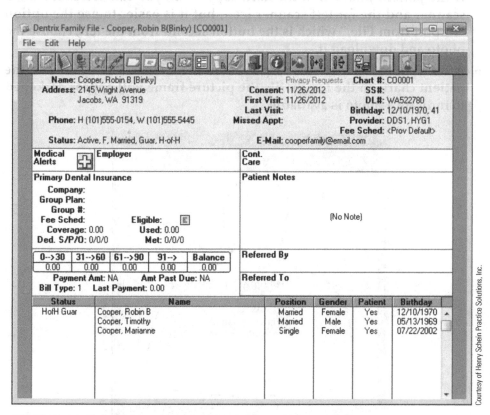

FIGURE 19-5 Addition of family members to a family file

Adding Patient Photos

Having photos of patients in the chart is becoming a valuable part of treatment planning. It can also be helpful to put a name to a face as you are taking a phone call or to identify patients as they arrive for appointments. Adding a photo takes just a few minutes. If you are just looking for nontechnical facial recognition photos it will only require a simple digital camera. Detailed intra-oral photos require a special camera and lighting.

1. **Take photos and download them into a file where they can be edited. Even if the photo is good, you'll probably want to be able to crop it and adjust the lighting.**

2. **Select a patient either by using the patient with the arrow icon or you could also use the file drop-down menu at the upper left.**

3. **Look for the icon of the patient in a picture frame on the toolbar.**

4. **Selecting that icon will open the Dentrix Patient Photo dialog box (Figure 19-6).**

5. **If the patient photo is in the hard copy form, you can access it from a scanner and the far left scanner icon, but it is easier to use the option "Import from File," which is the button second from the left; choose the photo and download it.**

6. **After a photo is added it is displayed on the toolbar when you open the patient chart; on the family file the picture frame will appear darkened to indicate a photo is available.**

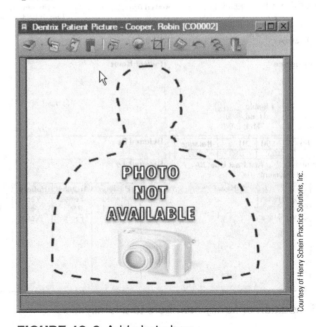

FIGURE 19-6 Add photo box

Adding Medical Alerts

It is the responsibility of every member of the dental team to keep patients safe and a part of doing that is adding medical alerts to a chart. Staff members can't assume someone else will add important changes in medical history. It is fast and easy.

1. **Go to the family file and select the correct patient, use Pat Abbott.**

   The Medical Alert area is clearly marked with a cross right under the box containing the patient's name. When the cross is red, there is an alert on the patient chart; when it is uncolored no alert exists.

2. **When you click on the cross icon the medical alert dialog box will open (Figure 19-7). If an alert already exists you will see what it is, and you can add an alert or edit one.**

   Pat Abbott has an excellent example of an alert that will need editing. She is currently pregnant. When the office becomes aware of her delivery that medical alert will be removed.

3. **By clicking on "Edit" a list of medical conditions will open; highlighting the appropriate condition and clicking OK will add the alert or**

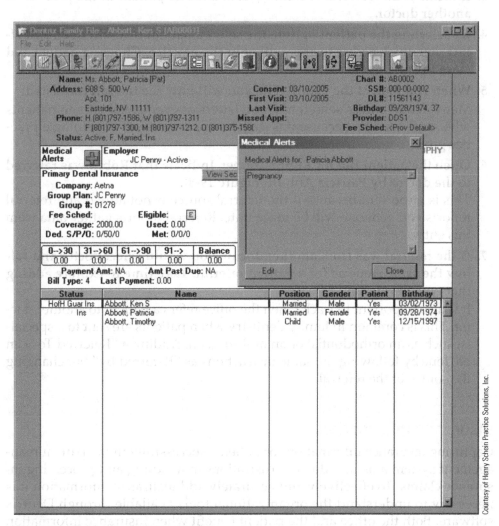

FIGURE 19-7 Medical Alert box

highlight the condition you would like to eliminate, clicking "Clear" will remove it.

Please note this is different from the patient alert icon on the toolbar that is illustrated by a patient with a white or yellow flag.

For practice: add the condition of fainting to Pat Abbott's chart. Confirm it is part of the chart, and then remove it and the pregnancy alert. Confirm that they are gone.

4. **Add the medical alerts for Robin Cooper from her information.**

Adding a Patient Referral

Referral information is one of the most important parts of helping the practice grow. Tracking referrals helps gain an understanding of how new patients are finding the practice. Patient management software provides an easy method of capturing and tracking this data.

1. **Double click on the "Referred By" box on the Family File screen (it is located just under patient notes) to add the information.**

2. **Select "Add Referral."**

3. **Indicate if this referral is coming from another patient in the practice or another doctor.**

4. **By selecting the patient option, the select a patient box will open and allow you quick access to any patient in the practice. Choose a patient and close this dialog box.**

5. **When you look at the Family File you will now see the referral listed.**
   Many dental offices send thank you letters or even small gifts to patients who send referrals because it is such an important part of helping a practice grow.

6. **Open the patient file for Robin Cooper. Indicate that Robin was referred to the doctor by Patricia Abbott (Figure 19-8).**
   This is important because if the referral source is not added any referral reports you generate will be inaccurate. Referral reports gather data from this entry.

7. **If the referral was from another doctor, you would select doctor and follow the same steps as for a patient referral. Take time to explore adding that type of referral.**
   It is also important to track when the office refers a patient to another doctor. This is common in family dentistry when patients are sent to a specialist such as an orthodontist or an oral surgeon. Adding a "Referred To" can be done by following the same instructions as "Referred By" but changing the source of the referral.

Insurance Information

Capturing insurance information for patients successfully in the patient management system aids in reducing frustrations in handling and processing insurance claims. To effectively and accurately add insurance information it is necessary to understand the organizational tools available through Dentrix software. Both the office and the patient benefit when insurance information is accurate.

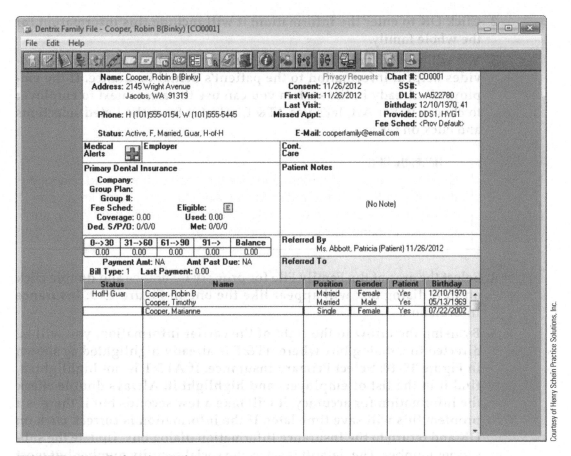

FIGURE 19-8 Referral notations

Adding a Primary Insurance Carrier

The first step in assuring accuracy of insurance claims is when adding insurance information to the Family File. If family members have insurance with different carriers, make sure all carrier information is included.

> ┌─ **HELPFUL HINT**
>
> Look for multiple insurance companies when both parents are insured. It would not be uncommon for the husband and wife to each carry policies through their employers and any children could be insured with either parent or even both. Dual insurance is less common now than in the past; however, you still may run into families who have dual insurance and should be aware of how to capture the information.

1. **Start by going to the Family File and selecting Arthur Blank as your patient.**

   Begin by adding his personal details:

   Preferred name: Art

   Address: 4527 Main St.

   Centerville, NV 55555

   Birth date: 09/05/1967

   SS#: 222-33-8407

   Email: blankfamily@gmail.com

   Home phone: 602-555-1212

2. Click OK to enter the information; it will include this information for the whole family.

3. You will want to enter the employer information because often this provides helpful information to the patient's dental insurance. If the employer is already in the system you can use the arrow next to employer to choose it. For Art, let's use AT&T; select it from the listed selections and click on OK.

> **HELPFUL HINT**
> Changing the address information for the head of household changes that information for the entire family. Adding something like an employer only adds it for the individual family member whose file you are working in when you make the addition.

4. Select the area of the Family File for primary insurance and double click on it. A dialog box will appear like the one in Figure 19-9: Insurance Information.

5. By using the arrow to the right of the carrier information, you will be directed to a dialog box where AT&T is already highlighted as shown in Figure 19-10: Select Primary Insurance. If AT&T is not highlighted, find it in the list of employers and highlight it. Always double check the information for accuracy, it will take a few seconds but if there is a problem this will save time later. If the information is correct, click on OK and return to the Insurance Information dialog box. Update the subscriber number. The default is set as the social security number but most

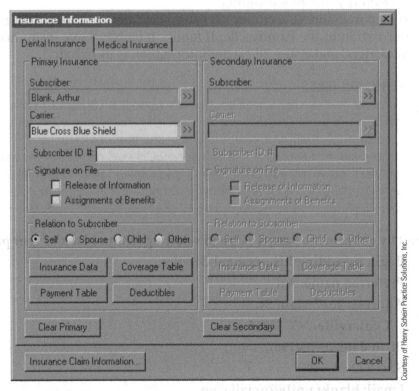

FIGURE 19-9 Insurance box

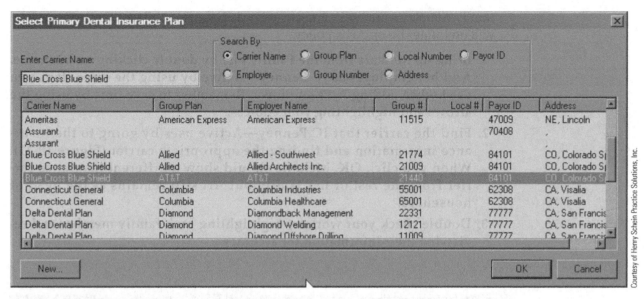

FIGURE 19-10 Primary Insurance selection box

patients will have another identifier on their insurance card to comply with privacy laws.

6. **If your patient has signed a form for:**

Release of Information **allowing for the office to submit the claim on the patient's behalf or to speak to the insurance company if there are questions regarding treatment. Make sure to check that box.**

Or

Assignment of Benefits, **which means that the insurance payment is sent directly to the dentist. Make sure to check that box unless the patient has already paid you directly.**

> **HELPFUL HINT**
>
> Always remember the contract with the insurance company is between the insurance company and the patient. You are filing as a courtesy to the patient but the policy and responsibility for payment belongs to the patient. This is different if you are working on a claim for a patient on public assistance.

Currently you have created the primary insurance for the head of household; we need to determine who else is covered under this policy. Art also carries the children as dependents on this policy.

7. **To add the children to this carrier: from the Family File screen highlight the child's name (we'll use Kendra) and double click. You will see the name at the top of the file is now Kendra. To add the insurance for her, double click the primary insurance box (it is currently empty) to bring up the Insurance Information. By using the arrows to the right of subscriber you will see Arthur's name highlighted. If you click OK, Kendra now has Blue Cross/Blue Shield insurance as part of her record.**

For practice: We'll add JC Penney as Melanie Blank's employer and add the company's dental insurance for her. It is an individual policy and no other family members are on it. For our records because she has this coverage, she will no longer be on Art's policy.

1. Bring up Melanie from the Family File by double clicking on her name. Add her employer as JC Penney—Active by using the same steps you used when adding Art's employer. Remember to save time by using the arrows and highlighting your choices.

2. Find the carrier that JC Penney—Active uses by going to the insurance information and finding the appropriate carrier (Figure 19-11). When you click OK, Melanie should show a different insurance carrier from the rest of her family but Art still remains as the head of household.

3. Double check your work by highlighting each family member and reviewing their information for accuracy.

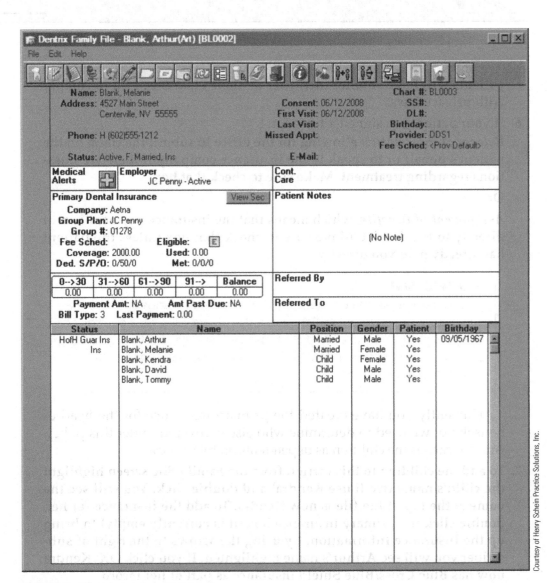

FIGURE 19-11 Adding Child to Insurance

> **HELPFUL HINT**
>
> To the right of insurance information is the patient note area. You can add reminders about things that are important to this patient or that may be useful in the future. One thing you might want to note is if a college-age child is still a full-time student. Within the patient note area you can insert a dateline and select hide or view.

4. **Add a note for Kendra Blank that the insurance company has her name spelled incorrectly (Figure 19-12). Remember the chart is a legal document; make sure your notes are professional.**

Adding Secondary Insurance

1. **Adding a secondary insurance company follows the same pattern as adding a primary company. For this exercise, we'll add Melanie Blank's**

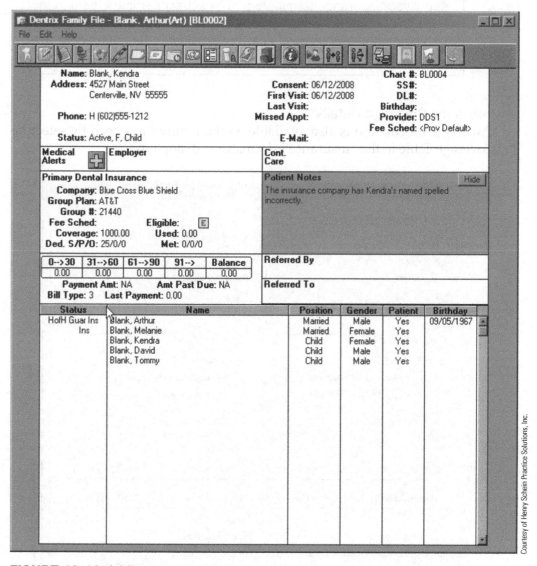

FIGURE 19-12 Adding a note to a record

Courtesy of Henry Schein Practice Solutions, Inc.

insurance as a secondary insurer for Art. Start by bringing up Art Blank from the Family File because his information is what we are changing. Double click the primary insurance box on the Family File sheet to access the insurance information dialog box. You will see the primary insurance information completed on the left and an area for secondary insurance information on the right.

2. On the secondary insurance side, use the subscriber arrow to see the choices for coverage. Melanie and Art will both be listed. For secondary coverage, you should, use Melanie's policy so highlight her name and click on okay. When you return to the Insurance Information dialog box for Art Blank you will see Melanie's Aetna policy added as the secondary carrier (shown in Figure 19-13: Adding secondary insurance). Also notice, Dentrix has automatically added the relationship to subscriber for you.

> **HELPFUL HINT**
>
> Know your insurance terminology. The subscriber is the person that owns the policy. This may or may not be the patient. The carrier is the company providing coverage. The provider is the doctor or professional who treated the patient.

Insurance Coverage Details

Coverage information is also available on the family file screen by selecting Coverage Table in the "insurance information" dialog box.

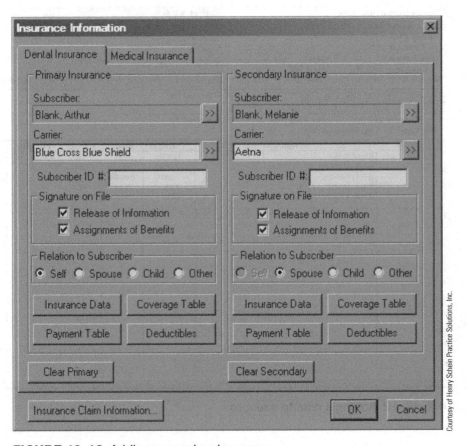

FIGURE 19-13 Adding secondary insurance

1. Bring up Art Blank in the Family File information and look at his primary dental insurance. It will show Art's annual coverage and how much of the allowable amount has already been used. His deductibles are also listed in categories of: standard, preventive, or other (s/p/o).

   It is quick and easy to see how much of each of those deductibles have been met. Because you have added secondary coverage for Art you will see a "View Sec" box in the upper right corner, by clicking it you can see the same information for the secondary carrier.

2. Double click on the primary insurance information. When you see the Insurance Information dialog box you will be able to find specific information for both primary and secondary.

3. Explore the insurance information seen in Figure 19-13: Insurance Information, by clicking on each of the following:
   - Insurance Data
   - Coverage Table
   - Payment Table
   - Deductibles
   - Insurance Claim Information

> **HELPFUL HINT**
>
> To clear the primary or secondary insurance you could use the clear buttons at the lower edge of the screen. If you hit one of the clear keys by accident, the information will disappear but if you choose to cancel the action it will not be deleted. If you click OK instead of cancel you will need to reenter it.

Entering New Insurance Information

It is likely that you will need to add new insurance carriers for some patients.

1. Choose Shawna Nelson as your next patient in the database. Currently she doesn't have insurance so you'll be able to add a company for her. Under her employer, add self-employed. Shawna has an insurance card with her for Assurant Dental. Access the insurance information by double clicking the primary insurance area of the Family File.

2. Click on the carrier search arrows. Take a moment to look down the list to make sure Assurant is not already listed before adding it. The easiest way to search is by carrier name so choose that as the "Search By" feature. Once you are sure you want to add a company, click the "New" button at the bottom of the dialog box.

3. At this point, assuming Shawna was your patient you would have her insurance card available to add the information for this screen as seen in Figure 19-14: Dental Insurance Plan Information. For this exercise just use Assurant as the carrier and leave other fields blank. Drop down to payer information and use the arrow to see a list of insurance companies. There are three Assurant Insurance companies so find the one that matches the patient's information and add the payer number to the plan information. For this exercise choose Assurant Employee Benefits. Leave the options unchecked, click OK, and return to the Insurance

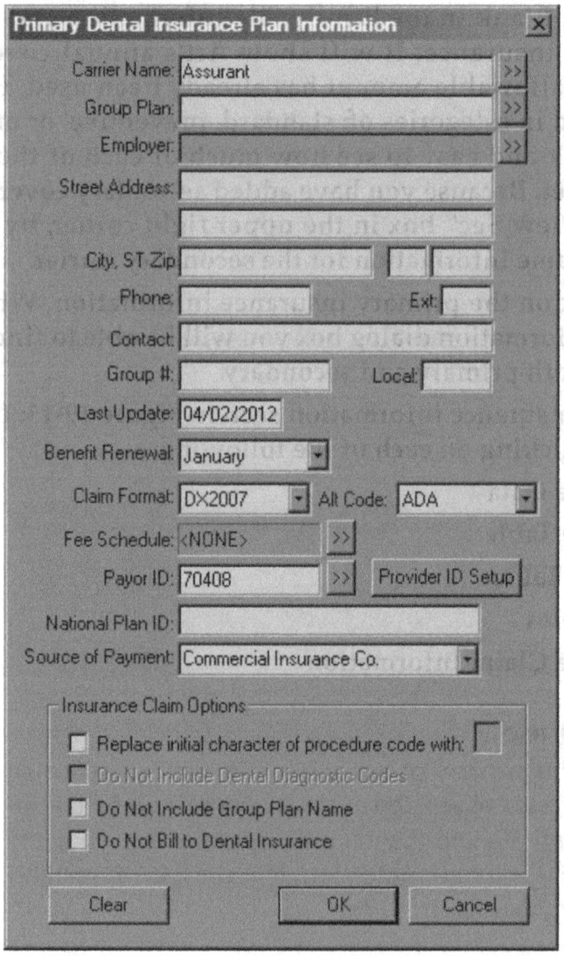

Courtesy of Henry Schein Practice Solutions, Inc.

FIGURE 19-14 Adding a new insurance company

Information dialog box and follow the steps to add an existing carrier until you see Assurant in the carrier information.

4. Now practice modifying the Coverage Table by clicking on it so you can add deductibles and maximums. To an annual individual deductible of $50 and Annual Maximum of $2,000 Individual and $4,000 Family. You do not need to include the $ sign when entering the information.

5. On the coverage table (Figure 19-15): Insurance coverage table, we'll change the coverage on crowns from 50 percent to 60 percent. Highlight the coverage line for crowns to see it displayed at the top of the list; make the change. At the right of the dialog box, click on the change button to change the coverage. When you click OK to exit the dialog box, Dentrix will tell you that coverage has been edited and all the patients with this plan will be affected. In this instance, go ahead and click OK to make the change.

6. Take a moment to verify that Shawna's insurance is exactly the way you want it. Congratulations you have just added a new insurance company to your carrier selections.

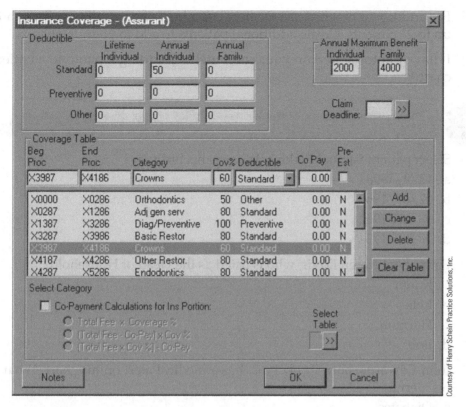

FIGURE 19-15 Insurance coverage table

Summary

Accessing existing patient information and creating accurate complete patient charts are tasks that are done repeatedly throughout the day in a dental office by administrative and clinical staff. Mastering these skills will increase your value to the dental team and will have a personal reward of reducing job stress.

Learning dental software can at times seem overwhelming; however, consider that it eliminates locating paper charts and looking through notes, that at times may be illegible, and it will make it worthwhile. Your success with dental practice management software is up to you.

 Skill Building

1. If you have Internet access, watch the *"On Demand Training"* videos and take the quiz for each:
    *   An Introduction to Dentrix
    *   Viewing and Navigating the Family File
    *   Adding Patient and Family Information
    *   Adding Employers and Insurance Carriers
    *   Assigning Insurance to Patients

2. Using the patients from Appendix A at the back of your book, create family files for Rachel Anthony, Thomas Lane, Janet Bruce, and Clayton Lewis. Make sure you include family members and insurance information.

3. For additional practice, the Dentrix Learning Software allows you to add up to 21 patients. Create additional patients to add to your database.

4. If have photos stored on your computer, try adding a photo to a patient chart.

 Challenge Your Understanding

1. Select patient Samuel Perkins. When is his birthday?
   a. 12/4/1998
   b. 07/05/1960
   c. 08/05/1962
   d. 09/05/1954

2. For patient Karen Davis, who is listed as the Head of Household?
   a. Karen
   b. Lyle
   c. Harmon
   d. Bob

3. John Edwards, born 7/14/1962, has a medical alert on his chart. What is his alert for?
   a. Diabetes
   b. Epilepsy
   c. Heart Murmur
   d. High Blood Pressure

4. Your patient, Harmon Davis, would like to know what percentage of endodontic treatment is covered by his dental insurance plan.
   a. 50%
   b. 70%
   c. No endo coverage
   d. 80%

5. What is the group number for Kimberly (Kim) Edward's insurance plan?
   a. VC
   b. 88442
   c. 442
   d. 1500

6. Which of the following is Michelle Keller's maximum annual insurance benefit?
   a. $1,500
   b. $1,000
   c. $1,900
   d. $2,500

7. Spencer Kenner would like to get braces. What percentage of his treatment would be covered?
   a. 50% up to $1,000 per person or $3,000 per family annually
   b. 60% up to $1,500 per person
   c. 50% up to $1,900 per person
   d. 50% with a $1,500 lifetime max for orthodontics

8. Chad Little has dual insurance coverage. What is his annual maximum for the primary carrier?
   a. $1,000 per individual
   b. $2,000 per individual
   c. $1,500 per family
   d. $1,900 per family

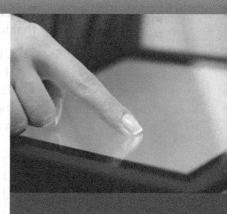

CHAPTER 20

Clinical Records

CHAPTER OUTLINES

- **Patient's Clinical Chart**
  Periodontal Charting
- **Making Treatment Plans**
- **Prescriptions**
- **Summary**

LEARNING OBJECTIVES

Upon completion of this chapter, the reader should be able to:

1. Demonstrate dental charting.
2. Demonstrate periodontal charting.
3. Successfully enter treatment notes into the clinical chart.
4. Successfully edit information within the clinical chart.
5. Accurately set up a patient treatment plan.

FIGURE 20-1
Patient Chart icon.
Courtesy of Henry Schein Practice Solutions, Inc.

Patient's Clinical Chart

To access Dentrix, open the family file screen and on the tool bar look for the single tooth icon on the far left representing the patient chart (Figure 20-1). Patient charts containing clinical information are accessed by clicking on that icon.

1. **Click on the icon now and start by examining the tool bar for this screen (Figure 20-2).**

   This tool bar has some additional choices when compared to the last toolbar used. Once again take a moment to move the cursor along each icon without clicking on them for a description.

   > **HELPFUL HINT**
   >
   > Dental offices can make changes to this toolbar to create one that works efficiently for them. If you are working in a new office, take a minute to look at the toolbar and familiarize yourself with their commonly used icons and their positions on the toolbar. However, don't make changes to the toolbar without discussing with other team members.

2. **On the tool bar, you will see the familiar "Select a Patient" icon so let's start by clicking there and selecting Robin Cooper (Figure 20-3).**

   The patient chart contains the patient clinical charting and a note page where in addition to the procedure the doctor, hygienist, or assistant can add comments regarding treatment. You can see the treatment notes, both progress and clinical, at the bottom of the chart. Figure 20-4 demonstrates the notes field on the chart.

   With paper charting, it is necessary to do the charting illustration and add treatment notes separately; a computerized system allows both tasks to be done at the same time as well as allowing creation of a treatment plan. Robin is an excellent candidate because her chart is blank so we will add some existing treatment for her. This would be treatment already done either in your office or by a previous dentist. We will use EO for existing other and Ex, in blue, for treatment done by this office. The other status choices are Tx, in red, for treatment planned, which would be assigned to any treatment needed and the check mark is for completed treatment.

   Charting with Dentrix is just like traditional charting except that instead of using a red and blue pencil you are using a keyboard.

3. First let's indicate that all her wisdom teeth or third molars were previously extracted by an oral surgeon not in this office. **Using the mouse, move the cursor (that now looks like an explorer) and highlight teeth numbers 1, 16, 17, and 32 by clicking on them.** When highlighting multiple teeth, hold down the control key on the keyboard while

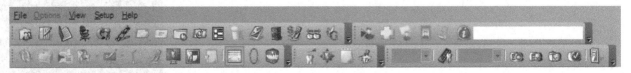

FIGURE 20-2 Tool bar on patient chart.
Courtesy of Henry Schein Practice Solutions, Inc.

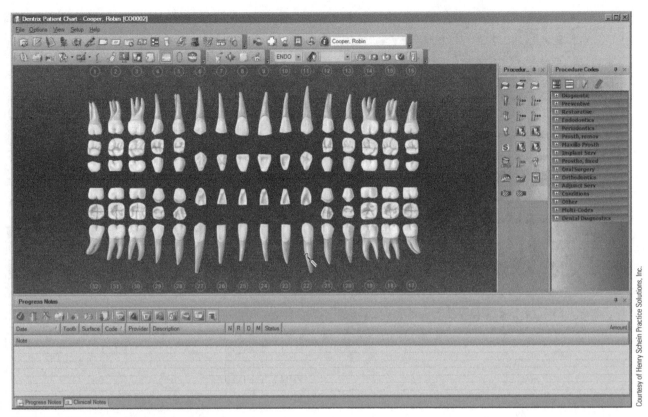

FIGURE 20-3   Patient clinical chart.

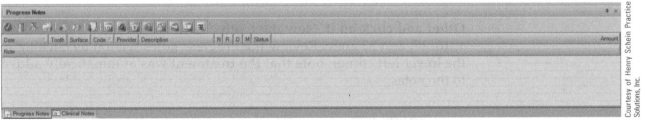

FIGURE 20-4   Progress notes.

clicking on the teeth in the illustration. If you are successful, those teeth will appear with a lighter aura around them as shown in Figure 20-5 (Patient Chart).

4. Now that the teeth are selected, choose a code or procedure. Because they were done in another office all that is known is they are gone. It is not possible to know the extraction procedure used to remove them. At the far right of the tooth chart graphic, there are procedures codes and short cuts we can use. To the immediate right of the chart are the shortcuts. The symbol for extraction is a tooth with 2 lines down it vertically and is found on the second row on the left. Directly above teeth 13 and 14 are the status codes. **Use the explorer to choose "EO" Existing**

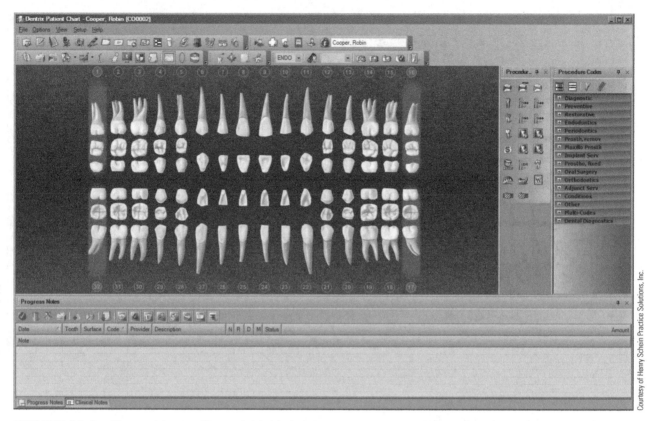

FIGURE 20-5   Chart with specific teeth highlighted.

Other and click on it. Now the tooth chart will show the third molars, 1, 16, 17, and 32 gone. Review the Progress notes section by clicking in the lower left corner, note that the treatment was automatically added to the notes.

> **HELPFUL HINT**
>
> Correcting an error and editing a chart is easy. In the progress notes double click on the line containing the incorrect procedure. A dialog box will automatically appear allowing you to make changes. You can change the status of the procedure, the fee charged for the procedure, and even the procedure code. These types of changes can be made by the end of the day quite easily. After you close the day the computer will automatically advance the date so any additional entries will show the new date. Think of it like writing in ink in a paper chart. Whenever an error is discovered, it must be corrected. Just add a line in the notes to specify the error, make the correction, and initial it.

Let's chart some work that needs to be done for Robin. She has caries on tooth #14 and will need an MOD restoration.

5. **First choose tooth #14 and highlight it just like in the previous exercise.**

6. **Choose MOD amalgam from your procedure short cuts followed by clicking on the Tx icon to indicate this is treatment needed.**
   Your tooth chart should now have an MOD colored in red.

7. See if you can figure out how to adjust the fee. **Remember to double click in the procedure notes to edit the chart and make a change.** What if Robin changed her mind and wanted a resin composite filling instead, this can also be done on that dialog screen. **On procedure code change it to the correct code if you already know it, or use the arrow prompt to find it. Click on the code you want and hit OK. You can check for the accuracy of the change by looking at the progress notes or on the graphic charting. On the graphic, it should now be outlined in red and filled with cross hatching (Figure 20-6).**

> **HELPFUL HINT**
> When working in Dentrix, if you don't understand a step go back and repeat the process until you do. This is your opportunity to learn. You will be able to build up speed after you know the basics. It just takes practice.

Periodontal Charting

Periodontal charting can be a bit complicated. Again, begin with the basics to build a strong foundation so that you can add skills later. Although periodontal charting is a clinical skill and not an administrative or management one, the

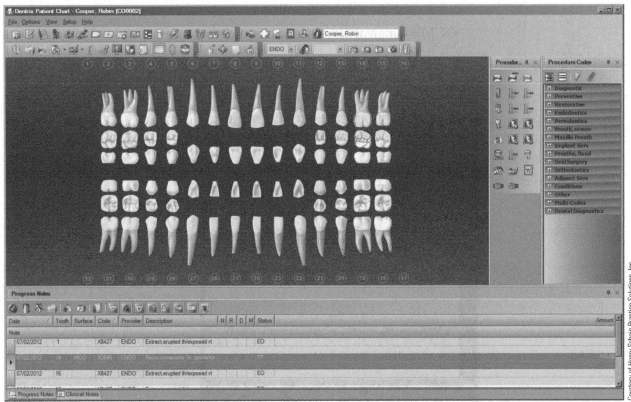

FIGURE 20-6 Charting a procedure.

office manager must be able to read and interpret the charting for treatment planning and insurance claims. With traditional charting on paper every tooth gets six measurements, three on the buccal or facial and three on the lingual. The same measurements are recorded in an electronic charting system. First a patient chart must be selected, then the periodontal charting is accessed from toolbar with the icon that is found along the second row (Figure 20-7). Choose Karen Davis as your example.

FIGURE 20-7
Periodontal chart
icon.

1. **Select Karen Davis as your patient.** Using your charting skills, confirm her third molars are missing. If you chart shows them present, indicate they are missing with the EO, existing other icon.

2. **Click on the perio charting icon; you should be looking at the chart shown in Figure 20-8. Again the toolbar has changed; take time now to run the mouse over the icons for their description. There are five icons that are important for perio charting; New Exam, Open Exam, Save Exam, Print Exam, and Delete Exam. Clicking New Exam will give you a dialog box to choose the date for the exam; click on OK. Open Exam opens a dialog box to allow you to select a past exam date. The icons for save, print, and delete are self-explanatory.**

   Note on Karen's chart that the third molars have been extracted. You will see they are missing on the perio chart by the red M. As you look at the perio chart, you will see the tooth numbers running along the top and bottom much like a non-computer chart. Along the far left column beginning at the top you will see some abbreviations:

   - F = Facial (this includes the buccal surfaces of posterior teeth)

   - PD = Probing depth measured in millimeters using a perio probe (this is by the dentist or hygienist)

   - GM = Gingival Margin indicates recession and is measured in millimeters

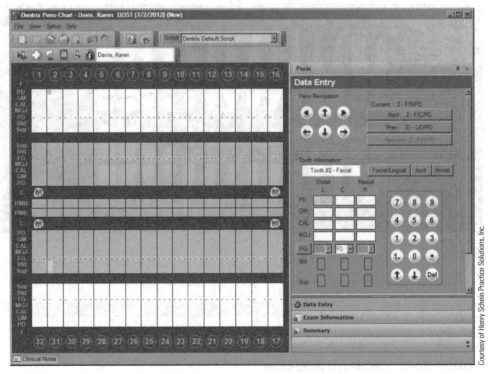

FIGURE 20-8 Periodontal chart icon.

- CAL = Clinical Attachment Level, which is measured in millimeters

- MGJ = Mucogingival Junction measured in millimeter

- FG = Functional Grade with furcation involvement for the tooth
  Thinking back to your tooth anatomy, you will remember the furcation is the point where the roots of the teeth divide. FG denotes furcation involvement and extent. By clicking on the square around FG you will see an explanation of the evaluation system.

- Bld = Bleeding, which is represented with a red oval at the point of bleeding

- Sup = Suppuration or an infection point is indicated by a yellow oval

As you continue to follow the column down on the left, you will see the abbreviations listed in reverse as they relate to the lingual side of the tooth. When charting, the maxillary teeth are on the top of the chart and the mandibular teeth are on the bottom, which is easy to remember because the top teeth in the mouth are the maxillary and the bottom teeth are the mandibular. Dentrix has also indicated facial tooth surfaces in white and lingual tooth surfaces in gray.

In the center, at the point where the maxillary and mandibular teeth meet you will find PMB (Plaque, Mobility, and Bone Loss), which are measurements specific to each tooth. Data entry for the PMB on each tooth is found at the bottom of the data entry box. Both maxillary and mandibular spaces for PMB are in gray.

The chart will look like a graph (Figure 20-9).

The perio chart also has a place for clinical notes, similar to the patient chart, when you click the lower left corner of the screen (Figure 20-10).

3. **Find the abbreviations, tooth locations, and area for clinical notes on the chart. It is important that you understand the chart before you continue with the exercise.**

Moving to the right side of the screen, you will see the Perio panel which includes data entry, exam information, and summary. (Figure 20-11).

4. **Click on each of the sections to see how you can move between them, click on data entry for our first exercise.**

5. **To enter periodontal probing for Karen, begin with the distal facial of tooth #2. You can verify your position on the date entry box at the top with current position. If you are not on tooth #2, use the navigation arrows until you get to the correct place. In the tooth information box you should see tooth #2 and the top left PD (perio depth) highlighted in yellow. Begin charting by using the key pad at the right and enter the depths 3 2 3 as your distal, facial, mesial readings. You will not need to select the next tooth just use the key pad or the PD on tooth #3 and charting system will automatically advance. If you want to jump to another tooth you can use the navigation system or just use your mouse to move the cursor to the tooth you want to chart. Go to tooth #14, notice the mesial measurement is now first. On tooth #14, chart the PD 6 5 6 and click the Bld (bleeding) box to indicate bleeding. Notice because these depths are outside of the normal range they are red. Add more PD if you like for practice.**

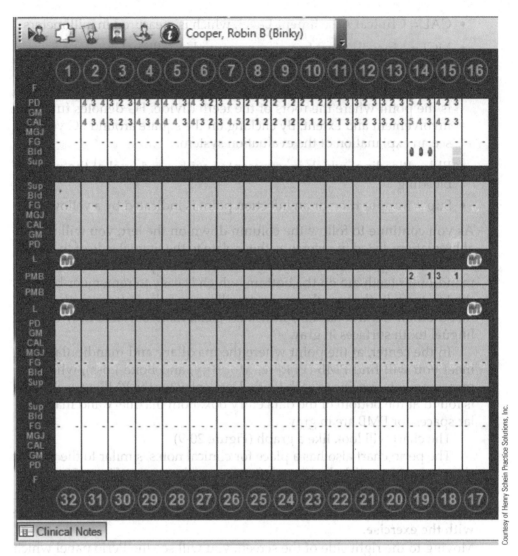

FIGURE 20-9 Sample of periodontal charting.

FIGURE 20-10 Clinical notes on periodontal chart.

When you have practiced entering as much data as you would like to; Click on the "exam information" button to add some description for Karen. As you highlight the term on the left you will have descriptive choices in a drop down menu on the right (Figure 20-12).

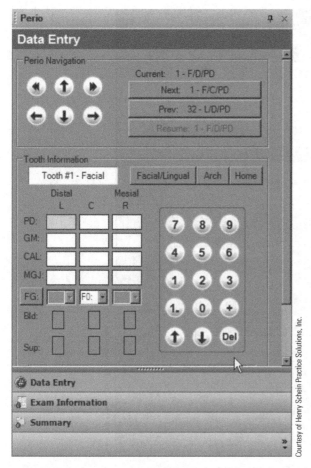

FIGURE 20-11 Data Entry.

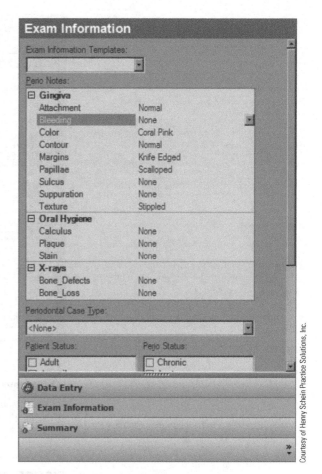

FIGURE 20-12 Exam Information.

6. **For practice visualize how Karen's soft tissue might look and choose the appearance on the small drop-down menu at the right. Since this is just practice navigating the perio charting system, make some changes. Click on attachment and choose enlarged to start and then choose any other observations you want to change.**

The summary allows you to see an overview of the patient and the information you have entered as shown in the Figure 20-13 (Perio Summary).

Because many patients prefer to see problem areas, use the perio Graphic Chart icon on the tool bar to convert your graph into an anatomical view (Figure 20-14).

7. **Make sure to hit the "Save Exam" before moving from the periodontal charting but if you forget Dentrix will remind you.**

You now have the basics of Dentrix-assisted perio charting; by practicing you will build speed and efficiency.

HELPFUL HINT

Charting is a great skill to practice with a partner because it simulates a dental office. The numbers and conditions being charted for practice are not as important as the pace. So your practice partner can be anyone.

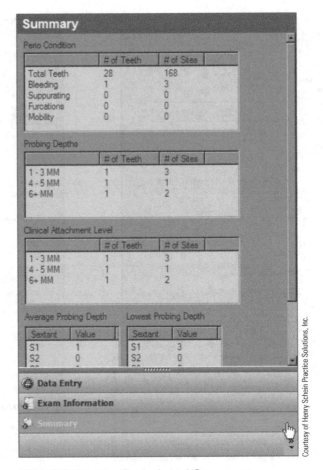

FIGURE 20-13 Periodontal Summary.

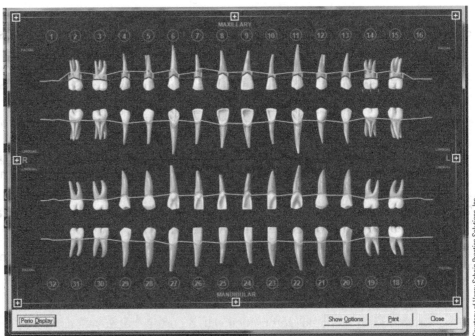

FIGURE 20-14 Anatomical representation of peridontal chart.

Making Treatment Plans

Every dental office faces the challenge of getting patients scheduled for treatment. It is the responsibility of the dentist and staff to educate the patient regarding the importance of making and keeping the treatment appointment. Dentrix Treatment Manager allows the patient to take home a visual of the treatment, as well as a fee and an insurance estimate. If team members have added accurate information to the patient chart, a treatment plan is automatically generated based on that information and contains the dentist's diagnosis for the patient and any treatment recommendations. Once the treatment plan is ready for the office manager, he or she is responsible for making sure the patient is scheduled for treatment or put into a follow-up system (covered in Chapter 21), understands the fee for treatment, and insurance details. These steps are the same as in an office without dental management software but the software just makes it much easier for the office manager and more understandable for the patient. Thorough treatment planning and follow up is an important part of informed consent.

1. **From the patient chart, we will select Brent Crosby as our patient. As you make that selection, you will see a pop-up alert. When you have read the alert, go ahead and close it by clicking OK.**

2. **Go to the icon on the toolbar for Treatment Planner; it looks like a green treatment chair (without the $ sign) (Figure 20-15).**

3. **You should see a screen similar to the one in Figure 20-16 (Sample Treatment Plan). At the upper left of the Treatment Planner screen is a toolbar that enables you to manage the information (Figure 20-17). Explore the icons on the toolbar.**

4. **At the lower left, highlight Treatment Plan Case Setup.** The case we are viewing has been created for Brent based on information that was added during his clinical exam and coded as Tx (treatment needed/planned).

5. **Click on the + signs next to the three treatment plans to expand the file to show treatment.** Brent has three options for treatment that he can choose from; look carefully and compare them to see the differences.

6. Details of the appointments are listed at the left of the Treatment Plan Case Setup. Dean's treatment will take multiple visits, the green number 1 indicates treatment for the first visit and the red number 2 indicates treatment for the second visit.

FIGURE 20-15
Treatment plan icon.
Courtesy of Henry Schein Practice Solutions, Inc.

> ┌─ **HELPFUL HINT**
> The ability to list appointments so clearly for a patient is really helpful. Many times patients have so many things to think about regarding treatment that timing is confusing.

7. You can include completed or rejected cases. This might be helpful if the patient had rejected smaller procedures and now is looking at substantial restorative work that is much more expensive. It is important the risk of rejecting treatment is shared with the patient.

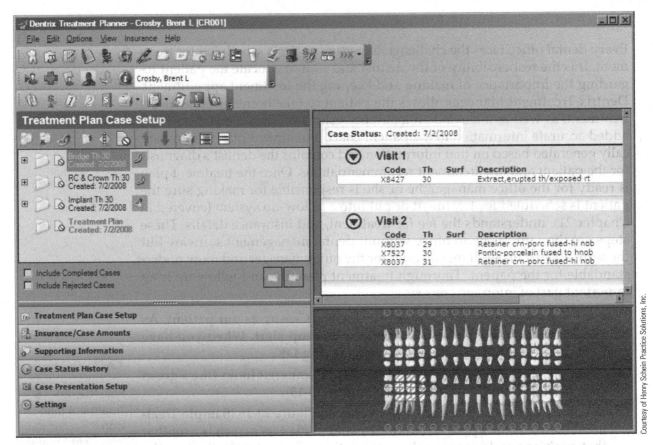

FIGURE 20-16 Sample treatment planner.

FIGURE 20-17 Treatment planner toolbar.

Courtesy of Henry Schein Practice Solutions, Inc.

8. Treatment Planner also allows you to set up a case presentation that includes educational material to assist you in explaining procedures to the patient.

9. **Click the Presenter icon and choose Root Canal (Guru) from Patient Education on the right side of your screen.**

10. **Use the circle with the green arrow to launch the visual presentation. This is a video so use the start arrow at the lower left.** Dentrix uses Guru for its education materials. When you have time, explore all of the patient education topics. Some are illustrations others are video. Notice at the lower right of your screen, there are draw and erase icons to personalize your patient presentation. Learning to use the patient education topics will assist you in presenting cases successfully to your patients.

11. **See if you can move through the previous steps and make a treatment plan for Robin (Binky) Cooper.**
    Treatment Planner is fun and amazingly informative but it will take practice to become proficient with it.

Prescriptions

As patients are dismissed, the doctor may also request that they receive a prescription for the treatment they received or to have before their next appointment. Even though Dentrix makes prescriptions easy they still need the doctor's approval.

FIGURE 20-18
Prescription icon.
Courtesy of Henry Schein Practice Solutions, Inc.

1. **Start by Selecting a Patient from the Patient Chart or the Family File, go ahead and choose Dean Little.**

2. **Click on the icon for prescriptions that looks like a pill bottle on the toolbar (Figure 20-18).**
   There are no previous prescriptions for Dean so click on the "New" button at the bottom of the dialog box and you will see a blank prescription.

3. **Use the prescription drop-down menu to see some of the most common prescriptions by this doctor. In Figure 20-19, Keflex was selected from the drop-down menu and the remainder of the prescription was completed automatically.**

4. **Explore the different prescriptions that could be selected by clicking on others from the drop-down menu.**

5. **In an office you would click the print button and have it ready and available for the doctor to sign. The prescription is also printed with instructions for the patient to call immediately if there is an adverse reaction (Figure 20-20). The prescription is automatically added to patient chart.**

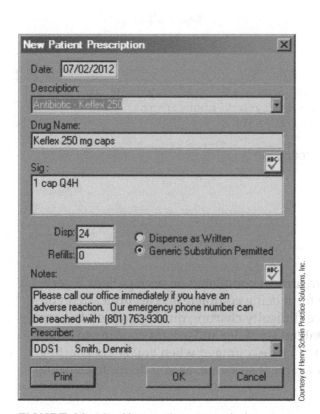

FIGURE 20-19 New patient prescription.

DENTRIX Learning Edition Licensed for Personal Non-Commercial Use	PRESCRIBER: Dennis Smith, D.D.S. TELEPHONE: - DEA No: DDS1_DrugID NPI: DDS1_NPI

PATIENT: Dean Little
ADDRESS: 650 N 650 W
          Southside, NV 33333

TELEPHONE: (111) 797-6241
DOB: 05/14/1973
DATE: 07/02/2012

R_x Keflex 250 mg caps

Disp: 24

1 cap Q4H

Refills: zero

☐ DISPENSE AS WRITTEN

☒ GENERIC SUBSTITUTION PERMITTED

_____
SIGNATURE OF PRESCRIBER

Copyright © 1967–2008 Henry Schein, Inc, RXo

---

cut here

PATIENT: Dean Little
PRESCRIPTION: Keflex 250 mg caps
PRESCRIBED BY: Dennis Smith, D.D.S.

DATE: 07/02/2012

Please call our office immediately if you have an adverse reaction. Our emergency phone number can be reached with (801) 763-9300.

FIGURE 20-20   Sample patient prescription.

© Cengage Learning 2014

Summary

Charting is a legal record of the treatment completed on each patient. Everyone in the practice is responsible for it being complete and accurate. In an office environment, it is easy to have difficulty charting quickly enough to keep up with the clinician. Never hesitate to speak up and ask for charting to be repeated to insure it is accurate. Don't be discouraged when you begin charting with Dentrix or any practice management software, as you do more charting your speed will increase.

Skill Building

1. If you have Internet access, watch the "On Demand Training" videos and take the quiz for each:
   - Using the Dentrix Presenter
   - Viewing and Navigating the Patient Chart
   - Customizing the Patient Chart
   - Charting and Editing Treatment
   - Viewing and Navigating the Perio chart
   - Charting and Comparing Perio Measurements
   - Viewing and Navigating the Treatment Planner

2. Using the patients from Appendix 1 (Patient Charts), add the clinical charting to the patient charts for Rachel Anthony, Thomas Lane, Janet Bruce, and Clayton Lewis.

3. For additional practice, work with a partner and write down charting for Peggy Perkins in your sample database and have your partner read the information off to you as you chart.

Sample of periodontal charting to use for practice for patient, Peggy Perkins:

Tooth # 1 is missing; beginning with #2 on the buccal: 423, 345, 423, 323, 312, 212, 212, midline, 212, 212, 213, 323, 323, 323, and 423; #16 is missing

On the lingual beginning with #15 on the distal: 424, 423, 434, 423, 312, 212, 212, midline, 212, 212, 213, 323, 323, 424, and 425

Tooth #17 is missing; Beginning with # 18 on the distal: 423, 435, 423, 323, 312, 312, 212, midline, 212, 212, 213, 313, 323, 434, and 423; # 32 is missing

On the lingual beginning with #18 distal: 433, 324, 434, 323, 323, 313, 313, midline, 313, 313, 323, 323, 333, 434, and 423

Bleeding on tooth numbers: 3, 15, 18, 19, 30, and 31

 Challenge Your Understanding

1. For patient Paul Olsen, which teeth have been extracted?
   a. All four wisdom teeth, 1, 16, 17, 32
   b. There are no missing teeth
   c. Paul is a non-patient
   d. All four bicuspids due to orthodontic treatment

2. When charting with Dentrix missing teeth are designated by:
   a. A blue X
   b. A red X
   c. A lighter blue aura.
   d. They are missing from chart

3. Which of the following is not already on Paula Pearson's prescription list? (hint: Paula Pearson is a doctor in the practice)
   a. Amoxicillin 250 mg
   b. Keflex 300 mg
   c. Tylenol # 3
   d. Clindamycin 300 mg

4. The charting for Thomas Lane would include:
   a. Tooth # 19 would have an MO with blue crosshatching
   b. Tooth # 32 would have an O with red crosshatching
   c. Tooth # 31 would have an MO with blue crosshatching
   d. Tooth # 9 would have an existing PFM crown

5. For Janet Bruce, the charting for tooth # 19 would show:
   a. The crown of the tooth outlined in red
   b. The crown of the tooth outlined and filled with blue crosshatching
   c. That the tooth has had root canal therapy
   d. The crown of the tooth outlined in blue.

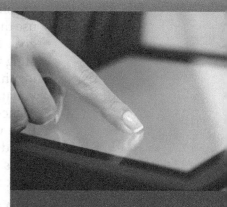

CHAPTER 21

Appointment Book

CHAPTER OUTLINES

- **The Appointment Book**
  Find an Appointment Time
  Scheduling Appointments for Existing Patients
  Scheduling Appointments for New Patients
  Rescheduling an Appointment
  Broken Appointments
  Tracking Patient Status
- **End of Day**
  Backing up Files
- **Summary**

LEARNING OBJECTIVES

Upon completion of this chapter, the reader should be able to:

1. Demonstrate setting up a new patient appointment.
2. Demonstrate setting up an appointment for an existing patient.
3. Demonstrate finding an appointment time, scheduling, and changing a patient appointment.
4. Create a "wait list" of patients wishing to schedule an appointment.
5. List the steps to close the day.
6. Successfully designate patient status.

The Appointment Book

The **appointment book** is the tool that determines office flow and keeps the office productive. The goal of good appointment book management is to help the office staff to reach maximum **production** with minimal stress. Learning to use the tools available to a practice management system will help achieve this goal. This module will cover an overview of setting up the appointments, creating wait/will call lists, and completing end of the day tasks. When progressing through an exercise, instructions will be numbered and in bold. Make sure you understand and feel comfortable with each task before moving to the next to increase your efficiency. As with most functions in Dentrix there are multiple ways to access information. All of them are correct. With practice you will determine which pathway is easiest for you. The exercises in this chapter focus on basics, but keep in mind it is possible to customize the appointment book to the needs of an individual dental office.

FIGURE 21-1
Appointment book icon.

Courtesy of Henry Schein Practice Solutions, Inc.

1. **After opening Dentrix find the appointment book by using the open book icon on the toolbar (Figure 21-1).**

   Your appointment book should be blank and look like a traditional paper appointment book (Figure 21-2). Dental offices typically work in 10- or 15-minute blocks of time called **units**. This appointment book is using 10-minute units but when the appointment book is set up, other time options are available. Offices generally do not change the amount of time they use as a unit without a lot of consideration because it means changing patient's appointment times and can cause confusion.

2. **Explore the toolbar by allowing the mouse to move over the icons revealing the labels.**

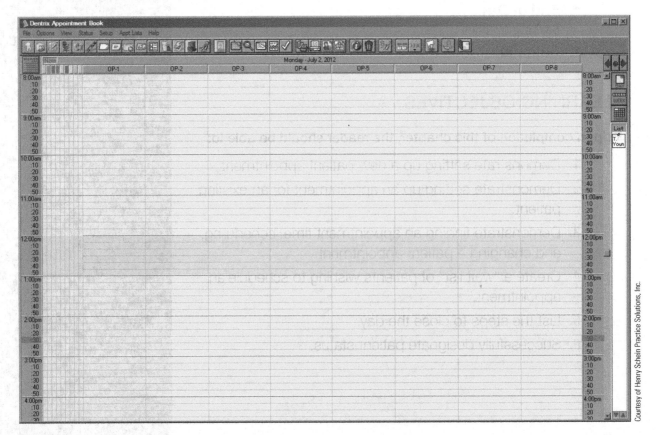

FIGURE 21-2 Sample appointment book.

Courtesy of Henry Schein Practice Solutions, Inc.

3. At the far right of the screen notice navigation arrows that allow movement forward and backward through the days of the week. Beneath those, there are icons to allow the view to be changed to a week or a month. The graph at the left of the appointment book is color coded at the top for each provider so you can see who is scheduled with a patient and in what treatment room. **Practice moving around in the appointment book.**

> ┌─ **HELPFUL HINT**
> │ Every member of the dental team plays a role in scheduling appointments either directly or indirectly.

Find an Appointment Time

First it is necessary to determine what type of an appointment is needed to find a space with enough time. As the patient charting was done, anything that was coded in red (treatment needed) automatically goes into the patient's appointment history as Tx, so a future appointment can be made. Average time requirements for the each procedure are predetermined but can be adjusted if necessary.

1. **Begin by adding an MOD amalgam on tooth number 14 as treatment needed to Pat Abbott's charting so we can observe how required treatment moves from the clinical area to the front desk.**

2. **Using the icon as in Figure 21-3 (Schedule Appointment) and then selecting Pat Abbott, you can see the "Appointment Information" for Pat. By selecting Tx in the box indicating "Reason" for the visit, you can see the treatment remaining on her treatment plan. Highlight it and close to indicate that this is the procedure you would like to schedule.**

   FIGURE 21-3
   Schedule appointment icon.
   Courtesy of Henry Schein Practice Solutions, Inc.

   If Pat had several items listed in her treatment plan you could schedule one or more than one. Under the reason for appointment is the appointment description and to the right of the description is the recommended appointment length. By using the arrow to the far right of Appt Length you can increase or decrease the time needed in 10-minute units. You will also see an estimate of the fee labeled as amount and to the far right you will see a list of scheduling options.

3. **To become acquainted with this dialog box and its functions, explore the dialog box now by using the drop-down menus and other buttons.** Practice by exploring some of the most frequently used buttons; the other options besides Tx that are frequently used are Initial, which is for treatment of new patients who would not have any existing treatment plans and Misc that could be used for existing patients that need to be scheduled for something not already diagnosed and in the treatment plan. In the appointment description area, you will find a button for status that gives information regarding confirmation of the patient and the status of the appointment once the patient is in the office; after you have appointments scheduled you will practice using this feature. There is a button for staff that tracks what staff member made the appointment. The Op button was abbreviated from **operatory**, which was an older name for treatment room and gives the option of which room to schedule for the patient. Date and time allow you to add preferences.

Along the right side of the dialog box are some additional choices, More Information will allow you to access general patient information directly from the appointment book. There is also access to other appointments by selecting that button, insurance claim information for the patient, and a schedule next to enter the appointment into a date in the appointment book.

Several of the right-hand buttons allow moving the appointment into a category where it can be placed for future follow-up. Wait/Will Call will add the patient to a list of unscheduled patients needing treatment. For example, Pat Abbott needs a three-surface amalgam, as seen earlier, when the office manager attempts to schedule treatment, Pat replies she doesn't have her calendar with her and she'll need to call back. To allow for follow-up, she should be placed into the wait/will call category. Find allows you to look for an appointment and when you are looking you can place the appointment on Pinboard to click and drag it into any available appointment space. If your appointment involves lab work you can even indicate that in appointment information.

4. **Click on wait/will call to save Pat's appointment to schedule when she is ready. Confirm you want to move her appointment by clicking yes in the pop up box.**

For practice, we will use what we've learned to add a patient to the appointment book.

5. **Go to the Schedule Appointment icon on the toolbar (Figure 21-3). Select Carol Little as the patient. An Appointment Information box pops up for Carol (Figure 21-4).**

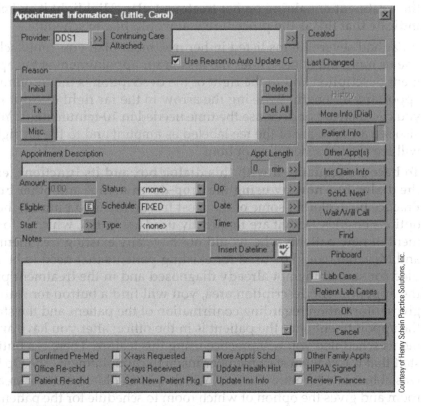

FIGURE 21-4 Appointment information.

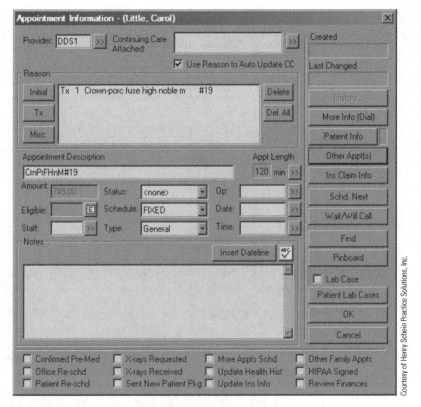

FIGURE 21-5 Adding the treatment.

6. **Look for and click on the Tx button. In the treatment plan box that opens you will see that Carol needs a crown on #19, click on the procedure and close the box.** The procedure will now be in the Reason box and you can see that the appointment will take 90 minutes. To change the appointment length, use the arrows to the right of the time button. Change the appointment length to 120 minutes (Figure 21-5).

> **HELPFUL HINT**
>
> Presetting appointment times takes the guesswork out of making appointments. The doctor and staff estimate how long procedures take to complete and it is set as a default in the computer. However, adjustments can be made; for example, if a patient with back problems must take a break during longer procedures, that has to be factored into the appointment time. This can be done at the front desk or by an assistant who is familiar with the patient.
>
> It is important to be precise with appointment times as even downtime of 10–15 minutes throughout the day adds up and affects production.

7. **Highlight the treatment, and then move it to the Pinboard by clicking on Pinboard to hold it until you are ready to put it in the appointment book.**

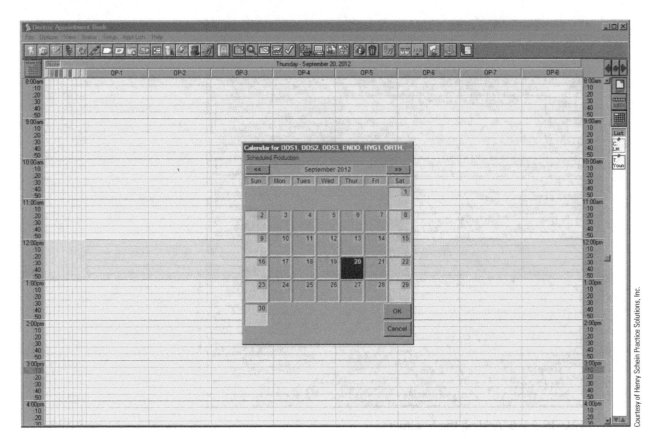

FIGURE 21-6 Looking up a date.

8. One way to find an appointment time is to search manually. This is efficient in cases where a patient has a very specific time requirement such as "I have the day off on September 20, do you have any time available." When this happens the fastest way to look is to go directly to the day in the appointment book. **Look up September 20 in the appointment book by clicking on the small calendar on the left under the toolbar to change the month and click on a specific day in that month (Figure 21-6).** By locating the date, you can see if you have appointments available or even if your office is open.

9. **To initiate a wider search, select the looking glass icon on your appointment book screen. It will open the New Appointment dialog box below (Figure 21-7).** The dialog box allows you to set parameters for searching for particular times or particular days. It is possible to choose dentist, treatment room, days of the week, where in the appointment book to start looking. The appointment length will be set but you can adjust it here also.

10. **As you look at your appointment book pages you will see Carol's appointment waiting for you "pinned" in the upper right hand corner as a New Appt, in the list as shown in Figure 21-8. From there you can drag it into the appointment book.**

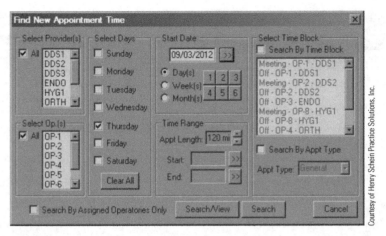

FIGURE 21-7 Find a new appointment time.

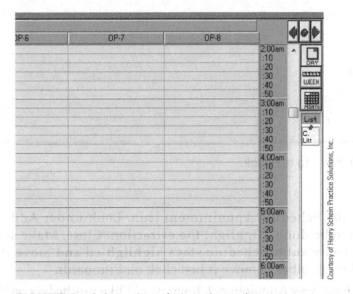

FIGURE 21-8 Location of pinned appointments.

11. Click and drag the appointment into the desired position. If after making the appointment it is necessary to move it, you can do that by clicking and dragging (Figure 21-9).

> **HELPFUL HINT**
>
> The click and drag feature is one that is often used. It is common for a patient to need to move an appointment. You can move it around on the same page visually or "pin" it in the upper right of the appointment book page and search for another date then drag it into place

Scheduling Appointments for Existing Patients

Repeat the steps above, using another patient.

1. Go to the appointment book icon from your current location.
2. Please schedule the extraction appointment for Brent Crosby.

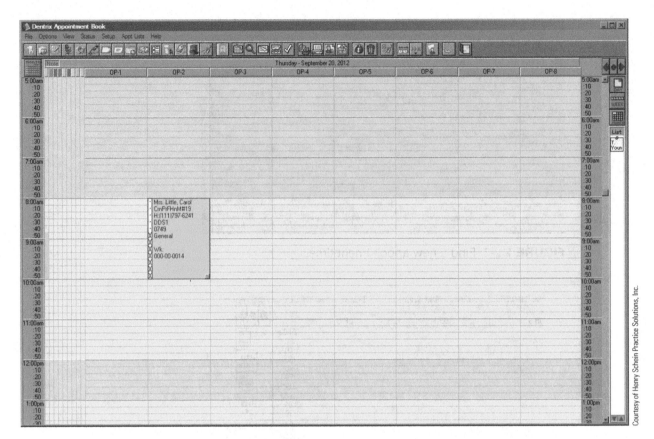

FIGURE 21-9 Adding an appointment to the book.

3. Click the Schedule Appointment icon. Look under Add Tx for what needs to be done. Highlight the extraction. Close. Make sure the treatment you want to schedule stays highlighted and move it to the Pinboard (remember to move it just click on Pinboard).

4. Go to Find New Appointment, Brent would like to schedule on September 15 in the morning with DDS 1. Use your tools for speed (e.g., calendar and drop-down menus).

5. Search/view possible options. Your appointment book should show that either treatment room 1 or 2 is available at that time with the doctor.

6. Select treatment room 1.

7. On the appointment page, you will see the time available indicated by an outline.

8. Click and drag Brent from the Pinboard's upper right.

9. Just for practice, move Brent's appointment around on the page. Notice that you are unable to move the appointment accidently because Dentrix asks for confirmation.

10. Want more practice? Choose other patients out of your database to schedule.

Scheduling Appointments for New Patients

Scheduling new patients is important because it is how the practice grows. When a new patient calls, it is their first impression of what the experience will be like in your practice. Depending on the practice, exactly how new patients are scheduled can vary but for this exercise we are going to make the appointment with the hygienist for one hour and include a cleaning.

1. **New patient, Susan Keller, calls and would like to set up an appointment for September 3 at 8** A.M.

2. **Go to the Appointment Book icon and click on it. Go the requested date of September 3, please use treatment room 5 as the hygiene room and double click on 8** A.M.

3. **The Select a Patient dialog box will open. Because this is a new patient, click on the New Patient button.** Complete the information for the new patient in the box that opens. Be as accurate as possible. You will need to fill in a referral source that can be another patient or another doctor. This is important information to get because you will want to thank the source of the referral.

4. **Once you have completed the patient information, a box will open for appointment information. This time you will want to select DDS 1 and indicate that it is an initial visit. By highlighting the procedures it will add them to the appointment. Choose adult prophy, pano, 4 BW, and periodic exam for this example (Figure 21-10).**

5. **Click the okay button to add this appointment (Figure 21-11).**

   NP next to the appointment will identify the patient as new to the practice. This patient does not have a family file and you will not be able to locate them in Select a Patient. New patient appointments are found by using the Locate Appointment button.

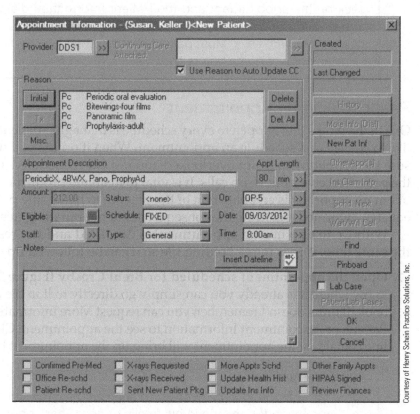

FIGURE 21-10 Adding a new patient appointment.

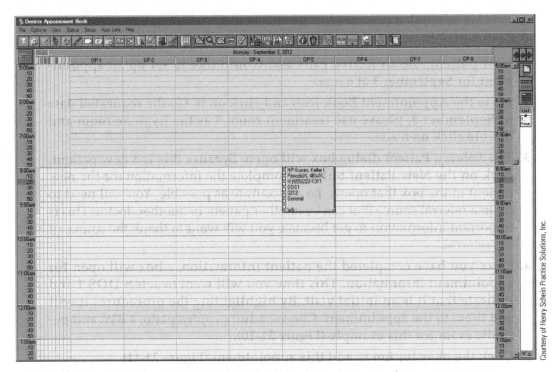

FIGURE 21-11 Posting appointment to appointment book.

HELPFUL HINT

If you find you have made an error with your appointment; for example, she will need more time. From the appointment book page, double click on the appointment and the Patient Information dialog box will appear and you can make corrections. Dentrix has made scheduling a new patient very easy. Most patients have some idea of when they like to make appointments before they call.

Rescheduling an Appointment

One of the things that happen to every schedule is managing patients that would like to change or reschedule an appointment. When it occurs you want to make sure the appointment is not overlooked and if it isn't scheduled again quickly the patient receives follow-up calls. It is vital to maintain production in the office but more important is an obligation of the practice to make sure patients are adequately informed regarding the consequences of not pursuing treatment.

With Dentrix, when an appointment is cancelled and not rescheduled at the same time, it goes into a holding file so it can be followed up on.

1. **Open the appointment scheduled for Brent Crosby (Figure 21-12);** if you know where it is already you can simply go directly to it in the appointment book. If Brent doesn't remember, you can request More Information in Select a Patient, or Appointment Information to see the appointment. Clicking on the line containing the appointment will bring up the appointment book page.

HELPFUL HINT

More Information also allows you to see Brent's information but also the information for anyone in his family or any other appointments he might need such as a cleaning and an exam. Monitoring more information helps you keep patients on schedule and your practice busy.

Courtesy of Henry Schein Practice Solutions, Inc.

Double check on the appointment directly from the appointment book and it will bring you back to the Appointment Information dialog box we used earlier. Brent needs to check his schedule before rescheduling so highlight the treatment you want to reschedule and move it to Wait/Will Call.

Tracking patients who need to schedule appointments is critical to fill last minute cancellations or simply to make sure schedules are full on a daily basis. So where did Brent's appointment go? The list of patients who need appointments can be retrieved by going to appt lists and looking through **wait/will call list** and **broken appointments** (Figure 21-13). The appointment lists can be found at the top of the toolbar. Clicking on the appointments list provides several options, and click on the unscheduled list. You should see Brent along with other patients who need appointments.

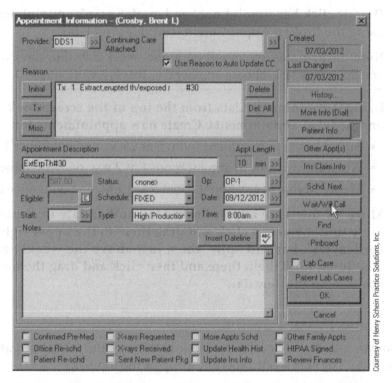

FIGURE 21-12 Opening patient appointment to reschedule.

Dentrix Unscheduled List

View   Appt   Refresh   Eligibility   Office Journal

Tue - Jul 3, 2012

Date	Status	Elig	Name	Prov	Reason	Ln	Pho
12/08/2008	Broken		Edwards, Anna	DDS1	4BWX, EmergEx	40	(801)
12/08/2008	Broken		Mr. Myers, Henry	DDS1	CompEx, ProphyAd	60	(801)
12/08/2008	Broken		Ms. Brown, Mary	DDS2	FMX	20	(801)
12/10/2008	Broken		Mr. Edwards, John	DDS2	Perio-Low	110	(801)
12/10/2008	Broken		Ms. Davis, Karen	HYG1	PeriodicX, 4BWX,	70	(801)
12/11/2008	Broken		Edwards, Anna	ENDO	CompEx, FMX, Con	70	(801)
12/11/2008	Broken		Mr. Edwards, John	ENDO	CompEx, FMX, Con	40	(801)
04/02/2012	W/Call		Taylor, Marri	DDS1	Consult	20	(801)
04/02/2012	Pboard		Mrs. Young, Tina	DDS1	2BWX	10	(801)
07/03/2012	W/Call		Mr. Crosby, Brent L	DDS1	ExtErpTh#30	10	(801)

FIGURE 21-13 Unscheduled list.

Broken Appointments

Broken appointments or appointments that patients do not show up for are another problem offices will need to handle. At the end of the day all the appointments need to be accounted for:

- As completed so they can be billed out
- Rescheduled and moved to a new position
- Moved to a list that can be followed up if not rescheduled
- Marked as broken so they appear on a follow-up list

1. **Move the appointment you made for Susan Keller to another position in the schedule.**
2. **Double click her appointment and mark Susan's appointment as broken using the Broken Appointment icon (Figure 21-14).**

   Note: If the dates above fall on a non–work day (Sunday) when you are practicing this task, choose another day that is a work day.

FIGURE 21-14
Broken appointment icon

Courtesy of Henry Schein Practice Solutions, Inc.

3. **Using Appointment Lists from the top of the screen look at the list of unscheduled appointments. Create new appointments for:**
   - Susan Keller in treatment room 5 at 2 p.m. on September 1
   - Anna Edwards in treatment room 1 at 2 p.m. on September 1
   - Henry Myers in treatment room 5 at 1 p.m. on September 1
4. **Move all the three appointments to another date in September at the same times. You can click and drag them to the upper right side of the vertical task bar and "pin" them just above the weekly and monthly schedules; hold them there and then click and drag them to the correct position on the new day.**

Tracking Patient Status

You can use the appointment book to convey the status of patients on the schedule. The status button is at the top of the toolbar.

1. **From the Appointment Book page, use the Status drop-down menu to see the options.**
2. **If you have already created an appointment book page use it; if you need a demonstration appointment page, you can use August 17, 2011.**
3. **To create a patient status, single click on the patient's appointment in the book, then go to status, and choose from the drop-down menu. On the appointment, a color code will appear on the left border. Try indicating that one of your patients was confirmed with a message left on voice mail. You will notice the color coding down the side of the appointment (Figure 21-15).**
4. **Status is how offices that have computer monitors in multiple areas track which patients have arrived in the office but may be completing paperwork or indicate which patients are actually ready to be seated in a treatment room.**
5. **You can click on a patient in the book and change the status.** For example, you left a message for this patient so that is the status; now the patient has arrived in the office you will click on the name and update the status. By using status, you will immediately see when patients are late for an appointment so you can call and verify if they are on their way.

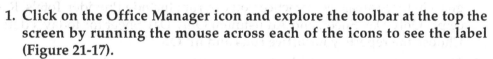

:20		
:30		
:40		
:50		
8:00am	X Reeves, Meredith	X Johnson, Adria
:10	X CompEx, FMX, Pano,	X LimitedEx, PA1st, Consult
:20	X H:(801)797-2729	X H:(111)797-8962
:30	X DDS1	X DDS2
:40	X 0296	
:50	X General	
9:00am		X Johnson, Rachelle
:10		X CompEx, 2BWX, Consult
:20		X H:(111)797-8962
:30		X Mrs. Little, Carol
:40	X Mr. Little, Dean	X PeriodicX, Consult
:50	X CompEx, FMX, EmergEx,	X Little, Kevin
10:00am	X H:(111)797-6241	X PeriodicX, Consult
:10	X DDS1	X Little, Matthew
:20	X 0426	X LimitedEx, Consult
:30	X General	X Mrs. Crosby, Shirley H
:40	X	X PeriodicX, 4BWX,
:50	X Wk:	X H:(801)797-5969
11:00am	X 000-00-0015	X DDS2
:10		X 0133
:20		
:30		
:40		
:50		
2:00pm		
:10		

FIGURE 21-15 Broken appointment icon.

End of Day

To close the day you'll need to go the Office Manager screen; you can find it by looking for the desk chair icon (Figure 21-16). It will allow you to run end of day reports.

FIGURE 21-16 Office manager icon.

1. **Click on the Office Manager icon and explore the toolbar at the top the screen by running the mouse across each of the icons to see the label (Figure 21-17).**

2. Before you get ready to close you will need to confirm that all information for the day has been entered.

   - Confirm all appointment information has been added and that all the patients have been checked out.
   - Make sure all payments have been posted so that you will balance.

   ─ HELPFUL HINT
   It is a good idea to make sure this has been done before clinical assistants start leaving for the day in case you need more information from them.

   ─ HELPFUL HINT
   On days when a large number of payments are received, you might consider doing a test close and balance at lunch. The sooner you identify a problem the easier it is to fix.

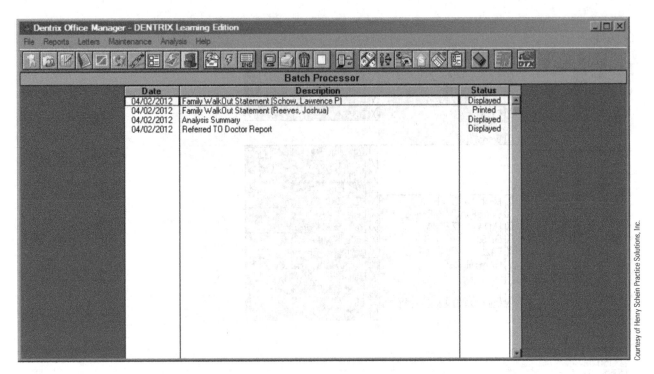

FIGURE 21-17 Office manager tool bar.

3. **When all information is entered, click on the Day Sheet Report, by going to the icon with the sun setting (Figure 21-18).**

4. There are lots of reports to choose from and not every practice wants to track the same information. Every office is going to be interested in the income for the day, how much money was received, and any adjustments such as family discounts that need to be accounted for. Some offices might also track daily referral or certain types of treatment if they have specific goals in those areas. For practice you can run: Include Provider Totals, Receipts Only Day Sheet, and Adjustment Only Day Sheet for today's date. **Choose the reports your office runs and hit OK.**

5. The reports you would like to print will appear as a list on the Batch Processor Screen of the dental office manager (Figure 21-19). **Find your reports.**

6. To print the pages that the practice uses, highlight them and send them to the printer. You should *not* print them now; just make sure you understand how to print from the Office Manager.

Backing up Files

It is important that the information in Dentrix is backed up daily to prevent it from being lost. This can occur onsite or offsite. If you back up onsite someone needs to be responsible for taking that copy away from the office in case of fire, flood, or earthquake. If an offsite location is chosen it must be compliant with HIPAA (Health Insurance Portability and Accountability Act) regarding patient privacy as discussed in Chapter 3 (Legal and Ethical Regulations in Dental Office Management).

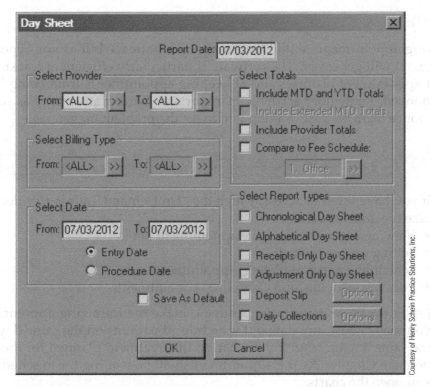

FIGURE 21-18 Day sheet report.

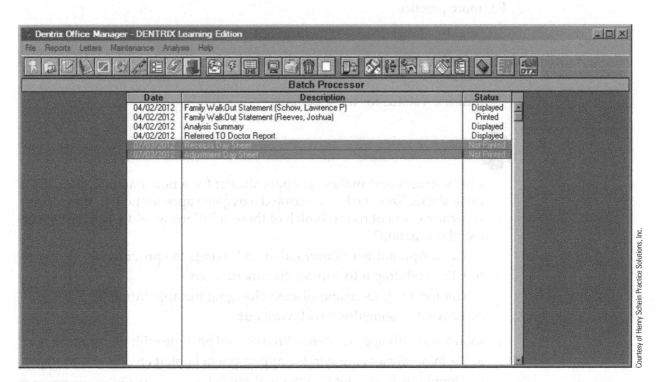

FIGURE 21-19 Printing reports.

Summary

Making appointments with Dentrix requires patience but as you repeat the process it will get easier. The software is particularly efficient at tracking patient appointment histories and at keeping appointments from being lost or overlooked. Remember accuracy is important. Correct any errors as soon as you notice them because waiting will make the problem bigger.

 Skill Building

1. If you have Internet access, watch the "On Demand Training" videos and take the quiz for each:
   - Viewing and navigating the appointment book
   - Setting up your schedule
   - Scheduling and completing Appointments
   - Locating, Moving, and Canceling Appointments

2. Using the patients from Appendix 1, make the following appointments you may choose any date but schedule all patients on the same day with the same doctor. *Hint*: If you charted the treatment planned for these patients in Chapter 20, the appointments will be waiting for to schedule as you open the charts.

   Rachel Anthony: Restoration of teeth #3, #14, and #30

   Thomas Lane: Root canal therapy #9

   Clayton Lewis: #19 Crown preparation

For more practice:

1. Schedule Janet Bruce for restorations on an appropriate date.

2. After the appointments are scheduled move them to different dates and times.

3. Indicate a status for these patients.

 Challenge Your Understanding

1. Cheryl enters and makes an appointment for a new patient. After she is done she realizes she has scheduled a hygiene appointment in the doctor's favorite treatment room. Which of these solutions would work best to correct the situation?
   a. Go to Appointment information and change the provider
   b. Click and drag it to another treatment room
   c. Contact the patient and discuss changing the appointment
   d. Leave it … something will work out.

2. John forgets his appointment. What should be done with the appointment?
   a. Nothing! By leaving it in the appointment book it creates a reminder
   b. Double click and put it in the will call list
   c. Single click and move it to broken appointments
   d. Move the appointment to another day and send him a postcard

3. Mary Brown has a broken appointment that was not rescheduled. What was it for?
   a. MOD amalgam filling
   b. Root canal therapy #18
   c. Full mouth survey
   d. Mary has no additional appointment requirements

4. Brent Crosby wants to move his appointment to next week. Where can you click and drag it to move it?
   a. The Appointment List
   b. To Broken Appointments
   c. Click and drag it to the day and time requested
   d. Use the Pinboard to park it

5. Appointment Status options include:
   a. Broken Appointment
   b. Ready for Operatory
   c. Rescheduled Appointment
   d. Appointment confirmed by mail

Financial Records

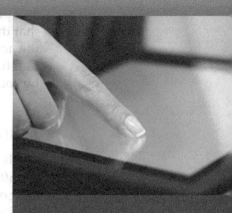

CHAPTER OUTLINES

LEARNING OBJECTIVES

Upon completion of this chapter, the reader should be able to:

1. Demonstrate how to post treatment fees to a patient account.
2. Demonstrate posting payments to a patient account.
3. Successfully make adjustments to patient accounts.
4. Successfully generate both hard copy and electronic insurance claim forms.
5. Accurately add a patient alert to an account.

Patient Accounts

Clinical and administrative staff need to make sure fees charged reflect the work that was done. Any adjustments or discounts that the patient received as a professional courtesy or because of prepayment must be categorized so that the management reports used to make decisions for the practice reflect the actual treatment. The ledger is the financial foundation for the practice. Careful attention and maintenance of the ledger is critical to the success of the business.

Managing the Patient Ledger

The ledger controls everything that involves the financial relationship between the office and the patient. Treatment is charged out and payments posted, fees can be changed or discounted, statements and insurance sent.

For offices using the Dentrix charting system, when treatment is completed and moves from the treatment plan to complete, the charges will automatically appear on the ledger.

If an office is using a paper chart, practice management software can still provide account management but it must be done manually.

Entering a Procedure

FIGURE 22-1
Ledger icon.
Courtesy of Henry Schein Practice Solutions, Inc.

1. **To go to the patient ledger, find the icon on the toolbar that looks like a pen and paper, and click on it (Figure 22-1). Explore the toolbar at the top of the ledger to see the labels for each icon (Figure 22-2).**
   The ledger contains valuable information. Once the treatment is added, the ledger automatically provides the total the patient owes for treatment and an estimate of the insurance portion as well as an estimate of the patient's portion.

   > **HELPFUL HINT**
   > As a dental office employee you can only *estimate* the insurance portion based on information provided by the patient and the insurance company.

   The ledger provides information about past account history including any past due charges and when insurance was filed.

2. **On the ledger page, use the icon on the toolbar to Select a Patient; choose Joshua Reeves for this exercise. Examine the ledger; you will notice that Joshua has an outstanding balance of $133 with no insurance filed (Figure 22-3).**

3. **You will be adding some additional treatment for Joshua. To Enter a Procedure you can click on the icon shown in Figure 22-4 or from the toolbar above the icons by going to Transactions and using the drop-down menu. The dialogue box in Figure 22-5 will appear.**
   Please note: Because of copyright issues Dentrix Learning Edition does not use CDT (Current Dental Terminology) Codes but substitutes them with generic codes.

Courtesy of Henry Schein Practice Solutions, Inc.

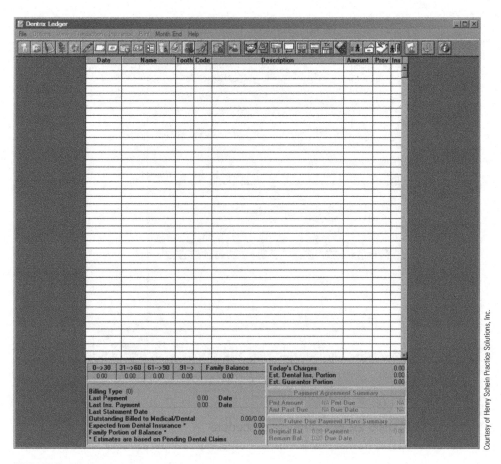

FIGURE 22-2 Ledger screen.

Courtesy of Henry Schein Practice Solutions, Inc.

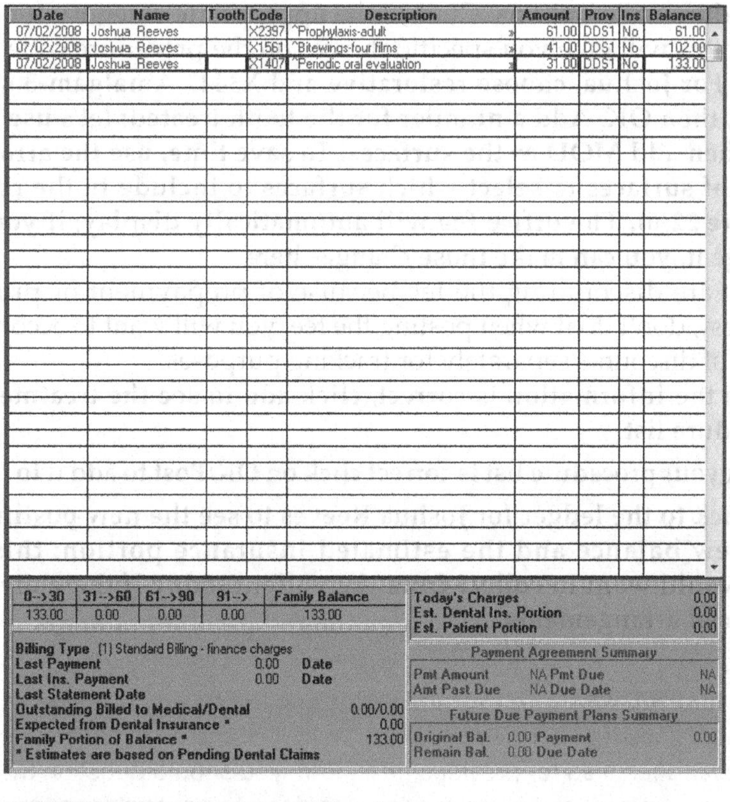

FIGURE 22-3 Patient ledger entry.

FIGURE 22-4
Procedure icon.

Courtesy of Henry Schein Practice Solutions, Inc.

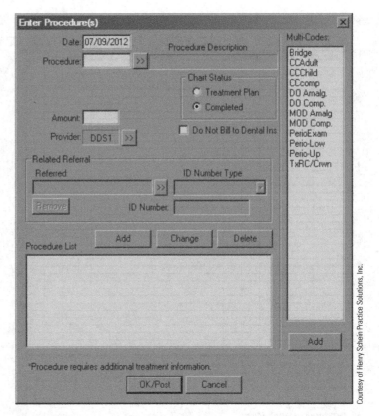

FIGURE 22-5 Entering a procedure.

4. The date is set as today's date by default. If you know the procedure code already enter it in the procedure code area; if not use the arrows to open procedure code options. Choose the appropriate category for the treatment; this will give you specific choices on the procedure code list to the right. **For Joshua, choose restorative and X3447 Amalgam-3 surf prim/ perm, then OK. Add a number for the tooth treated; let's use tooth #30 and then add MOD as the surfaces. To save time, use the arrows to the right of surfaces to select which surfaces to include in the restoration (Figure 22-6). The office fee will automatically display; if you want to change it, you can make those changes here.**

If you are discounting the fee because of prepayment or professional courtesy, don't do it when posting the fee, you will want to account for the types of discounts separately for tracking purposes.

When the information is correct, click add to see the treatment on the procedure list.

5. **When your procedure list is correct click on OK/Post to add it to the ledger.**

6. **Go back to the ledger for Joshua Reeves to see the new posting. Notice the new balance and the estimated insurance portion; this is what you would want to collect from the patient today if there are no other financial arrangements.**

HELPFUL HINT

In an office if you pulled up Joshua's ledger and saw that insurance had never been filed for previous treatment, you should question that. Try to figure out why and what needs to be done to get this account current.

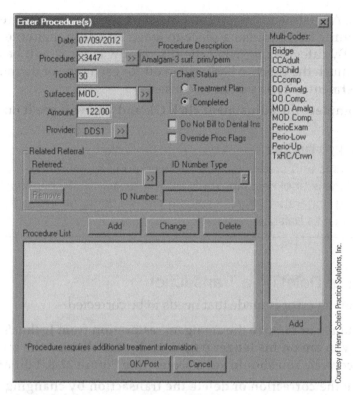

FIGURE 22-6 Entering a procedure.

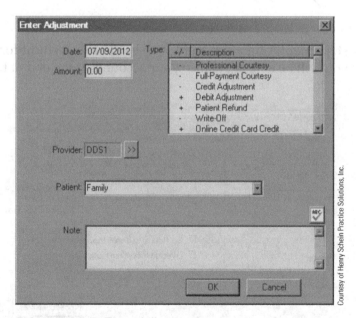

FIGURE 22-7 Enter Adjustment.

Adjusting an Account

For practice, let's give Joshua a Family/ Friend Courtesy discount of $25.

1. **To do that, you need to go to the Ledger screen; make sure you have selected Joshua Reeves as your patient. Highlight the transaction(s) you are going to adjust, then select transactions from above the icon toolbar. When you click on transactions, the drop-down menu will include Enter Adjustment; click on it. When you select the adjustment option you will see a screen like Figure 22-7 : Enter Adjustment.**

2. Enter Adjustment has options to select the amount and reason for the discount. There is also a place to leave an additional note for clarification. By categorizing what the discount was for, you'll be able to track how much the practice has written off for each type of discount. **Enter the adjustment criteria you have chosen.**

3. **To complete the adjustment click Ok and you will see it on the ledger.**

HELPFUL HINT

Debits and credits can be confusing unless your main function in the office is bookkeeping. You will see next to the description +/− to help you understand if your adjustment is adding or subtracting from the patient's balance.

Editing or Deleting a Transaction

Sometimes an error is made that needs to be corrected.

1. **To change or remove the amalgam restoration from Joshua's ledger make sure you are on his ledger page and double click on the transaction that is incorrect. You should see a screen like Figure 22-8: Edit or Delete.**

2. **Make the correction or delete the transaction by changing the incorrect field(s) or choosing delete in the lower left hand corner of the dialog box.**

Entering a Patient Payment

The first step in entering a payment is to be sure to account for it correctly; that way you will be able to balance your accounts at the end of the day.

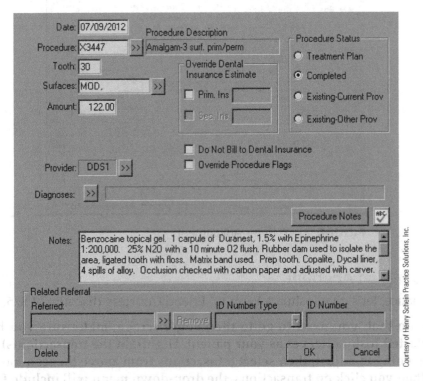

FIGURE 22-8 Edit or delete a payment.

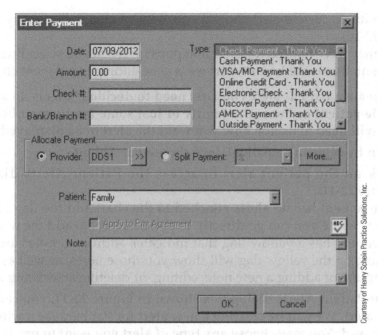

FIGURE 22-9 Enter a Payment.

1. To enter a payment, go to the ledger and select the correct patient, let's keep working with Joshua.

2. To get to the Enter Payment screen, shown in Figure 22-9: Enter a Payment, by choosing the icon that looks like a check with G $ under it or go to Transactions and choose Enter Payment from the drop-down menu.

3. We'll practice adding a $100 payment for Joshua in the form of a check #1550.

4. Add the information to the fields and when you are satisfied that it is correct, click OK to enter the payment.

5. To check the accuracy of your entry look at the ledger for Joshua.

6. Let's say your entry is incorrect. Correct it by double clicking on the ledger entry and Dentrix will bring up a correction screen.

7. Repeat steps 1–4 to enter the payment again.

> **HELPFUL HINT**
>
> When you make an error anywhere in Dentrix, first try double clicking on the incorrect entry, whether it is clinical, financial, or insurance; often you can make the correction right there.

Patient Alerts

Adding an alert, especially one concerning finances to a patient chart, can be very helpful in managing patient accounts. Patient alerts are designed to be noticed; so if you are working in an area where others can see your screen make sure your alerts conform to guidelines for privacy. Patient alerts are accessed through the patient alerts button, the icon with the patient, and the flag. On most of the screens you have been working with up until now, once you have selected a patient, you will see the alert icon with a white flag for a

FIGURE 22-10
Create a patient
alert.

Courtesy of Henry Schein Practice Solutions, Inc.

patient with no current alert and patients with an alert will have a yellow flag (Figure 22-10).

You may have noticed the alert that pops up when you select Brent Crosby as a patient; that is the type of alert we will be adding to a patient chart.

1. **To create a patient alert you first need to decide if this is an alert for a single patient or the entire family or just some family members. Then, you will need to decide how you want the alert to be displayed.**

2. **Begin by selecting a patient, let's choose Pat Abbott.**

3. **Click on the patient alert to access the Patient Alerts dialog box (Figure 22-11).**

   If the patient has no alerts attached to the chart and the flag on patient alert is white you can go directly to patient alerts to add the new alert. If the patient has a yellow flag that indicates additional notes are present, clicking on the yellow flag will show you those notes, as well as give you the option of adding a new note, editing, or deleting an existing one.

4. **From Patient Alerts dialog box shown in Figure 22-11, you can create a new alert. We will be creating a new alert for Pat because a white flag is displayed. You may choose any type of alert you want to practice.**

5. **Complete the fields shown in Figure 22-11: Create Patient Alert beginning with the start and end date. Select the other options for your alert.**

   • **Show symbol on appointments: if you want the alert to appear on the appointment book next to the patient's appointment information.**

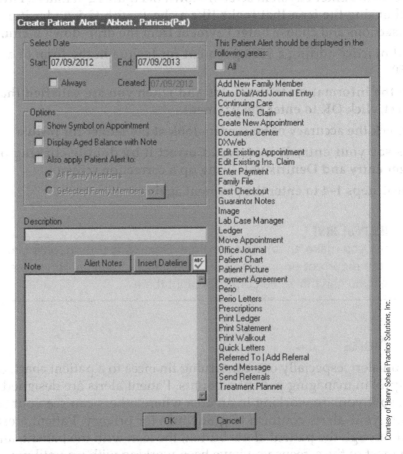

FIGURE 22-11 Adding a patient alert.

- **Display Aged Balance with Note:** this will create a pop-up with the family's aged account balance.

- **Apply Patient Alert to:** choose this if you want to select which family members to include in the alert.

6. **Enter Description:** You have 15 characters to describe the type of alert. For example, Collections or Financial or even a direction to see a specific note in the patient chart. You will probably have to abbreviate.

7. Enter a note or choose one from the template.

8. Choose the areas in Dentrix where the note should pop up by highlighting them or choose all if you want the note to appear everywhere.

9. When you choose OK the note will appear in the chosen areas (Figure 22-12).

To edit an alert, select the patient and access the alert dialog box like you did when the alert was created. Highlight the note to edit and the edit button. Make your changes and click OK to save. You can practice by editing the note on Pat's chart.

To delete, follow the process above and when you have highlighted the note you would like to delete, choose delete.

To suspend patient alerts on an individual workstation.

1. From Office Manager, select Maintenance.

2. Go to Practice Setup and then to Preferences.

3. When the Preferences dialog box appears, click on general options.

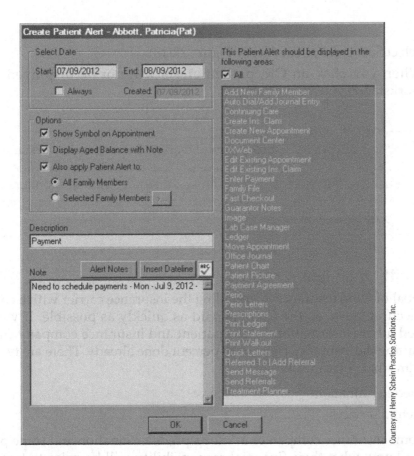

FIGURE 22-12 Alert in patient file.

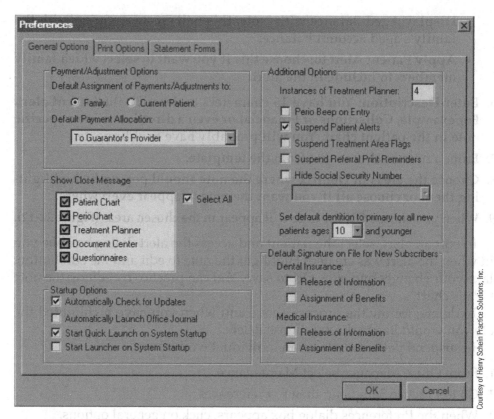

FIGURE 22-13 Suspend patient alerts.

4. Select Suspend Patient Alerts (Figure 22-13).

5. When you click on OK, patient alerts will not be displayed on the workstation you are working on.

> **HELPFUL HINT**
>
> Why would you want to suspend alerts? Sometimes a workstation is in an area where patients can easily see the pop-up. An office might suspend financial alerts from the chairside computer monitors in an orthodontic office because that isn't a time to concern young patients about family finances.

Submitting an Insurance Claim

The goal of filing insurance is providing the insurance carrier with a complete and accurate form so the claim is paid as quickly as possible. If you have entered all the information for the patient and insurance company correctly submitting the insurance claim is 80 percent done already. There are two types of claims that you can submit:

- Predetermination

- Actual services

Some insurance companies ask for a predetermination and some patients like to know what their financial responsibility will be prior to treatment. When you send a predetermination, it is very clear when it is returned that it does not guarantee coverage but with some companies it does speed processing of the actual claim. To send a predetermination, you will follow the same steps as for an actual claim. Dentrix will recognize the treatment as still in the Treatment Plan and not actually completed, so the claim will indicate it is a pretreatment estimate.

Actual services must be completed before including them on an insurance claim. It is easy to see on the charting by the red for work needed and the blue for work completed. By using a patient with completed work, you can file an insurance claim form.

1. **Bring up the Ledger and select Dean Little as a patient. His ledger will show root canal therapy for a total fee of $669.00.**

2. **Highlight the item you would like to submit to his insurance company, from the toolbar select the Insurance Selected Procedure Icon and click on it (Figure 22-14). The claim form is automatically prepared and you can see it in red on the Ledger as batched.**

   You may have noticed the option to use Insurance Today Procedure to the left of Insurance Selected Procedure Icon. If you were checking a patient out for treatment just completed, this would be an option for filing insurance.

3. **To check your work or see the actual form waiting to be submitted, click on the Office Manager icon. In the Batch Processor you can see the Dental Insurance for Dean Little (Figure 22-15). Highlight it, go to the Print Preview icon and you will see the claim form as it will be sent (Figure 22-16).**

FIGURE 22-14
Insurance Selected Procedure Icon.
Courtesy of Henry Schein Practice Solutions, Inc.

FIGURE 22-16
Print preview icon.
Courtesy of Henry Schein Practice Solutions, Inc.

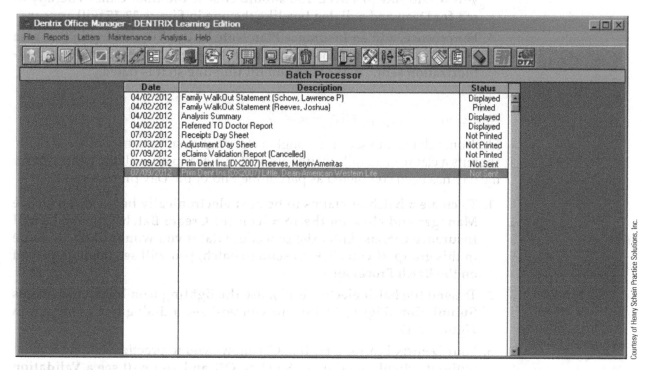

FIGURE 22-15 Claim for processing.

Primary Dental Insurance Claim (07/09/2012) Batched ☒

File Create Secondary Create Medical Enter Payment Remarks Submit Help

Patient: Little, Dean	**Carrier:** American Western Life
Subscriber: Little, Dean	**Group Plan:** Circuit City
Employer: Circuit City	(Release of Info/Assign of Benefits)(Secondary Insurance)
	eClaims Ready: (AHG01)

Billing Provider: Smith, Dennis	**Claim Information:** Standard
Rendering Provider: Smith, Dennis	**Diagnostic Codes:**
Pay-To Provider: Smith, Dennis	

Tooth	Surface	Description	Date	Code	Fee	Ins Paid
31		Root canal therapy - molar	07/02/2008	X4617	669.00	0.00

		Pmt Date	Pmt Amt	Bank/Branch #	Check #	Prov
Total Billed:	669.00					
Est Ins Portion:	535.20					
Itemized Total:	0.00					
Total Paid:	0.00					
Total Credit Adj:	0.00					
Total Chrg Adj:	0.00	Adj Date	Adj Amt	Type		Prov
Ded S/P/O:	0/0/0					

Status
Create Date: 07/09/2012 Tracer:
Date Sent : 07/09/2012 On Hold:
Re-Sent:
Claim Status Note:
· Mon - Jul 9, 2012 12:56:09 pm - >Batched

Insurance Plan Note
(No Note)

Remarks for Unusual Services
(No Note)

Courtesy of Henry Schein Practice Solutions, Inc.

FIGURE 22-17 Adding notes to a claim form.

4. **To add notes to the claim from the ledger double click on the procedure you would like to select. You should choose the Root Canal Therapy in red for Dean and a dialog box like the one in Figure 22-17 will appear.**

5. **For practice, add an Insurance Plan Note by double clicking in that area of the dialog box and inserting a note "emergency treatment, no preauthorization sent," make sure you hit timeline so it is dated.**

Electronic Claims Submission

Electronic claims are set up through a clearinghouse before an office actually submits a claim. Generally claims are sent in a group after all the treatment for the day has been completed as part of the End of the Day procedures.

1. **To create a batch of claims to be sent electronically begin at the Office Manager and click on the INS icon for Create Batch Primary Dental Insurance Claims. Enter the procedure dates you would like to include in this group. If you click on send to batch, you will see them displayed on the Batch Processor.**

2. **To send the batch electronically, use the lighting icon Electronic Claims Submission (Figure 22-18) and you will see a dialog box as shown in Figure 22-19.**

3. **Your Dentrix Learning Edition CD allows you to practice sending a claim without actually sending it. So click OK and you will see a Validation Report like Figure 22-20: Validation Report.**

FIGURE 22-18 Icon for submitting electronic claims.

Courtesy of Henry Schein Practice Solutions, Inc.

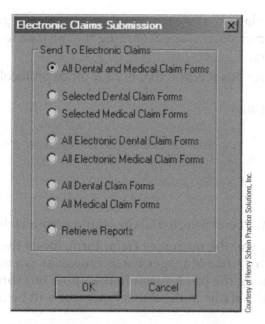

FIGURE 22-19 Submitting an electronic claim.

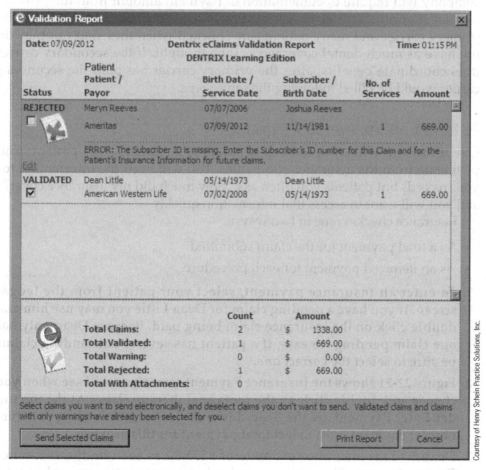

FIGURE 22-20 Validation report.

4. If you had a claim that was incomplete, you would get a rejected on its status with an error message regarding the mistake so it can be corrected before sending.

5. You could print this report if that is your office protocol.

> **HELPFUL HINT**
>
> Once your office is truly paperless you will want to do as little printing as possible. You save ink and paper but also benefit by not having to shred documents containing personal information. Anything with a patient's name must be disposed of according to HIPAA regulations.

6. By selecting the Send Selected Claims button, your claim would be sent.

7. **To print a copy of the insurance claim form, locate the claim you want to print from the Office Manager Batch Processor. Go to the Print Preview Icon; by clicking the printer icon in the upper left corner your form will be printed. The status in the Batch Processor will be updated to printed.**

Filing Secondary Claims

Filing a secondary claim is done after the primary claim is paid. The secondary company will require documentation of payment amount from the primary carrier. A secondary carrier doesn't have to coordinate benefits with the primary carrier and many patients are shocked when they find out they do not have as much dental coverage as they thought. If the secondary carrier does coordinate benefits, after the primary carrier has paid the secondary carrier would be billed following the same steps.

Entering an Insurance Payment

One thing you will want to keep separate is payments from patients and payments from the insurance companies. You will need the information for your records but patients will often ask "how much did my insurance cover?" and you will want to access that information quickly.

Insurance checks come in two ways:

- As a total payment for the claim submitted.
- As an itemized payment for each procedure.

1. **To enter an insurance payment, select your patient from the ledger screen. If you have a pending claim for Dean Little you may use him and double click on the insurance claim being paid. Because Dean only has one claim pending it's easy, if a patient has several outstanding claims be sure to select the correct one.**

2. **Figure 22-21 shows the Insurance Payment screen you will see when you choose and double click on the root canal therapy claim. At the top under Enter Payment are the drop-down choices of itemize by procedure or total payment only. Select total payment for this exercise.**

3. Dean had an insurance estimate of $535.20 as seen on the Insurance Payment screen. The coverage dialog box appears after you select total payment only.

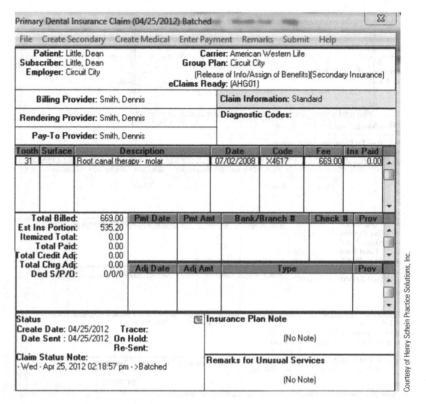

FIGURE 22-21 Insurance payment.

4. **After entering the check and bank numbers, select add to enter the amount paid; for this exercise we'll assume that the payment was $530.20.**
   Some insurance companies send funds by electronic payment. If the payment was by electronic funds be sure to check Electronic Payment so you aren't looking for a check you don't have at the end of the day.

5. **When your entries are complete and accurate. Click on OK/Post to complete the transaction.** If you were working in Dean's account, you can return to his ledger to check your work and his family file to see how it changed the balance on the account.
   By managing patient accounts and payments correctly, it is very easy to see at a glance if the balance is the patient's responsibility and if additional insurance payments are expected.
   Now we'll repeat the process with an account where the payment is by procedure.

1. **Open the ledger for Joshua Reeves.** If insurance has not been filed for his prophylaxis, bitewings, and oral exam, do so by highlighting all three and selecting the Insurance Selected Procedure icon, this was the icon you used in a previous exercise and can be found on the toolbar. To highlight all, hold down your shift key when selecting. This will file a claim quickly so we can see how a claim for multiple procedures can be itemized.

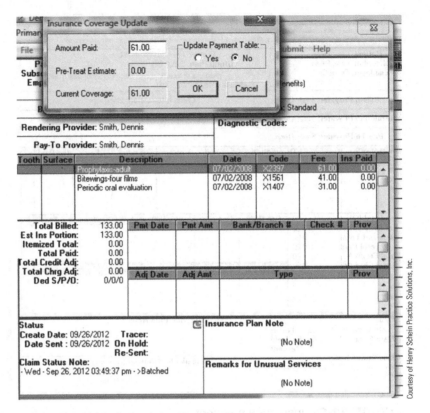

FIGURE 22-22 Submitting itemized claim.

2. **From the ledger double click on the claim in red and enter payment.** This is the same as for Dean in the previous exercise.

3. **Select itemize payment for this exercise. You will see a screen similar to the one in Figure 22-22: Insurance Coverage Update.** Directly behind that screen you will see the insurance estimates on each procedure.

4. **When an insurance check comes in an itemized format each procedure will have a payment amount instead of just a total.** Because Joshua had three procedures enter each separately and for this assignment make sure they were all paid at 100 percent or $61 for prophylaxis, $41 for bitewings, and $31 for his exam. **Enter those amounts and click OK.**

5. **You have returned to the total payment screen and from here you complete posting the payment exactly as you did with Dean in the previous exercise.**

Walkout Statements

A walkout statement is an update for the patient regarding their account. It can be used as a receipt or a bill. Within any dental office, the best way to receive payment for the treatment done is the same day as the visit. This saves staff time and the cost of printing and mailing statements. It also eliminates possible collection problems at a later date. If the patient's financial arrangement allows him or her to pay the fee after the appointment, or for some reason the patient is unable to pay at the time of the appointment, a walkout statement is a good alternative. Some offices even give patients an envelope to send payment to encourage them to do so promptly.

1. **Go to Patient Chart and Select Pat Abbott as your Patient. By charting completed treatment, you will be able to see one way the statement system works. Highlight with your explorer tooth #18 in her clinical chart and choose MOD amalgam from your procedure short cuts. Because we are only interested in the statement part of her treatment, go to completed, which is shown as a check mark at the right of EO, Ex, Tx. Now you have a completed procedure so you can create statements.**

2. **From the toolbar, click on the ledger icon.**

3. **Use print from the line above the graphic icons and choose walkout from the options under the print drop-down menu. You will see a dialog box like Figure 22-23: Print Walkout.**

4. **You have several areas that allow you to customize the walkout statement including a place to include a message, try including your own message or use mine.**

   - Enhanced or plain is determined by the printer the office uses so once this is set, it does not need to be changed.

   - Family walkout will include any charges pending for family members as well as the patient. Then Dentrix prints appointment reminders for upcoming appointments for each family member.

   - The walkout/doctor's statement is used by offices that ask patients to do their own insurance billing. This form gives them the information needed.

   - You can also print an appointment card or an appointment label.

   - The additional fields are optional but could be added if it is your office protocol.

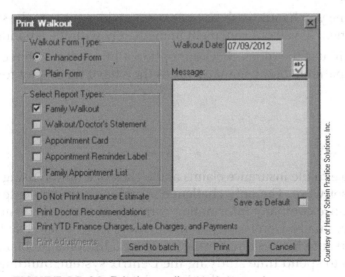

FIGURE 22-23 Printing walk out statement.

If you had a message you wanted to print on all your walkout statements you would save it as default; a general message like "Our office will be closed on Fridays beginning in June." When you are ready you would print it from the dialog box or send it to batch.

> ┌─ **HELPFUL HINT**
>
> When you send an item to batch, you will see it on the Office Managers Desk. Doing that enables you to print everything at the end of day or a later date. From the Managers Desk, you can view an item, print an item, or send it electronically. To view any of the items in the batch processor, highlight it and use the icon to the left of the printer that looks like a monitor screen.

5. **For practice: send your walkout statement to batch. Go to the Office Manager, highlight it and then view it by using the monitor icon for print preview. Can you see your message? Figure 22-24 shows a printed statement.**

FIGURE 22-25
Fast checkout
icon.

Quick Checkout

Once you understand the checkout system and the individual steps in checking a patient out you can graduate to the quick checkout. This will enable you to quickly post treatment, payments, and file insurance.

1. **From the Ledger, choose Brent Crosby as your patient and go to the fast checkout icon, which looks like a little man going out the door (Figure 22-25). You may click OK on the alert since you are aware of it.**

2. Brent had no new treatment today but if he'd had something done the insurance for that treatment would automatically go to the Batch Processor, so click OK to acknowledge that you understand.

3. **Enter any payment he needs to make, for example, the $133 he still owes for past treatment. Let's say he gives that to you in cash so go ahead and post it.**

4. Anytime you handle cash payments, you will want to make sure you give the patient a walkout statement immediately with the amount on it.

5. You will use the quick checkout option all the time with recurring care/recall patients because many times they have no co-pay for preventive work.

Summary

You are able to file insurance claims at the click of a button using dental management software. The only challenge is making sure you enter the patient and insurance company information correctly at the initial visit and update it at least annually. Don't guess at information, leave a field blank rather than enter errors into the system. Errors can cause additional problems to crop up later. Plan to spend time studying the Dentrix system, building speed, and then find ways to incorporate that into a dental practice.

STATEMENT OF SERVICES RENDERED					

DENTRIX Learning Edition
Licensed for Personal
Non-Commercial Use
,

CHART NO.	PAGE NO.
AB0001	1

BILLING DATE
07/09/2012

GUARANTOR NAME AND MAILING ADDRESS

Mr. Ken S Abbott
608 S 500 W
Apt. 101
Eastside, NV 11111

PATIENT	TOOTH	SURF	DESCRIPTION	CHARGE	CREDIT
Patricia	18	MOD	Amalgam-3 surf. prim/perm	122.00	

PRIOR BALANCE	CURRENT CREDITS	CURRENT CHARGES	NEW BALANCE	DENTAL INS, EST.	PLEASE PAY
0.00 −	0.00 +	122.00 =	122.00 −	0.00 =	122.00

PATIENT	DATE	TIME	REASON

Our office will be closed on Fridays beginning in June

FIGURE 22-24 Sample walk out statement.

Skill Building

For exercise number 2, these payments may create a positive balance.

1. Enter the following payments:
   - Post a personal payment for Rachel Anthony in the amount of $50 received by check number 1220.
   - Post an insurance payment for Thomas Lane in the amount of $75.
   - Post a personal payment from Clayton Lewis in the amount of $100 received by MasterCard.
   - Enter an adjustment for Clayton Lewis of $25 as a professional courtesy.

2. Using the patients from Appendix 1
   - Print insurance claims for Rachel Anthony, Thomas Lane, and Clayton Lewis.
   - Print statements for Rachel Anthony, Thomas Lane, and Clayton Lewis.

Challenge Your Understanding

1. Corey Hansen has an outstanding balance of $377.00. How much of it is expected from the insurance company?
   a. Insurance should pay the entire amount
   b. Insurance was not filed, no estimate on file
   c. Insurance should pay $155
   d. This patient does not have insurance

2. What is the balance for Adria Johnson?
   a. $300
   b. $150
   c. $75
   d. No balance

3. What is the patient alert for Peggy Perkins?
   a. There is no alert
   b. She has been sent to collections
   c. She has a privacy request
   d. Her alert is suspended

4. Types of print options from the ledger would not include:
   a. Walkout
   b. Family ledger
   c. Patient with discounts
   d. Statement

5. Mary Brown has a balance on her account of $377.00. On which date were the fees posted?
   a. July 2, 2008
   b. April 5, 2005
   c. July 8, 2008
   d. June 2, 2008

CHAPTER 23

Communication Using Practice Management Software

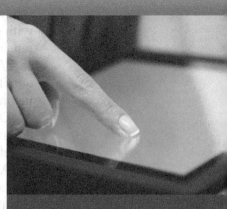

CHAPTER OUTLINES

- **Communicating with Patients**
- **Writing Quick Letters**
- **Recurring Care/Recall**
- **Letters**
  Changing an Existing Letter
- **Office Journal**
- **Email**
- **Statements**
- **Documenting Patient Contacts**
- **Summary**

LEARNING OBJECTIVES

Upon completion of this chapter, the reader should be able to:

1. Write letters using templates in Dentrix.
2. Set up contact communication for recurring care.
3. Use electronic communication to contact patients.
4. Demonstrate modifying and generating account statements.
5. Successfully document patient contacts.

KEY TERMS

statement
email
recurring care
template

Communicating with Patients

Written communication to patients can assist in building a dental practice by using letters of welcome to new patients or letters of congratulations to new parents. Communication maintains a practice by keeping accounts current with perfectly worded collection letters. Best of all it is easy to use the prewritten letters in Dentrix. Letters can be generated automatically such as recurring care/recall or individually with personalization. Electronic communication, email, is how many patients manage their lives so Dentrix can also make contacting them via the web fast and easy.

Dentrix uses Microsoft Word to create and merge correspondence. Before beginning any letter writing process Dentrix recommends opening Microsoft Word and minimizing it.

As you work on writing letters, printing is an option but is not necessary. All exercises can be done without making a hard copy so don't be concerned if you are not connected to a printer. If you do have access to a printer, it is fun to have some samples of your work.

In this chapter you will work with **recurring care** to see how written communication can track your patients encouraging them to have regular visits. You will also see how sending effective statements can help keep accounts current. With practice management software and a few clicks you can send letters, postcards, and statements out in minutes.

As we work on correspondence, it is important to be aware of patient privacy requests, such as no correspondence. As the Patient Information is entered into Dentrix, any privacy requests the patient has made should be noted in the privacy request fields. To access patient information from the Family File, select the patient then double click on the top part of the screen that contains the patient's name and make additions or changes (Figure A 23-1 and B 23-1). Protecting a patient's privacy isn't just a good idea, it's the law.

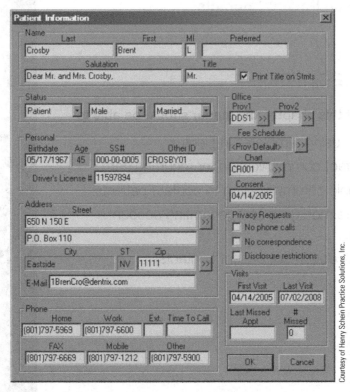

FIGURE 23-1(A) Patient information box.

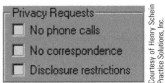

FIGURE 23-1(B)

> **HELPFUL HINT**
> One of the goals of patient communication is making it appear personal, not computer generated.

Writing Quick Letters

Quick letters are easy so it is a good place to begin practicing.

1. **After accessing the Dentrix program, go to Family File to begin exploring the quick letter writing process.**
2. **Choose Dean Little from Select a Patient.**
3. **Click on the icon for quick letters (Figure 23-2). You should see a dialog box like the one in Figure 23-3: Quick Letters**
4. **To view what each letter looks like before the actual patient information is added, highlight the letter name and open the template.**
   Please take the time to open each letter and see the variety of prewritten letters available.
   Now let's personalize the letter.

FIGURE 23-2
Quick letters icon.

Courtesy of Henry Schein Practice Solutions, Inc.

> **HELPFUL HINT**
> It is always a good idea to view any letter before you print it to proofread it and make sure it represents the professionalism of your office. For example, recently I received a "thank you for visiting us" letter from a car dealer. It was obvious it was computer generated without taking time to double check it because of capitalization errors in the salutation. Small things can make an impression. Make sure your written communication makes an excellent impression.

5. **For this exercise choose the New Patient Welcome letter and highlight it.**
   - To create the letter as it is, simply click print and Dentrix will merge the patient information and print the letter.

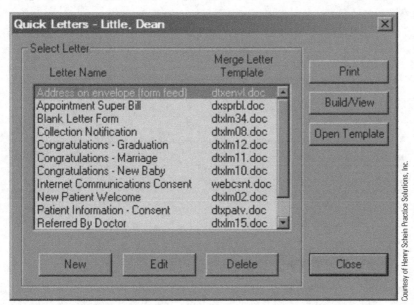

FIGURE 23-3 Quick letters list.

- To see the letter before printing it, click on Build/View. Your letter will be merged with the patient's information and you can make any changes necessary.

6. **Use the Build/View button to see your letter to Dean Little. There are some things you will want to correct before you print.**
   - **First, this letter is to Dean so you should make sure the salutation is to Dear Dean or if it is more appropriate Dear Mr. Little,**
   Please note this can be set in patient information under salutation to make writing letters even quicker. How you address patients will depend on the personality of the practice and where it is located.
   - **In the body of the letter, in the third line is the term reasonable prices, please change that to reasonable fees.**
   - **When you have made the changes you are ready to print the letter. Go to print and your letter is ready to be sent.**

7. **A dialog box will ask if you want to save the changes to the letter. You could save it to a file to print later. Otherwise, once you have printed the letter you can hit no to saving it.**
   You also have an icon on your toolbar (next to the quick letters icon) to allow you to create a label.

8. **Continue using Dean Little as your patient and open Quick Labels from the toolbar. You will see the dialog box shown in Figure 23-4: Quick Labels.**
   As you read through the list of possible labels, note how each would be used. If we were sending a letter to the person financially responsible for the account or guarantor you wouldn't want to click on quick label for the patient.

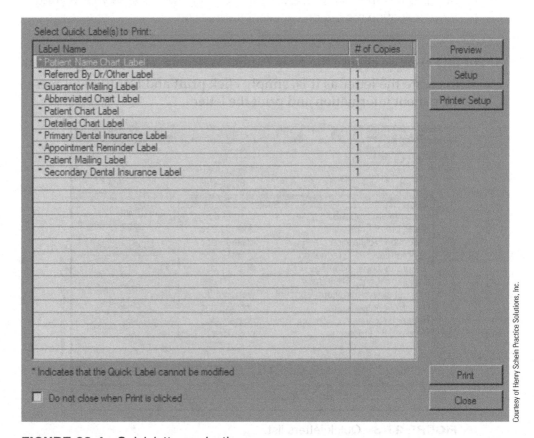

FIGURE 23-4 Quick letters selection.

9. Once you have selected to whom the correspondence should be addressed, highlight the label and if you want to print, click on the print key.

Recurring Care/Recall

It is common for offices to send out reminders to patients that have or need appointments for routine cleaning and check-up appointments. Offices often use postcards to save on printing, paper cost, and also postage. To do this, we will be merging a list of patients with the postcard we want to send.

1. Go to Office Manager and from the toolbar above the icons choose and click on Letters.

2. A dialog box should open with choices of several types of letters.

3. Choose Continuing Care by clicking on it; then clicking on Cont. Care Cards—Appointment. Click on the Edit button to customize who should get these postcards.

   This series of selections will bring up the dialog selection box with criteria for sending cards as seen in Figure 23-5: Patient Report View.

> **── HELPFUL HINT**
>
> Most offices have a regular protocol for making recurring care contacts. If you chose not to edit the group you were sending postcards to, the system will send out cards to everyone. According to office protocol, you will want to be specific. For example, if you send cards one month ahead, in December you set the system to send for January, and so on.

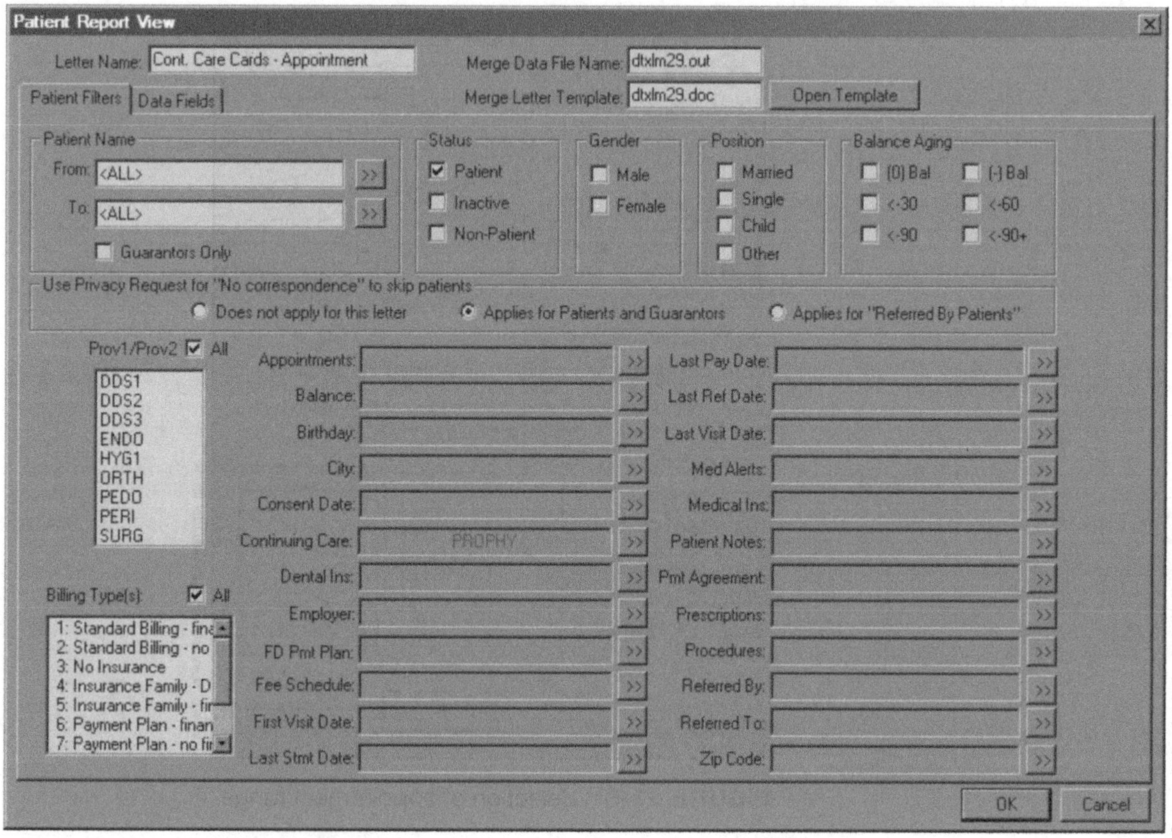

FIGURE 23-5 Patient report view.

4. The Patient Report View dialog box will enable you to select the patients to receive cards. For this exercise, Cont. Care Cards—Appointment should appear in the letter name field because we chose it from Continuing Care Letters.

   To the right of the letter name is the selection for Merge Letter Template. In an office you would make this selection based on the type of postcards the office has purchased.

5. At the top right of the file name and template is an open template; for this exercise open that to investigate the wording on your postcard. When you are sending this out in an office, this step would be omitted unless you needed to make changes. After you read the template you may close it at the upper right X.

   In the Patient Report View, just underneath the Letter Name you will see Patient Filters; these allow you to narrow the group of patients you are sending postcards to. You can send to only the responsible party or guarantors, select to send only to patients or inactive patients, further eliminate patients by choosing only a letter to patients based on gender or marital status. Under patient filters you can use privacy requests to skip some patients.

   For this exercise create Continuing Care postcards for January 2012 to patients with appointments, click on the arrow next to the appointment information box and a selection box will open enabling you to choose your date range (Figure 23-6). Then, under search, choose Existing Patients with appointments in date range in Appointment Date Range.

6. Because you want to send these reminders to all patients who have appointments, you won't want to limit your mailing but you could by

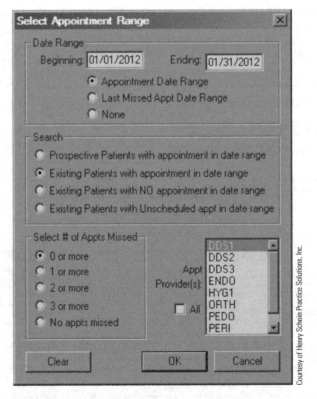

FIGURE 23-6 Selection of appointment range.

using other fields available. Go ahead and look through all the ways you could control who receives any mailing you produce.

An example of limiting a field for correspondence would be to send to only patients in a specific zip code. In that selection box you would enter the zip you want to mail to. Or you could mail only to a group of patients who all work for the same employer by customizing that field. **After you have looked through all your fields, click the OK button.**

7. **As you return to the Continuing Care Letters dialog box (this happens after you click okay) check to make sure the Cont. Care Cards— Appointment line is still highlighted.**

   If it is, click on the bottom left button for Create/Merge.

8. **Under Create/Merge options select Create Data File and Merge Letters along with Add to Journal.**

9. **There are probably no patients in our tutorial database that fit these exact criteria so to practice: we'll repeat with different information.**

┌─ HELPFUL HINT

By covering the basics of what Dentrix is able to do with correspondence, you will be able to transfer your knowledge to a dental office. Just remember each office has its own procedures and they may be slightly different than we have practiced. When you are confident with the basics the transition will be effortless.

Repeat the steps above with the exception of:

- **Use Cont. Care Cards—Appointment Cards—Reminder**
- **Use edit to set your criteria.**
- **Under Select Appointment Range "search" use Existing Patients with appointment in the date range and all providers.**
- **Use a date range of 1/1/2005 to today's date.**
- **Hit OK until you return to Continuing Care Letters, confirm that Cont. Care Cards—Appointment Cards—Reminder is still selected, then go to create/merge.**
- **There are several patients within this broader search range. You will see what would be printed on postcards to those patients.**
- **At this point once you are happy with your results you would print your postcards.**

Letters

Sometimes you will want to send a letter to a group of patients. While quick letters works great for single pieces of correspondence, it is not practical for larger mailings.

We will follow the same basic steps for letters that we did for the continuing care postcard mailing.

1. **We will be sending out birthday letters using the create/merge function; go to the Office Manager and use the drop-down menu for letters from above the icon toolbar.**

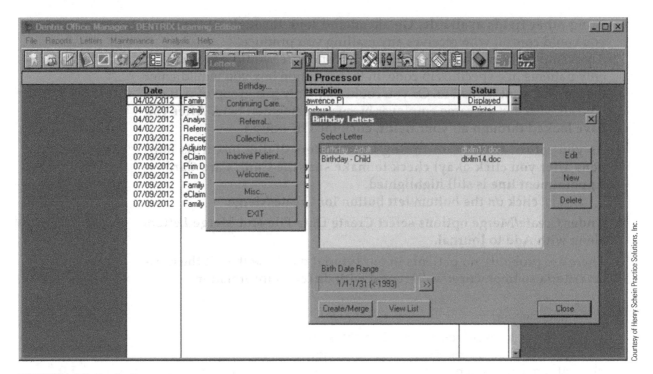

FIGURE 23-7 Letters.

2. Look at the letter choices shown in Figure 23-7: Letters. Choose birthday at the top of the list. You will see a dialog box for Birthday Letters that shows you there are actually two versions of the letter; an adult letter and a child letter.

3. For this exercise choose the adult letter by highlighting it. You can complete your date range from this dialog box or go to edit. We are sending out a January birthday letter to adults so our date range is 01/01 to 01/31; then select the years to include as adults. Because we want to include any of the oldest patients in the practice, we'll choose a date well before the year anyone was born so put 1900 as the beginning date and let's include anyone up to 2003 as an adult and check search as date range

   Who you include as an adult may depend a lot on the wording of the letter and your practice so adjust your dates accordingly. Don't offend the teens in your practice by sending a juvenile letter.

4. Instead of using the fast date selection box you could also use the edit function to add the dates included in this birthday mailing. The edit function allows you to make other choices such as; do you send the letter just to patients? Or do family members that are non-patients also get a birthday greeting? Do you want to send this to inactive patients as well as active patients?

5. When you are satisfied with your "birthday group," go to create/merge, create a data file, merge letters, and add to journal.

6. You will be able to see the letters in the group and you are ready to print.
   Practice using the different letters and different criteria available until you feel comfortable.

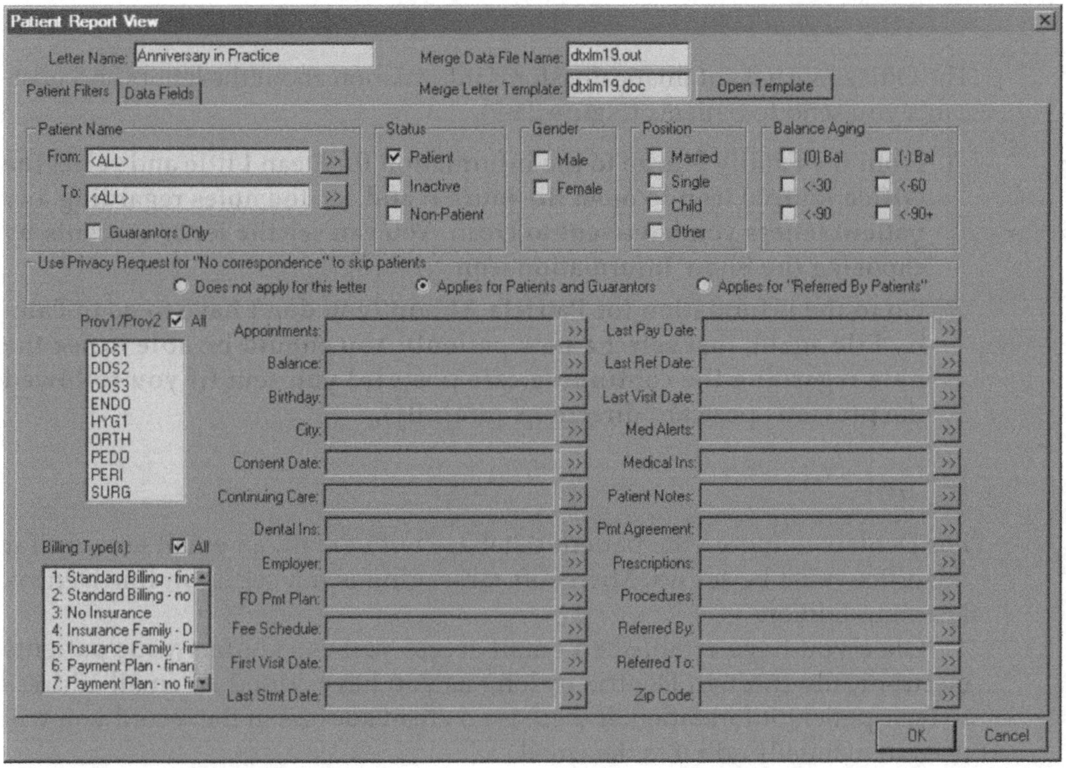

Courtesy of Henry Schein Practice Solutions, Inc.

FIGURE 23-8 Patient report view.

Changing an Existing Letter

While Dentrix has carefully chosen the wording in the letters available occasionally you may want to change a letter to make it reflect your practice. When you change the **template** you will be doing so for all future letters so make sure you want to make the change and, if needed, that you have permission to do so.

1. **Go to the Office Manager and open the letters from the drop-down menu.**
2. **Select Anniversary in the Practice from the Welcome group to change.**
3. **Select edit to access the Patient Report View (Figure 23-8). This time in the upper right corner Open the Template. The template is like the recipe for the letter so you will want to be careful.**
4. **Find the line in the letter that reads "reasonable prices" and change it to "reasonable fees."**
5. **Close the letter from the upper right X, and when asked, say Yes to save the change.**
6. **From now on this letter will include that change. For practice, repeat the steps and confirm the change then try making another one.**

It is possible to create custom letters in Dentrix but it takes an excellent knowledge of word processing. Practice for now with the letters available in quick letters or from the drop-down menu under letters. When you have mastered those you can refer to the User's Manual for step by step instruction on custom letters.

Office Journal

FIGURE 23-9
Journal icon
Courtesy of Henry Schein Practice Solutions, Inc.

The Office Journal automatically stores information about the letters and postcards you send to patients (Figure 23-9).

1. **From the Family File go to the information for Dean Little and select the Office Journal icon to open the journal and see the notes regarding any patient letters you have sent to Dean. You can see the letter contents by choosing the Show Information icon.**

2. **Go to the information for Patricia Abbott (you don't have to go to Family File again, just select a new patient). You should be able to see the note regarding the continuing care postcard you sent (if you followed the previous postcard directions carefully).**

Email

For Dentrix to merge the patient database with email, an email account for the office must be set up. Microsoft messaging is not set up in this Dentrix Learning Edition.

Once you have established email access you can contact your patients electronically through Dentrix as long as you have added an email address to their patient information. If there is no email address in the record you will need to manually add it to the email.

> **HELPFUL HINT**
> It is very important to make the patient information as accurate and complete as possible. When you need to contact a patient and you have missing information it can be extremely frustrating.

There are several patient screens where you will find an email icon; it looks like a letter with an @ symbol in the middle and the icon will identify itself as Send Message.

Email needs to be treated like any other professional correspondence and checked for spelling and grammatical errors.

> **HELPFUL HINT**
> If you are unsure of yourself when it comes to proofreading the contents of an email ask for assistance from another dental team member. They should be happy to assist you because an email full of errors reflects poorly on the entire office.

Statements

FIGURE 23-10
Process billing statement icon
Courtesy of Henry Schein Practice Solutions, Inc.

A billing statement can be printed immediately by choosing the patient, going to the Ledger and selecting Statements from the Print drop-down (Figure 23-10). So if a patient contacts the office requesting a copy, this is one quick and easy way to access a statement.

Mailed statements are sent by either regular post or electronically. Most practices do this once a month, the same time of the month. Before sending statements, all payments received are posted. Many offices wait until the second week of the month to send statements so that any checks mailed on the first have time to be received and processed. Checks would not only be coming from the patients but also insurance companies.

1. **To print the month's statements, go to the Office Manager and select Reports from the drop-down menu and then choose billing. The dialog box shown in Figure 23-11 (Billing Statements) should be visible.**

2. **As you have done in other exercises, you need to choose who and what should be included in your statement mailing.**

3. **Let's choose a statement date of 5/15/2011 and the balance forward of 4/15/2011. Choose all guarantors (these are the people financially responsible for the account) and all providers. Let's only send statements to patients or families that owe more than $5.00. Select to put them into batch. Under options, check skip accounts with claim pending and with a patient portion of $20.00 or less. Also print account aging, so the patient can see how long they have owed the balance. Sort by patient name and select billing statement. There is currently a message on the screen that is very appropriate so leave it.**

4. **Save as default and click OK.**

5. **By returning to the Office Manager, you will see Billing Statements on the Batch Processor. Highlight the billing statements line and go to the Print Preview icon to look at what the statements will look like.**

6. **Close the preview and either send them electronically or by regular post.**
    To clarify, statements can be sent electronically, much like insurance claims, but there are fees associated with doing both of those things because they go through a clearinghouse. Fees are small but electronic doesn't necessarily mean free.

7. **To send electronically, highlight that you would like to send from the Office Manager batch processor. Then select the lightning bolt icon for electronic billing submission. You will see a dialog box like Figure 23-12; Click OK to send. You will see the electronic submission.**

> **HELPFUL HINT**
> Anytime a billing statement is produced for a patients account it is automatically recorded in the Office Journal.

Documenting Patient Contacts

Whenever you contact a patient it is a good idea to leave a detailed notation in the patient chart. Notes of this nature are recorded in the Office Journal so that they don't appear in the clinical care portion of the patient's file.

1. **Go to Dean Little's family file and select the Office Journal icon and click on it.**

2. **Open Add Journal Entry at the upper left and add a contact regarding by phone call to Dean Little's chart journal as is shown in Figure 23-13 (Add Journal Entry).**

Documenting these contacts is important if you would ever need to prove that you had been regularly contacting a patient and had not abandoned them.

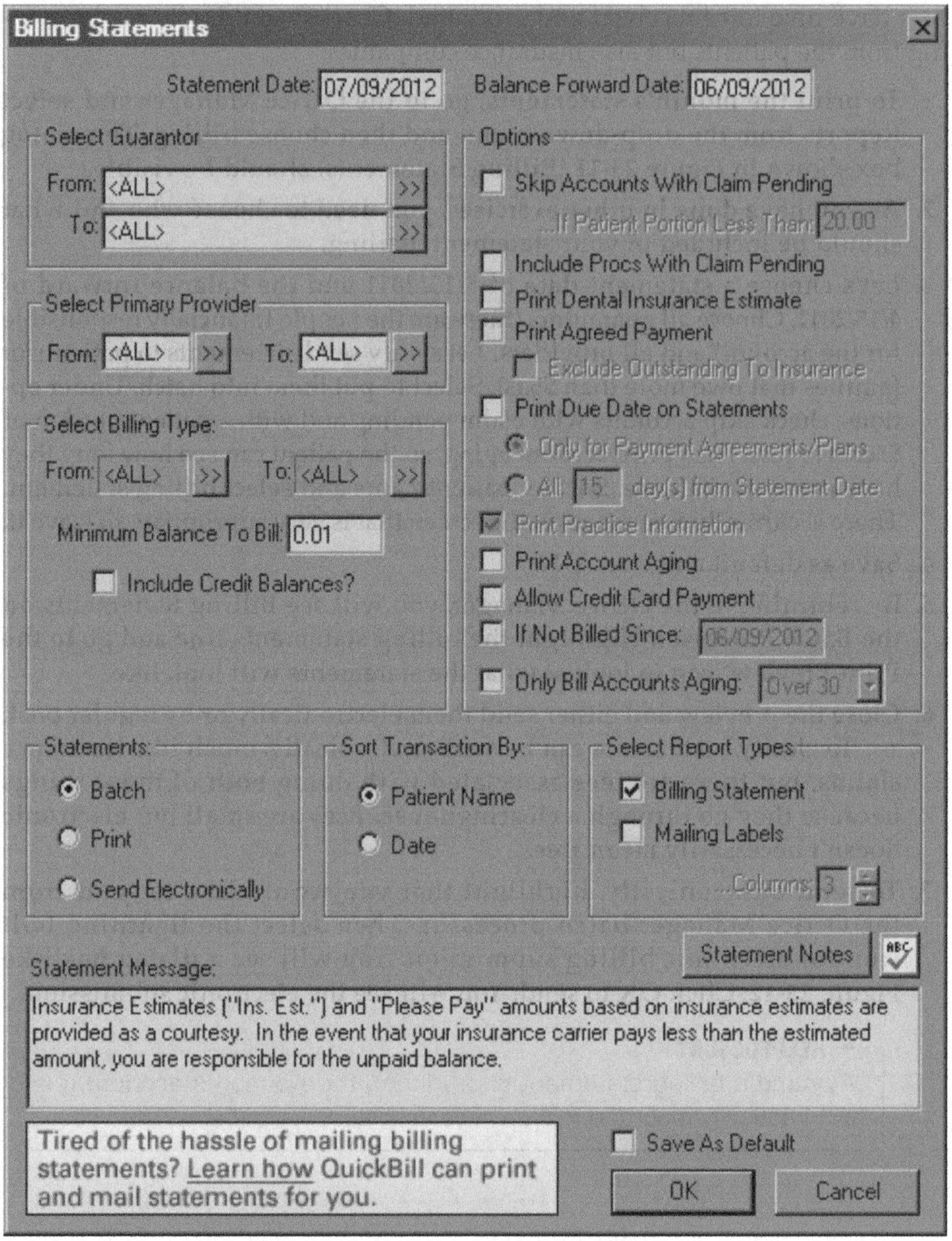

FIGURE 23-11 Billing statement.

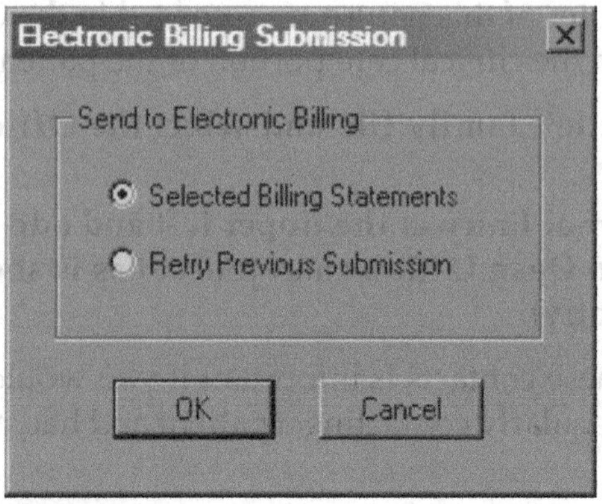

FIGURE 23-12 Electronic billing.

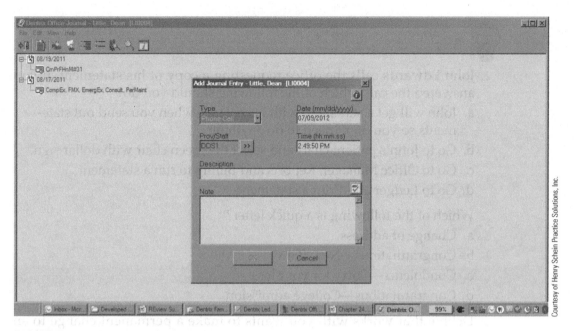

FIGURE 23-13 Journal entry.

Summary

Communication can build or break a dental practice. Whether you are sending a letter or an email, make sure the message reflects the practice. If your correspondence is sloppy, patients may assume your dental work is too. Dentrix makes all communication easier but dental software is only as accurate as the user.

 Skill Building

1. **Using the patients from Appendix 1, write the following letters:**
   - To Rachel Anthony: Please write a "Congratulations on your Marriage" letter to Rachel.
   - To Thomas Lane: Please write a "Collection Notification"; this is just for practice so don't be concerned that Tom isn't a delinquent account.
   - To Janet Bruce: Please write a referral letter to David Jones DDS, MS, an oral surgeon, for extractions indicated in her treatment plan. Make sure you include any health restrictions.
   - To Clayton Lewis: Please send an "Internet Communications Request" form.

2. Print statements for Rachel Anthony, Thomas Lane, Janet Bruce, and Clayton Lewis. Include all balances.

3. View or print "Patient Information-Consent" for Rachel Anthony, Thomas Lane, Janet Bruce, and Clayton Lewis.

Courtesy of Henry Schein Practice Solutions, Inc.

Challenge Your Understanding

1. John Edwards calls the office requesting a copy of his statement. If you answered the call, which of the following should you do?
   a. John will get a statement with his balance when you send out statements so you don't need to do anything.
   b. Go to John's patient chart and select the green chair with dollar sign.
   c. Go to Office Manager, Reports and Billing to run a statement.
   d. Go to Ledger and Print a statement.

2. Which of the following is a quick letter?
   a. Change of address
   b. Congratulations—New Baby
   c. Condolence—Sorry for your loss
   d. Congratulations—College admission

3. Debbie that works with you wants to make a permanent change to an existing letter within your system. Where should she start?
   a. Go to Office Manager and open letters from the top of the page
   b. Ask the doctor or office manager if they object to the change
   c. Use the edit function from Quick Letters because it is a small change
   d. Letters in Dentrix cannot be changed

4. Statements should be?
   a. Sent electronically because it's free
   b. Sent on the first of the month
   c. Sent the same time of the month
   d. After 60 days with no payment

5. To track correspondence it is important to do which of the following?
   a. Print an additional copy for your records
   b. Make an entry in the patient treatment notes
   c. Verify a copy was added to Office Journal
   d. For patient privacy no record should be kept

Beyond the Basics

CHAPTER OUTLINES

KEY TERMS

LEARNING OBJECTIVES

Upon completion of this chapter, the reader should be able to:

1. Describe the process to add additional staff members.
2. Demonstrate how to clock in and out using Dentrix and how to gather personal work history.
3. Successfully use Dentrix to gather practice management information and create reports.

4. Demonstrate adding fees and procedures to the Dentrix system.

5. Produce reports using Practice Assistant.

Making the Most of Dentrix

Lots of dental offices use practice management software but very few offices take advantage of everything it can do. This chapter will cover a few things that are beyond the basics in Dentrix. All of these functions are easy to learn and use but they do take practice.

Time Clock

The fastest way to get to the time clock is to use Dentrix **Quick Launch**. You can reach it from your programs menu and then going to Dentrix by choosing quick launch. Check your computer toolbar for the quick launch icon shown with an arrow on the Figure 24-1 (Quick Launch).

1. **Double clicking on this icon will bring up the time clock. Right clicking on it will allow you to access other Dentrix functions. Go ahead and double click.**

2. **The staff within the Dentrix Learning CD cannot be changed so for this exercise clock in as Sally Hayes; highlight her name on the list and click OK (Figure 24-2).**

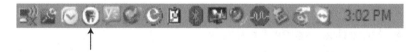

FIGURE 24-1 Quick launch from programs toolbar.

Courtesy of Henry Schein Practice Solutions, Inc.

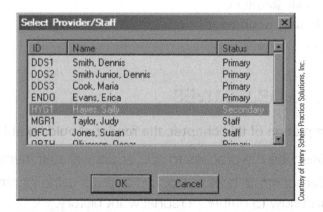

FIGURE 24-2 Selecting staff from time clock.

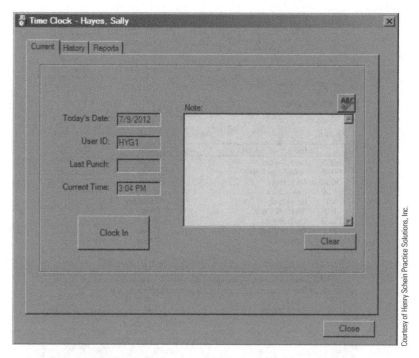

FIGURE 24-3 Clocking in.

3. After selecting Sally, you will see the Time Clock dialog box (Figure 24-3).

4. To clock in click on the button, it will then become the clock out button.

5. Next to the Current tab at the top of the dialog box are the options to view the History and/or Reports.

6. Check out and explore the information on the tabs. In an office, there would be passwords and limited access protocols set up with the time clock for privacy; however, it allows the individual with payroll responsibility to clock staff members in or out when they forget.

Practice Setup

Understanding how to customize many aspects of the practice is important but it isn't usually something you will be asked to do on your first day. Practice set up is accessed from Dental Office Manager and the maintenance drop-down menu at the top of your screen. From that menu there will be a list of options.

Take the time to go through the entire list so you are familiar with the screens and in the next exercises you will be guided through some of the more commonly used tasks.

> **— HELPFUL HINT**
>
> Remember if you are working in an office and you don't know how to find something in Dentrix you can ask the software itself by using the Help button at the top or referring to the User's Guide. One of the reasons Dentrix has maintained its popularity in dental offices is its ease of use.

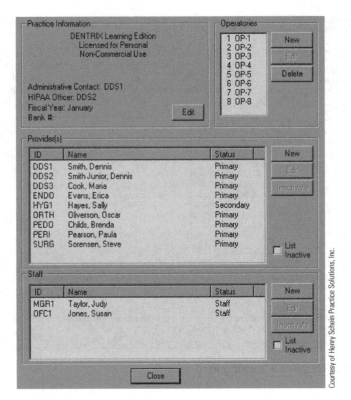

FIGURE 24-4 Practice information and set up.

Adding New Staff Members

To add a new staff member you will use Practice Resource Setup from the Practice Setup List and select new (Figure 24-4). The Dentrix G4 Learning CD has a practice in place that cannot be altered but you will be able to see how it is done.

The practice resource setup will also allow you to edit the information for current staff members by highlighting the name and choosing edit. When a staff member leaves the practice you will inactivate them rather than delete. Because they have worked with patients in your practice they need to be maintained as part of the practice record.

Adding Fees and Procedures

ADA/CDT codes do not change often but when they do you need to be able to make the modification. Adding a code is easy but deleting it again may require assistance from Dentrix. This is because once a code is added it could have been used in a patient chart so deleting it will leave an inconsistency in the record. When a code is no longer being used a note could be added to it indicating the code is obsolete. To keep your system accurate let's talk through adding a code without actually doing it.

1. To add a new code go to add a procedure code from the practice setup drop-down menu and you will get a dialog box (Figure 24-5A); select a category for your new code; review existing codes to made sure you aren't adding this code twice then click on new for a new code or edit. If you are setting up a new code you will see the Procedure Code Editor—New box with all the fields blank (Figure 24-5B).

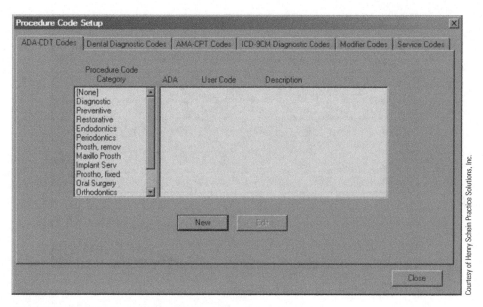

FIGURE 24-5A Procedure Code Set up.

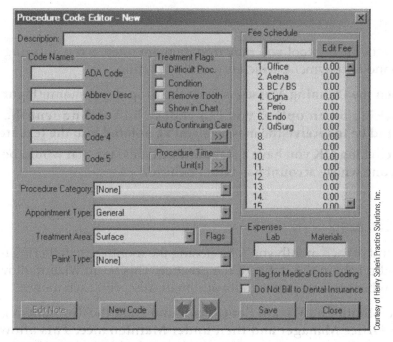

FIGURE 24-5B Procedure code editor.

2. US offices and insurance companies use ADA/CDT codes so select that tab. Remember the codes you are seeing in this Dentrix Learning Edition are generic and not actual CDT codes. Enter a description, code, and complete any field that applies. On the right side of the box you can enter a fee for the procedure.

3. To see what existing codes look like for comparison follow the first direction, highlight a category, an existing code, and hit edit instead of new. After examining how a code is entered, hit close to exit.

This may seem complicated right now but once you have experience with practice management software it becomes very easy.

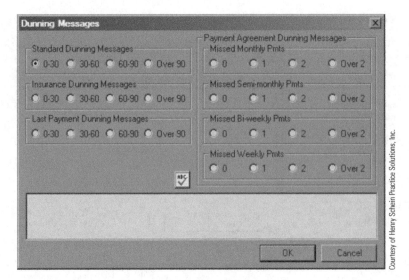

FIGURE 24-6 Dunning messages.

Dunning Messages

One practice setup tool you may update more often is the dunning message or demand for payment, which is usually in writing.

1. Open the Dunning Messages from the drop-down menu (Figure 24-6).
2. Clicking on an option you can choose how delinquent the account would be to receive the message you've entered into the text area.
3. By clicking OK you have a standardized message that would be used for anyone whose account has fallen behind.

Month End Wizard

At the end of each month you'll be closing the month and gathering important information about the status of the practice. This setup wizard allows you to choose which reports you want to automatically print each month.

1. The Month End Wizard Set Up is found from the drop-down menu under Office Manager and then under Maintenance. This allows you to request the reports that will run at the end of every month.
2. Beginning with start at the top; click on each square and carefully read the information. To change your selection, click on the correct response and go to next to continue. To keep the report or action the same, just go to next (Figure 24-7).
3. Once you have made your selections, all you will need to do each month is close the month; the reports and actions will be automatic.

Changing the Fee Schedule

Let's look at an overall fee increase for the practice. To keep it simple, we'll imagine our practice has had a significant increase in sterilization and PPE supplies that we need to add to the office fee.

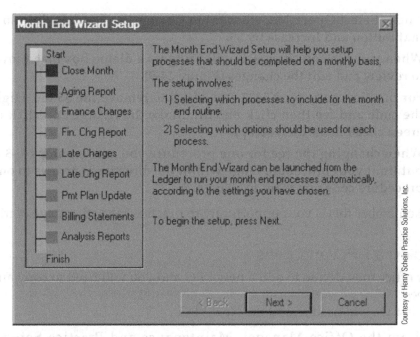

FIGURE 24-7 Month end wizard.

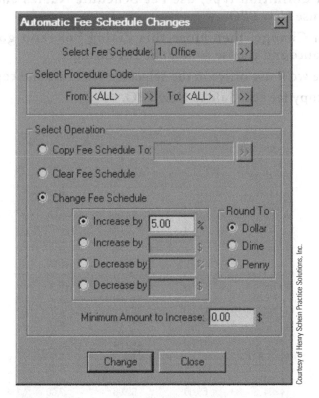

FIGURE 24-8 Fee schedule change.

1. From the Office Manager go to Maintenance to Practice Setup and from the drop-down menu go to Automatic Fee Schedule Changes (Figure 24-8).
2. We would like to increase the office fee for every procedure by $5.
3. Beginning at the top we want to select office as our fee schedule.
4. We want all procedures, which is already the default.

5. Under Select Operation, we want to Change the Fee Schedule so select that button and Increase by $5.

6. When you click on change, it will bring up a dialog box that allows you to review and edit the changes (Figure 24-9).

7. For practice, go to fee X3427 and edit it to remove the $5 fee. Highlight the code and fee then click on edit. Make the change and click on the green check mark then accept.

8. When changing the fee for one procedure you can use steps 1–3 above but limit your procedure range within the directional arrows to only the procedure code you want to change.

Remember this is your opportunity to practice, take advantage of it!

Adding a PPO and Fees

Your office may decide to add a new PPO and you will need to copy and edit its fees.

First we will need to add the New PPO.

1. From the Office Manager, Maintenance and Practice Setup; find Definitions.

2. For your definition type; use Fee Schedule Names and in an open position use New PPO.

3. Click on Change, then close this dialog box, and go back to the Maintenance and choose Automatic Fee Change.

4. This time we'll use office in the select fee schedule and copy all fees.

5. Choose copy fee schedule to New PPO.

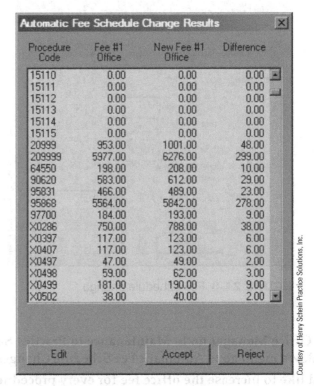

FIGURE 24-9 Review fee schedule change.

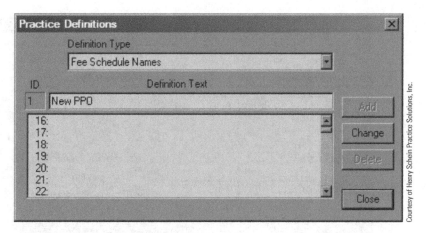

FIGURE 24-10 Practice definitions.

6. When the fees are copied you will see the office fees as well as a column for the PPO fees. Currently they are the same. Where the fees differ you will need to edit the PPO fees to make them correct.

Running Reports

If you have entered information completely and correctly, Dentrix can put it together for you in just about any report you would want to see.

1. To run management reports: from Office Manager, go to Report from the top of your screen, then to Management, and a list of possible reports will appear.

> **HELPFUL HINT**
>
> Some of these you may have already chosen to run automatically with the Month End report but let's look at running a few of these manually. Often doctors want specific information and they want it now and not at the end of the month. If your employer is having a meeting with colleagues, it is nice to have information about referrals that were sent to the office. Maybe there are financial decisions being made, for example, a large equipment purchase, the doctor may want a practice analysis.

2. Let's begin by running a practice analysis. Choose Analysis Summary from the list displayed to get the dialog box with the specific information you would like to include in your report (Figure 24-11).

3. If you are working in a multiple doctor office, you can choose to run the report for all of the providers or just one or a group; for example, just the information for the specialists in the practice.

4. Because the sample practice in the Dentrix Learning CD is small, you'll want to select dates for an extended time to get more information. For this exercise choose 9/1/2008 to today's date. For an actual report, choose the dates that are important to the report. For example, if the dentist asks for information from the last 6 months, those are the dates you would want to include.

5. On the right side of the dialog box, you can choose billing types; choose Daily Summary, Provider Summary, or both. Go ahead and choose both.

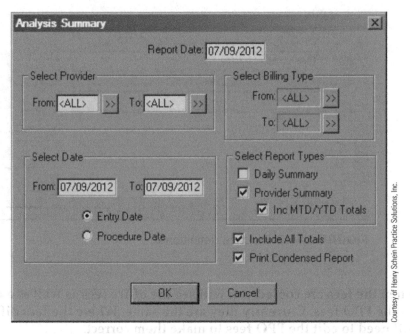

FIGURE 24-11 Running a practice analysis.

> ┌─ **HELPFUL HINT**
> │ If you are asked to run an analysis for your employer, ask what infor-
> │ mation is needed and be ready to give options. It will save you running
> │ a report that includes too much or not enough information.

6. Once you are satisfied with your report criteria, click OK.
7. To find the report, look at the batch processor on the Office Manager screen. When you find it, highlight it and use the print preview icon from the toolbar to view it.

   Try running other management reports on your own to see the information available. Give your reports a big date range because the data base we are using is small.
8. Start by running a referred to doctor report from 2005 to 2011 (Figure 24-12).
9. Continue looking at different reports.

Practice Goals Analysis

Another type of report that is helpful when evaluating the production of a practice is the Practice Goals Analysis.

1. From the Office Manager, go to analysis and begin with practice. Because the end of month reports were not run for this practice last month you will get a pop-up reminder, just click OK to continue for now.
2. With the screen shown in Figure 24-13 (Practice analysis report), each practitioner is able to set production goals and then evaluate their achievement.
3. Go to setup and choose goals; setting up a goal will help to see this report. For practice, set up a monthly goal in June 2012 of $10,000 of production.

REFERRED TO DOCTOR REPORT
DENTRIX Learning Edition
Referral Date: All Referral Sources

Date: 07/09/2012   Page: 1

| DOCTOR'S NAME | PHONE | | |
| | REFERRED PATIENT NAME | REFERRAL DATE | |

Dr. Clark, Robert S (Oral and Maxillofacial S   (111)222-3333 Ext: 1234   Total Referrals: 2
1750 N College Ave   Listed Referrals: 2
Suite 12
Northside, NV 22222

                    Mary Brown   07/02/2008
                    Joshua Reeves   07/02/2008

                                        TOTAL REFERRALS: 2
                                        TOTAL LISTED REFERRALS: 2

Courtesy of Henry Schein Practice Solutions, Inc.

FIGURE 24-12 Referred to doctor report.

Dentrix Practice Analysis (All)				
File Reports Setup Change Page Comparison Help				
Production Analysis	07/09/2012-07/09/2012	MTD-Cur	AVG 04/2012-06/2012	YTD-Cur
Beginning Balance		2,735.00	0.00	2,735.00
Charges				
Non-insured Charges	122.00	(425.00)	0.00	(425.00)
Insured Charges	669.00	1,460.00	0.00	1,460.00
Sub-total	791.00	1,035.00	0.00	1,035.00
Finance Charges	0.00	0.00	0.00	0.00
Late Charges	0.00	0.00	0.00	0.00
Adjustments: Additions	0.00	25.00	0.00	25.00
Total Charges	791.00	1,060.00	0.00	1,060.00
Credits				
Patient Payments	(100.00)	(200.00)	0.00	(200.00)
Insurance Payments	(535.20)	(592.80)	0.00	(592.80)
Sub-total	(635.20)	(792.80)	0.00	(792.80)
Adjustments: Reductions	0.00	0.00	0.00	0.00
Total Credits	(635.20) 80%	(792.80) 74%	0.00 100%	(792.80) 74%
Ending Balance	155.80	3,002.20	0.00	3,002.20

Production Analysis is calculated according to the provider and entry date attached to transactions.

Contract Analysis				
Future Due Payment Plans		0.00	0.00	0.00
Payment Agreements		0.00	0.00	0.00

Contract Analysis is calculated according to the provider attached to payment plans.

Courtesy of Henry Schein Practice Solutions, Inc.

FIGURE 24-13 Practice analysis report.

Using Practice Assistant

Dentrix Practice Assistant provides you with reports and graphs that are automatically scheduled to print or are printed on demand. The Practice Assistant can also send these reports via email when set up to do so.

FIGURE 24-14
Practice assistant icon.

Courtesy of Henry Schein Practice Solutions, Inc.

1. **Find the icon for Practice Assistant and click on it or go to Office Manager, find analysis and choose Practice Assistant from the drop-down menu (Figure 24-14).**

2. **There are three tabs: Reports, Scheduled Reports, and an Address Book for storing email; click on each tab to explore the contents.**

3. **View the list in the Reports tab. Highlight each report and to the right use the view button to see the type of report it generates (Figure 24-15).**

4. **Highlighting and viewing Adjustment Summary Report should show you a report similar to Figure 24-16 (Example Report).**

5. **To create a report, double click on the folder and fill in the desired criteria.**

6. **Report in the Practice Assistant can be scheduled to print automatically by following the directions in your User's Guide.**

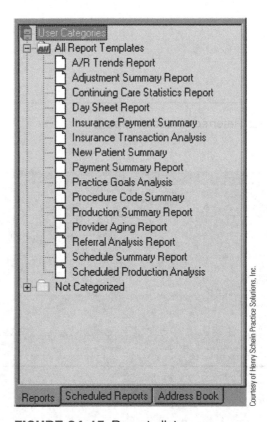

FIGURE 24-15 Reports list.

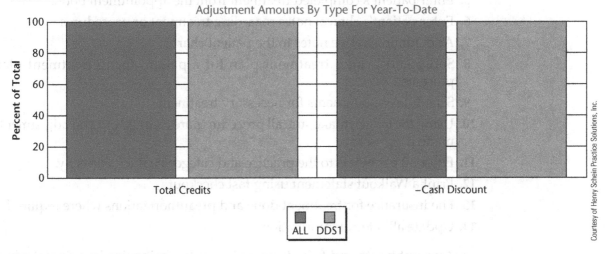

EXAMPLE REPORT
Adjustment Summary (By Provider) (Include YTD Totals)
Date 01/01/2002–01/25/2002
All Providers, All Billing Types

Date: 7/29/2009   Page: 1

	Prov	Quantity	Total	Average	Percent	YTD Quantity	YTD Total	YTD Average	YTD Percent
–Cash Discount									
	ALL	1	–34.00	–34.00	100.00	1	–34.00	–34.00	100.00
	DD 81	1	–34.00	–34.00	100.00	1	–34.00	–34.00	100.00
Total Credits									
	ALL	1	–34.00	–34.00	100.00	1	–34.00	–34.00	100.00
	DD 81	1	–34.00	–34.00	100.00	1	–34.00	–34.00	100.00

Adjustment Amounts By Type For Year-To-Date

ALL DDS1

FIGURE 24-16 Example report.

Management Routines

Every dental office needs to establish regular routines that they perform daily, weekly, monthly, and annually. Being consistent means tasks are not overlooked. In large dental practices, several staff members often share these responsibilities but everyone should be able to accomplish all of them. This list covers many of the jobs assigned to dental staff but every office is different and practices might vary this list depending on need and staffing. As you look down the list of activities, ask yourself if this was your job and could you access the information in Dentrix to complete it.

Daily Routines

Because so many tasks are done on a daily basis to make them easier to see they have been divided into patient care, appointment scheduling, and tracking insurance. Everyday these are going on simultaneously. While the list may seem overwhelming at first glance, practice management software assists the administrative dental staff by adding reminder messages of incomplete information during the day or of unfinished tasks before allowing the day to be closed.

Daily "To Do" List

- Patient Care: The following administrative and clinical tasks are required on a daily basis when working with patients.

1. Create a family file for a new patient or access patient records for an existing patient.
2. Determine if a "new" patient is new to the practice or coming back after an absence by using patient archive.
3. Update patient's personal and financial information including insurance.
4. Chart existing conditions and treatment needed using the patient chart or enter treatment needed through the ledger.
5. Enter patient's completed treatment from the appointment book.
6. Enter patient's clinical notes regarding treatment or procedures.
7. Add administrative notes to the patient chart.
8. Setup and print a treatment plan for a patient using treatment plan presenter.
9. Schedule appointments for necessary treatment.
10. Using the ledger, make sure all procedures are charged out and adjustments made if necessary.
11. Enter all payments to the practice and categorize them correctly.
12. Print a Walkout statement using fast checkout.
13. File insurance for treatment done and preauthorizations where required.
14. Update all referral information.

- Appointments and Scheduling: One of the priorities in a dental office is keeping the schedule full so being diligent about follow-up calls to patients is critical. Your appointment book reflects the production for your practice. Not maintaining it on a daily basis can result in financial losses. Practice management software organizes your information and maintains lists of patients that need to be rescheduled because of cancellation or scheduled after diagnosis but the lists require the administrative team to follow through on a daily basis.

1. Confirm the appointments for the next day.
2. Use Office Journal to make any notes regarding the contact.
3. Note broken appointments so they move into a call list.
4. Use call list ASAP to try and fill the schedule.
5. Follow-up with the Continuing Care Lists to make sure patients are returning for preventive visits.
6. Follow-up with patients on the broken appointment list to schedule appointments.

- Tracking Insurance: At any time a significant amount of income for a practice is waiting for insurance claims to be paid. Making that happen as quickly as possible by following up on claims benefits the entire staff.

1. Enter insurance checks received; make sure deductibles are updated.
2. If the primary insurance claim is received for a patient with dual insurance, submit the secondary claim.

3. Note reasons claims were not paid. If the claim was rejected because of an error or oversight, file again with an explanation.

4. Update insurance payment tables if/when new fees are received.

5. Enter the information regarding pretreatment authorizations when received and inform the patient.

6. Batch the day's insurance.

Weekly Routines

Weekly routines are things that need to be done soon but not immediately. Productive offices start this list on Monday and don't wait until the end of the week to begin these jobs. However, it is nice to have a few things you don't have to do before you leave to go home at the end of the day.

Weekly "To Do" List

1. Run weekly reports.

2. Write letters. These might be congratulation letters or collection letters. Most offices do birthday postcards once a month.

Monthly Routines

Monthly Routines are extremely important because many of them provide financial guidance for the practice. Included here are the reports that assist the practice in making decisions for the future. Monthly routines can be tasks done anytime during the month and some that may be done at a certain time during the month.

Monthly "To Do" List

Sometime during the month:

1. Statements are sent. This does not have to be on the first of the month but it should always be done at the same time of the month.
   Make sure you have applied finance or late charges before sending statements; you can do this automatically during the month end process.

2. Update any payment plans.

On the first of the month before entering any new transactions:

1. Do monthly backup of the Dentrix database. Dentrix has specific recommendations to make this a legal document. Make sure you know office policy regarding backup and storage of data.

2. Close everything except the Ledger.

3. Close the month using Month-End in the Ledger.

4. Print aging reports so delinquent accounts can be followed up on.

5. Print collection letters.

6. Print any reports that are part of your dental practice's routine.

Summary

The amount of information you can access from Dentrix reports makes setting realistic goals for the practice much easier. Reports can take on personality by adding graphics from Practice Assistant. Aging and delinquent reports make collecting past due accounts almost effortless by allowing you to keep them current. You can evaluate your proficiency in using Dentrix by using the Management Routines as a check list for additional practice.

 Skill Building

If you have Internet access, watch the "On Demand Training" videos and take the quiz for each:

- Practice Advisor
- Viewing and navigating the Office Manager
- Entering Office, Provider and Staff Information
- Generating Key Reports
- Storing Documents in the Document Center
- Using the Questionnaires Module

 Challenge Your Understanding

1. Where are reports viewed before printing?
   a. The Ledger
   b. The Batch Processor
   c. View Reports
   d. Office Journal
2. The Daily Appointment List includes which of the following?
   a. Balance due
   b. Patient's address
   c. Patient's phone number
   d. Health status
3. To print a list of current insurance carriers, you would access it through:
   a. Ledger and Insurance Claims
   b. Reports and Reference
   c. Reports and Management
   d. Reference Insurance Maintenance
4. Which of these is not found in the Practice Assistant?
   a. Email addresses
   b. Scheduled Production Analysis
   c. Archived Patient Summary
   d. Procedure Code Summary
5. Susan needs to clock into Dentrix, where can she find the Time Clock?
   a. Office Manager
   b. Quick Launch
   c. Ledger
   d. File/Document Manager

Patient Charts

RACHEL ANTHONY

Patient Personal Information

Address:	76021 Hillside Dr. Westside, UT 44444
Person Responsible for Account:	Rachel Anthony
Phone:	805-345-8081
E-Mail:	ranthony87@yahoo.com
Birth date:	8-24-1987
Sex:	Female
Marital Status:	Married
Office status:	Patient
Employer:	AT&T
Social Security #:	123-77-6767
Preferred Provider:	Maria Cook, DDS
Preferred Provider 2 (hygienist):	Sally Hayes, RDH

Family Information

Spouse:	Cameron Anthony
Birth date:	6-2-1985
Sex:	Male
Office status:	Patient
Preferred provider:	Maria Cook, DDS
Employer:	Unemployed

No other family members

Financial Facts

Note: Rachel and Cameron are both covered under Rachel's insurance policy

Primary Insurance Company:	Blue Cross/ Blue Shield
Insurance ID #:	321-88-6767
Group Number:	21440
Subscriber:	Rachel Anthony

Health History

Note: Rachel is a healthy adult. No prescription medications. She has a history of fainting when standing up quickly.

Dental History

Existing dental work done in this office:	Simple extraction of #s 1, 16, 17, 32
	#3 MO Amalgam
	#14 MO Amalgam
	#18 O Amalgam
	#19 O Amalgam
	#30 O Amalgam

Treatment Planned

Replace existing amalgam restorations with composite
Oral hygiene instruction to minimize further gum recession

Treatment Notes

Gingiva is healthy pink and stippled, no bleeding.

Slight gum recession approx. 2 mm on buccal of #3 probably the result of orthodontic treatment
6-month recall for preventive care

THOMAS LANE

Patient Personal Information

Address:	7886 Main St
	Northside, UT 22222
Preferred name:	Tom
Person Responsible for Account:	Thomas Lane
Phone:	805-651-3451
Email:	tomlovesaparty@hotmail.com
Birth date:	7-4-1985
Sex:	Male
Marital status:	Single
Office status	Patient
Employer:	Chevron
Social Security #:	012-76-0987
Preferred Provider:	Dennis Smith, DDS
Preferred Provider 2:	None

Family Information

No dependents

Financial Facts

Primary Insurance Company:	MetLife
Insurance ID #:	210-0987
Group Number:	87663
Subscriber:	Thomas Lane

Health History

Note: Tom is a diabetic controlled with insulin.

Dental History

All existing dental work done in another office. Patient had orthodontic treatment as an adolescent

Existing Dental Treatment:	Missing #s 1, 5, 12, 16, 17, 21, 28, 32
	Sealants on #s 3, 14, 19, 30
	#18 O Amalgam
	#31 O Composite/Resin

Treatment Planned

#9 is nonvital and needs root canal therapy

Treatment Notes

#9 sustained traumatic injury during a pickup basketball game with friends;
No evidence of fracture to crown or root; no discomfort to patient
Gingiva is healthy, pink stippled with 1–3 mm pockets
6-month recall for preventive care

JANET BRUCE

Patient Personal Information

Address: 34 Morning Glory Circle
Sunnyside, UT 88888

Person Responsible for Account: David Bruce
Phone: 805-877-5678
Email: brucefamily@hotmail.com
Birth date: 3-18-1983
Sex: Female
Marital Status: Married
Employer: Homemaker
Social Security#: 555-21-9878
Preferred Provider: Dennis Smith

Family Information

Spouse: David Bruce
Birth date: 4-25-1986
Sex: Male
Office status: Patient
Preferred provider: Dennis Smith, DDS
Social Security #: 001-88-9876
Spouse Employer: Consumer Advocate Group
Child: Sarah Bruce
Sex: Female
Date of Birth: 1-19-2008
Office status: Patient
Preferred provider: Dennis Smith, DDS

Financial Facts

Note: All family members are covered under Bruce's Aetna policy.
Insurance Company: Aetna
Insurance subscriber number: 010-87987
Group Number: 01278
Subscriber: David Bruce

Health History

Note: Janet is 6 months pregnant; no complications. Normal health. No medications with the exception of over the counter pre-natal vitamins.

Dental History

Existing done in this office: #3 MOD Amalgam
#14 DO Amalgam
#15 MO Amalgam
#19 PFM Crown (fused to base metal)
#31 MO Amalgam

Treatment Planned

The restorations on #14 and #15 have recurrent decay and should be replaced. Janet would like them replaced with composite.
#1, 16, 17, 32 should be extracted

Treatment Notes

No restorative treatment until after delivery. Emergency treatment in third trimester with approval of her physician.

CLAYTON LEWIS

Patient Personal Information

Address:	2437 Skyline Dr.
	Centerville, UT 55555
Person Responsible for Account:	Clayton Lewis
Phone:	805-345-4556
Email:	clayton@lewisfamily.com
Birth date:	5-23-1975
Sex:	Male
Marital status:	Married
Office status:	Patient
Employer:	Central City Clinic
Social Security #	555-22-3344
Preferred Provider:	Dennis Smith, DDS
Preferred Provider 2 (hygienist):	Sally Hayes, RDH

Family Information

Spouse:	Mary Lewis
Birth date:	9-06-1976
Sex:	Female
Marital status:	Married
Office status:	Patient
Spouse Employer:	American Express
Child:	Jason Lewis
Sex:	Male
Birth date:	10-15-2003
Office status:	Patient
Preferred provider:	Dennis Smith, DDS
Child:	Justin Lewis
Birth date:	12-05-2005
Sex:	Male
Office status:	Patient
Preferred provider:	Dennis Smith, DDS
Child:	Jamie Lewis
Birth date:	3-13-2008
Sex:	Female
Office status:	Non-patient

Financial Facts

Note: Clayton is primary for himself and the children, and secondary for Mary
Mary is primary for herself and secondary for Clayton and the children

Primary Insurance Company:	American Western Life
Insurance subscriber number:	63324- 546
Group Number:	41336
Subscriber:	Clayton Lewis
Secondary Insurance Company:	Ameritas
Insurance subscriber number:	63324- 546
Group Number:	11515
Subscriber:	Mary Lewis

Health History

Note: Allergy to penicillin, High blood pressure-no medication required

Dental History

Previous treatment done in another office: Extraction #'s 1, 16, 17, 32

Existing treatment done in this office:
- #2 MOD Amalgam
- #3 DO Amalgam
- #7 DL Composite/Resin
- #13 DO Amalgam
- #14 PFM Crown
- #15 MOD Amalgam
- #18 O Amalgam
- #19 MOD Amalgam
- #30 MO Amalgam
- #31 O Amalgam

Treatment Planned

#4 DO Composite/Resin	New caries
#10 DL Composite/Resin	New caries
#19 PFM Crown	Recurrent caries around older amalgam restoration
#28 DO Resin	New caries

Treatment Notes

Gingiva appears healthy, pink, and stippled with normal pocket depths with the exception of the following:

Abnormal (3 mm+) pocket depths:
- #19 4 mm MF and ML
- #20 5 mm DF and DL
- #30 6 mm MF and ML

Slight bleeding on probing 19, 20, and 30 in area of deeper pockets.
Possible cause older failing restorations and lack of flossing
3-month preventive care recall until periodontal pockets are resolved; oral hygiene instruction

Answer Key

CHAPTER 1 The Dental Office Manager

1. d
2. b
3. a
4. b
5. d
6. c
7. b
8. a
9. d
10. c

CHAPTER 2 The Dental Team

1. a
2. c
3. a
4. b
5. d
6. a
7. a
8. b
9. a
10. d

CHAPTER 3 Regulations in Dental Office Management

1. d
2. b
3. d
4. b
5. d
6. d
7. d
8. b
9. c
10. c
11. c
12. d
13. d
14. b
15. d
16. c
17. c
18. d
19. d
20. b

CHAPTER 4 Hazard Communications and Regulatory Agency Mandates

1. d
2. d
3. d
4. b
5. d
6. d
7. a
8. c
9. d
10. d
11. a
12. d
13. c
14. d
15. d
16. d
17. d
18. d
19. c
20. c

CHAPTER 5 The Dental Office Manager as a Patient Relations Specialist

1. d	10. d
2. c	11. c
3. b	12. b
4. c	13. d
5. a	14. b
6. d	15. d
7. c	16. d
8. b	17. b
9. b	18. a

CHAPTER 6 Marketing the Practice

1. b	10. a
2. d	11. a
3. b	12. d
4. d	13. c
5. a	14. a
6. a	15. a
7. d	16. b
8. d	17. c
9. a	18. a

CHAPTER 7 Printed Communications

1. d	9. d
2. d	10. b
3. d	11. d
4. c	12. d
5. a	13. d
6. a	14. d
7. a	15. d
8. d	

CHAPTER 8 Business Office Equipment

1. b	9. d
2. c	10. b
3. d	11. c
4. b	12. d
5. d	13. d
6. b	14. a
7. c	15. a
8. b	16. d

CHAPTER 9 Dental Nomenclature and Related Terminology

1. d	11. d
2. b	12. a
3. a	13. b
4. c	14. b
5. d	15. a
6. a	16. a
7. c	17. d
8. d	18. c
9. d	19. a
10. a	20. b

CHAPTER 10 Charting the Oral Cavity

1. a	11. a
2. d	12. d
3. c	13. b
4. d	14. c
5. b	15. d
6. b	16. a
7. d	17. b
8. b	18. c
9. a	19. b
10. a	20. a

CHAPTER 11 Patient Records, Diagnosis, and Treatment Planning

1. d	11. b
2. b	12. c
3. d	13. b
4. c	14. b
5. a	15. b
6. a	16. d
7. c	17. d
8. d	18. b
9. a	19. b
10. d	20. c

CHAPTER 12 Scheduling to Optimize Practice Efficiency

1. d
2. b
3. d
4. c
5. b
6. b
7. a
8. d
9. a
10. c
11. a
12. b
13. b
14. b
15. a
16. a
17. d
18. d

CHAPTER 13 Managing Accounts Receivable

1. d
2. a
3. b
4. b
5. b
6. a
7. d
8. c
9. d
10. a
11. b
12. a
13. b
14. b
15. d
16. a
17. d
18. b
19. a
20. d

CHAPTER 14 Managing Accounts Payable

1. a
2. d
3. a
4. c
5. d
6. c
7. c
8. a
9. d
10. d
11. b
12. c
13. d
14. d
15. a
16. a
17. d
18. d
19. d
20. c

CHAPTER 15 Supply Ordering and Inventory

1. c
2. b
3. b
4. a
5. b
6. d
7. a
8. d
9. d
10. a
11. a
12. d
13. d
14. a
15. c
16. a
17. a
18. d
19. b
20. d

CHAPTER 16 Employment Opportunities

1. b	11. b
2. d	12. d
3. a	13. b
4. d	14. d
5. a	15. a
6. d	16. b
7. c	17. d
8. d	18. a
9. b	19. c
10. a	20. b

CHAPTER 17 Hiring a Dental Team

1. c	11. d
2. b	12. b
3. d	13. a
4. b	14. d
5. b	15. b
6. c	16. b
7. a	17. c
8. b	18. d
9. a	19. d
10. b	20. a

CHAPTER 18 Dental Practice Management Software

1. c	4. b
2. d	5. d
3. d	

CHAPTER 19 Entering, Updating, and Maintaining Patient Information

1. a	5. b
2. a	6. d
3. a	7. a
4. d	8. b

CHAPTER 20 Clinical Records

1. b	4. c
2. d	5. d
3. b	

CHAPTER 21 Appointment Book

1. b	4. d
2. c	5. b
3. c	

CHAPTER 22 Financial Records

1. b
2. d
3. c

4. c
5. a

CHAPTER 23 Communication Using Practice Management Software

1. d
2. b
3. b

4. c
5. c

CHAPTER 24 Beyond the Basics

1. b
2. c
3. b

4. c
5. b

A

abandonment – failure to provide necessary dental treatment.

abuse – any care relationship that harms, pains, or causes mental anguish to another.

abutments – the natural tooth that is prepared as an anchor or attachment to hold a bridge in place

accounts payable – the system of distributing money owed by the practice.

adjustment – a change in accounting often due to a discount received by a patient for payment in full or as a courtesy.

advertising – the promotion of products or services provided by a business or organization through a variety of media.

alphabetic – one type of filing system used in dental offices; patient files are organized by first letter of the patient's last name.

amalgam – soft alloy that hardens into a silver colored dental restoration; contains mercury

amenities – gestures of comfort or convenience.

American Association of Dental Office Managers (AADOM) – an organization of professional office managers, practice administrators, patient coordinators, insurance and financial coordinators, and treatment coordinators of general and specialized dental practices.

Americans with Disabilities Act (AwDA) – a law that prohibits discrimination in access to services and employment against persons who are disabled.

anatomical dental chart – shows the anatomic landmarks of the teeth and some supporting oral structures.

anaphylaxis – a severe allergic reaction.

anaphylactic shock – a severe allergic reaction that overwhelms the body's ability to defend against the antigen; this is a medical emergency.

anomaly – any deviation from the normal.

anterior – toward the front of the mouth.

anterior sextant – comprises the six front teeth in each dental arch

anxiety – a normal but enhanced feeling of concern.

appointment book – a record of times set aside for scheduled patients to receive treatment; it can be hand written or computerized.

appointment card – a courtesy to remind patients of their next appointment. It typically contains the business card information on one side and the specifics of the appointment on the reverse.

assignment of benefits – a request from the subscriber to pay benefits received to another person; generally, a patient is requesting payment directly to the dentist.

audit – method used by third parties to check for accuracy of records. Clinical records are matched with dental claims submitted.

automatic payment system – a system whereby the payer's bank automatically deducts a specific amount owed to a third party.

automatic shipments – the delivery of products or supplies on a regular basis eliminating the need for frequent ordering.

B

backorder – occurs when an item ordered is not in stock with the vendor/supplier and will be shipped separately to the dentist's office when it becomes available.

beneficiary – the person receiving the payment of the benefit.

benefits – incentives to employment that may include paid vacation, sick days, and compensation for reaching production goals, health insurance, or pension plan contributions.

bicuspid/premolar – a permanent tooth having two cusps. The adult dentition contains a first and second bicuspid/premolar in each quadrant. *Premolar* is the more contemporary term.

bid – an offer extended to a number of suppliers to provide all dental supplies at a lower price.

bioburden – a contaminated hazardous or infectious material.

biofilms – microorganisms that accumulate on surfaces inside moist environments such as dental unit waterlines, allowing bacteria, fungi, and viruses to multiply. This can significantly increase a patient's susceptibility to transmissible diseases.

biohazard warning label – a label or tag affixed to hazardous waste items; it must be readable from a distance of five feet.

birthday rule – a method used by insurance companies to determine which company is considered the primary carrier when a child is covered by more than one dental insurance policy.

block/unit appointment scheduling – specific units of time allocated for scheduling dental appointments; most often 10- or 15-minute units.

Bloodborne Pathogens Standard – an OSHA regulation that covers all dental employees who could *reasonably anticipate* coming into contact with blood, saliva, and other potentially infectious materials (PIMs) during the course of employment.

bloodborne pathogens – infectious microorganisms present in blood that can cause disease in humans.

Board of Dental Examiners – a group of individuals that have the authority to grant dental licenses and monitor the practice of dentistry among the licensees.

bridge – connects two or more local networks together.

broken appointments – appointment that the patient fails to keep without calling to cancel; sometimes called failed appointments or "no shows."

buccal/facial – the surface of the tooth facing *toward the cheek* in the posterior region of the mouth; it is named for the buccinator (chewing) muscle.

burden of proof – the patient seeking to impose liability against the dentist must supply the more convincing evidence that the dentist's action caused resulting harm or injury.

business card – a marketing device that contains all of the information found on the letterhead stationery in a condensed size.

byte – computer memory that corresponds to one location, usually capable of storing one character.

C

call list – a handy reference that the office manager uses to fill an available appointment in the schedule on short notice.

canine/cuspid – the tooth used to tear and break off food. It is an older term that is being used less in practice. The more current and descriptive term is *cuspid*. Older patients may also identify this tooth as an eye tooth.

capitation – a form of contracted care, usually by a corporation, institution, or other group; the provider receives a set fee per patient per a given timeframe and provides all or most of the services covered in the program to subscribers.

caries – tooth decay.

carrier – the insurance company providing coverage.

case presentation – a non-treatment appointment when the dentist or office manager meets with the patient (and often an accompanying family member) to explain an extensive case.

cash on delivery (COD) – a form of cash payment made for goods at the time of delivery. If the purchaser does not make the payment for the goods, they are returned to the seller.

cementum – the yellowish-white outer covering of the root portion of the tooth that is normally below the gum line.

Centers for Disease Control and Prevention (CDC) – a federal agency that sets guidelines for health care practitioners; CDC's guidelines are enforced by OSHA.

central processing unit (CPU) – the brain of the computer.

Certified Dental Assistant (CDA) – a dental assistant who has completed the requirements for certification through the Dental Assisting National Board.

Certified Orthodontic Assistant (COA) – a dental assistant who has completed the requirements for certification in infection control and orthodontics assisting through the Dental Assisting National Board.

Certified Preventive Functions Dental Assistant (CPFDA) – a dental assistant who has completed the requirements for certification in coronal polishing, sealants, topical anesthetics, and topical fluorides through the Dental Assisting National Board.

chairside dental assistant – an employee who helps the dentist with the clinical needs of the patient; depending on the state of employment this person may be required to be certified or registered.

chronological – a filing system based upon the date of the office visit.

clinical attachment level – point at which the hard tissue (tooth) and soft tissue (gingiva) are connected.

closing – the courteous ending to a letter. Examples of closings would include Sincerely, Yours Truly, and With Regards.

code of ethics/ethics – a moral obligation that encompasses professional conduct and judgment imposed by the members of a particular profession; considered a higher standard (moral) than jurisprudence (legal) requirements.

compact disc (CD) – a device used to store digital files.

compensation – financial remuneration in the form of wage, salary, or paid benefits.

composite/resin – tooth colored material used for dental restoration.

consumable supplies – those that are completely used up or consumed with use.

contract – a formal or legally binding agreement. For example: an agreement between the dental practice and a patient, or the dental practice and a vendor of dental supplies.

coordination of benefits – submitting dual coverage claims according to the instructions provided by two insurance companies.

continuing education (CE) – additional instruction received by dental professionals to maintain competency; often required by a state for registration or licensure.

copayment – the portion of a health care charge that must be paid by the patient per their agreement with the insurance company.

cosmetic dentistry – a branch of dentistry not yet recognized as a specialty that is particularly concerned with the appearance of the teeth.

cover letter – accompanies a résumé; introduces the candidate and explains the reason for the inquiry, the job desired, and the source of the notification.

credit check – examination of person's history of paying accounts used as a predictor for payment of future accounts.

credit invoice – a credit or refund issued against a statement.

crown – a prosthetic replacement of the coronal portion of a natural tooth; a crown may be three-quarter or full.

Current Dental Terminology (CDT) – A group of codes, standardized by the American Dental Association, to consistently report services to dental benefit companies.

cusp – the pointed or rounded eminence on the surface of a tooth.

cuspid – tooth used to tear and break off food. It is a newer more descriptive term for the tooth sometimes referred to as the canine. Older patients may refer to this tooth as an eye tooth.

customary fee – the fee for a specific dental service that is recognized by third-party dental payers.

deciduous/primary dentition – the first set of teeth, consisting of 10 teeth in each arch. The deciduous dentition is eventually replaced by the secondary (succedaneous) or permanent dentition.

deductible – the portion of the fee that the patient pays before insurance starts its coverage.

dental anesthesiology – a branch of dentistry not yet recognized as a specialty concerned with the need for deep sedation and general anesthetic to manage pain and anxiety in patients for whom local anesthetic and lighter levels of sedation are ineffective or inappropriate.

Dental Assisting National Board (DANB) – the national credentialing organization for dental assistants.

dental hygienist – a member of the dental team whose primary duties include the prevention of dental disease through patient education and dental prophylaxis. The dental hygienist must be licensed in the state of employment.

dental laboratory technician – a member of the dental team who fabricates crowns, bridges, dentures, and orthodontic appliances.

dental office manager – employee in charge of all business aspects associated with operating a dental practice.

Dental Practice Act – the laws that govern the practice of dentistry in each state.

dental public health – dental specialty that develops policies and programs, such as health care reform, that affect the community at large.

dental radiograph (x-ray) – an image of the tooth, teeth, mouth, jaws, and/or related oral structures on film.

dental supply representative – a salesperson who provides the office with products, information, and services to help the practice run smoothly.

dentin – the layer of tooth surface below the enamel and cementum; it comprises the bulk of the tooth and affects the color of the tooth.

dentofacial orthopedics – the dental specialty that involves the repositioning of teeth to create a functional bite that will improve the appearance of the smile and make the teeth last longer by reducing abnormal biting stresses. It is concerned with the alignment of not only teeth but jaws.

dependents – persons who are covered under the primary subscribers insurance coverage.

diagnosis – the clinical conclusion reached by the dentist resulting from an oral examination and review of additional aids including radiographs, study models, periodontal disease susceptibility, and the intraoral camera.

diagnostic code – a numeric code used to clarify why a procedure was done; example, International Classification of Disease (ICD) codes

digital radiography – a computerized method of projecting and freezing dental radiographic images onto a computer screen for examination and storage in a database.

digital versatile disc (DVD) – an optical disk that can store a very large amount of digital data, as text, music, or images.

direct marketing campaign – a specific promotion directed to a defined target audience.

direct reimbursement – a self-funded program in which the individual patient or employee is reimbursed based upon a percentage of dollars spent for care provided; it allows beneficiaries to seek treatment from the provider of their choice.

direct supervision – duties legally delegated by the dentist to be performed by qualified staff; the dentist must be physically present in the office while these duties are performed.

disability – a person who has a physical or mental impairment that substantially limits one or more major life activities, a person who has a history or record of such impairment, or a person who is perceived by others as having such impairment.

disposable supplies – supplies that are used and discarded.

distal – the surface of the tooth that is facing away (distant) from the midline of the mouth, following the line of the arch.

Doctor of Dental Surgery (DDS) – degree awarded after completion of all educational requirements for the dentist.

Doctor of Medical Dentistry (DMD) – degree awarded after completion of all educational requirements for the dentist.

double booking – a method of appointment scheduling in which two patients are booked at approximately the same time; it is commonly used for patients who are chronically late or likely to fail their appointment.

duel insurance coverage – a system of insurance participation that permits spouses who both carry dental insurance to cover each other as dependents, increasing the amount of the benefit up to the actual cost of the treatment. Children that have insurance coverage from both parents would also be considered to have duel coverage.

dunning – the process of communicating with patients to ensure the collection of accounts receivable; can range from a gentle reminder to a warning of being sent to a third-party collection company.

E

edentulous – having no natural teeth.

electronic charting – the chairside assistant directly inputs all clinical findings of the dentist into the treatment room computer.

electronic claims processing – insurance claims that are sent to the carrier through the Internet.

electronic funds transfer – transfer of funds from one account to another, usually via the telephone.

email – electronic mail is communication sent through the Internet.

embezzlement – the fraudulent appropriation of money entrusted into one's care.

emergency patient – patient of record or first-time patient, without a scheduled appointment, who calls the office in pain or for an urgent problem.

employment ad – a written announcement regarding job availability can be found in a newspaper or through various Internet sources.

employment plan – detailed outline for finding a job.

enamel – the hardest structure in the human body; forms the outer covering of the crown of the tooth.

endodontics – the field of diagnosis, cause, prevention, and treatment of diseases of the dental pulp and related tissues.

endodontist – a dental specialist who performs root canals and related procedures.

engineering controls – specific equipment or devices that facilitate prevention of accidental exposure.

Environmental Protection Agency (EPA) – regulates and registers certain products used in dental practices, including surface disinfectants; requires products to undergo and pass specific testing requirements prior to approval for registration.

Equal Employment Opportunity Commission (EEOC) – responsible for ensuring all individuals have the right to compete for employment opportunities, as well as to reduce the potential for hiring discrimination based upon a variety of factors.

equipment – major items that are used for five or more years and may be depreciated by the office over a number of years.

esthetics – a pleasant or cosmetic appearance.

etiquette – practicing good manners, knowing how to behave in a given situation, and knowing how to interact with people.

ethics – a moral obligation that encompasses professional conduct and judgment imposed by the members of a particular profession.

event marketing – a form of internal marketing that acknowledges specific events or occasions according to information contained in the individual patient's attribute profile.

exclusion – dental service or procedure not listed under the dental plan.

expanded functions (duties) dental assistant – a dental assistant whose additional training and education allow the performance of more independent patient care. The expanded duties allowed are defined by the State Dental Practice Act.

expendable supplies – those items that are relatively low in cost and are replaced frequently.

explanation of benefits (EOB) – a detailed description showing payment or denial of a dental insurance claim.

exposure-control plan – identifies tasks, procedures, and job classifications where occupational exposure takes place.

exposure incident – specific eye, mouth, or other mucous membranes, non-intact skin or parenteral (through the skin) contact with blood or OPIMs that directly results from the performance of an employee's duties.

external marketing – marketing efforts or campaigns directed to people outside of the office who may desire to become patients.

extraction – surgical removal of a tooth; an extraction may be classified as either simple or complicated.

F

facial/labial – the surface of the tooth that faces toward the face or lips.

failed appointments – appointments not kept or cancelled by the patient; often referred to as a "no-show" or "broken appointment."

Fédération Dentaire Internationale System – the tooth numbering system that combines quadrant number as the first digit with the tooth number in the quadrant as the second digit; this tooth numbering system designates tooth #11 through #48 in the adult dentition and tooth #51 through #85 in the primary dentition.

fee – the amount requested as payment for a dental service.

fee-for-service – the financial relationship between a patient and the practice in which the patient pays the dentist's fee without discounts or negotiated fees from a third party.

fee schedule – a list of fees for procedures performed in the office that is established by the dentist or those fees that the dentist and a dental benefits provider have agreed on.

fellowship – a period of training leading to an advanced credential or expertise in the field.

file extension – the suffix at the end of a filename that indicates what type of file it is.

filing systems – either manual or computerized; a system of office records management.

fixed bridge – a prosthetic replacement for one or more missing teeth that is cemented into place.

fixed expenses – office overhead expenses that remain approximately the same from month to month.

flagging system – an organization method used to alert the office manager that it is time to reorder a supply product.

flash drive – uses flash memory and a USB connection to store data.

focus group – a small group or representative cross-section of the patient base that share their opinions regarding the practice.

Food and Drug Administration (FDA) – a federal agency that regulates marketing of medical devices, including equipment and disposable items; it also reviews product labels for false or misleading information and sufficient directions for use.

foramen – an opening or hole in the tooth or bone that allows nerves and blood vessels to pass through

forensic dentistry – a branch of dentistry not yet recognized as a specialty that deals with the identification of bite marks or the identification of an individual by use of dental records.

G

general supervision – duties legally allowed to be performed by qualified staff; the dentist need not be physically present in the office while these duties are performed, but should be available by telephone.

generic equivalent – a drug that is not a name brand but has the same formulation as that of a name brand drug.

geometric dental chart – depicts the teeth as round graphic elements with lines differentiating the surfaces and edges.

gingiva – the tissue that surrounds the teeth. Known in lay terms as the gums.

group practice – a dental office consisting of multiple practitioners. Financial arrangements between the dentists within the practice can vary.

H

hardware – physical or visible computing equipment.

hazard communication program – a written program outlining the methods and procedures used in the office to reduce risks to staff associated with hazardous substances, diseases, chemicals, blood or OPIMs.

Hazard Communication Standard – the *Employee Right to Know Law,* that addresses the right of every employee to know the possible dangers associated with hazardous chemicals and related hazards in the place of employment; this law also requires employers to provide methods for corrective action.

heading – the part of a prescription that includes the dentist's contact information.

head of household – a designation within Dentrix to denote the person responsible for the family account. Often this person is the primary subscriber on the insurance policy.

health history form – a document completed by the patient that identifies all the patient's current and past medical/dental conditions; drugs being taken; and any allergies to materials or medications.

Health Insurance Portability and Accountability Act (HIPAA) – a federal act consisting of several parts including the requirement that dental offices and insurance companies protect the patient's privacy. It also protects health care coverage for people that change or lose their jobs. By simplification and standardization of administrative procedures it is designed to reduce costs.

Hepatitis B vaccination – a vaccine to prevent hepatitis B that must be provided by the employer to all full-time employees who may have potential for occupational exposure; the dentist must provide this at no charge to employees.

I

International Classification of Disease (ICD) – a standard series of alphanumeric codes used to describe the diagnosis, epidemiology, health management and clinical care for patients. It is a part of the 2012 ADA insurance claim form.

impacted (tooth) – a tooth covered by soft tissue or bone.

impairment – any physiological disorder or condition, cosmetic disfigurement, or anatomical loss; or any mental or psychological disorder, such as mental retardation, emotional or mental illness, or specific learning disabilities.

impression – the traits and characteristics of the dental office as experienced by the patient.

incisal edge – the biting edge of the anterior teeth.

incisor – an anterior tooth used for biting and cutting.

indemnity – a type of insurance plan where the patient can visit any dentist they choose and after paying their deductible are responsible for a percentage of the usual and customary/reasonable fee.

informed consent – the agreement of the patient to treatment after disclosure of the ailment, disease, or problem; the recommended treatment and the risks involved; alternative treatments and their risks; inadequate or non-treatment risks; and fees.

information packet – provides a number of pieces of information about the practice.

injury/accident log – a record that must be kept on file to reflect occupational exposure incidents and corrective/follow-up methods.

input device(s) – computer components consisting of the keyboard and/or mouse. These input devices interpret commands in a manner that allows the computer to process specific information.

inscription – the portion of a pharmaceutical prescription that contains the name of the drug, dosage form, and the amount of the dose.

insured party – any person covered under the insurance plan.

internal marketing – promotional efforts targeted to existing (active) patients of the practice.

interview – when two or more parties meet face-to-face to discuss the nature of the job and to obtain additional information from each other.

intraoral camera – a computerized device that uses a camera wand inside the mouth to enlarge dental images onto a color monitor, print color photographs, or film a video of an oral examination.

inventory – a written or computer-printed list of all supplies on hand, the amount ordered, the manufacturer/supplier, and the per unit price.

invoice – a statement requesting payment for merchandise purchased.

J–K

job description – a written list of duties to be performed by an employee.

jurisprudence – a set or system of laws; dental jurisprudence is set forth by each state's Legislature in the Dental Practice Act.

L

label – the part of the prescription that describes the contents.

laboratory prescription – the specific written directions to the dental laboratory regarding fabrication of a dental restoration, prosthesis, or orthodontic appliance.

ledger – the record keeping sheet (written or electronic) for recording services and payments.

letterhead stationery – paper and envelopes imprinted with the logo, name of the practice (if used), the doctor's name and credentials, the office address, telephone number, and fax number; if the office is online, it may also contain the practice's *email address* or *website address*.

liable/liability – being held legally responsible for an act.

license – identifies the members of a profession that have met the requirements to practice as outlined by the Dental Practice Act.

licensee – the holder of license to perform specific duties within the dental office, issued by the State Board of Dental Examiners. The dentist and dental hygienist must be licensed in the state in which they perform dental procedures.

lingual – the tooth surface facing toward the tongue.

link – an electronic connection from one digital page of content to another.

logo – a design or symbol that represents a business.

M

malpractice – professional negligence; failure to perform one's professional duties, either by omission or commission.

managed care – a cost-containment system that directs the utilization of health benefits by restricting the type, level, and frequency of treatment; limiting access to care and controlling the level of reimbursement for services.

mandible – the lower jaw.

marketing – creating the need or demand for, or awareness of, a product or service the consumer may have been unaware was available, or that he or she may have been unaware that he or she desired; dental practices may ethically promote their services through a variety of internal and external marketing strategies.

Material Safety Data Sheets (MSDSs) – the written information about the content and potential hazard of specific products used in the dental office. Each product that has a potential hazard must have a corresponding MSDS on file in the office.

maxilla – the upper jaw.

media – forms of advertising including telephone directories, newspapers, magazines, radio, television broadcasting, and billboards.

medical alert – a warning attached to a patient record or chart regarding a medical condition that could affect treatment.

medical waste – liquid or semiliquid body fluid, including any items in the dental office that release *bioburden* when compressed; items caked with dried body fluid that have the potential to release bioburden during handling; contaminated sharps; and pathological and microbial wastes containing body fluid.

mesial – the tooth surface facing *toward the midline* of the mouth.

midline – an imaginary vertical line down the middle of the face that determines right and left sides

mixed dentition – a set of teeth that includes both deciduous and permanent teeth.

mobility – the amount of movement a tooth is capable of; part of the screening for periodontal disease.

modem – is an output device that sends and receives computer information over a telephone line or high-speed cable.

molar – a posterior tooth; the adult permanent dentition has three molars in each quadrant.

mucogingival junction – meeting point of mucosal and gingival tissue.

N

National Practitioner Data Bank (NPDB) – established in 1986 as a national reporting entity to track and monitor complaints against licensed health care professionals, including dentists and dental hygienists.

National Provider Identifier Standard (NPI) – a unique and distinctive number issued by the federal government that replaces the provider's social security number or individual tax ID or other identifiers on dental insurance claim forms.

negligence – performing a procedure that a reasonable professional would not do, or not providing treatment a reasonable professional would in similar circumstances.

newsletter – communicates information about the practice and the services it provides; it may also profile interesting developments and advances in dental techniques or treatments and offers professional advice to patients.

noncompliance – failure to adhere to laws, rules, or regulations set forth in the State Dental Practice Act or the patient's unwillingness to follow treatment plans or directions from the dentist or another party.

non verbal communications – communication that takes place using facial expression, body language or other gestures.

numeric – a filing system that uses assigned patient identification numbers for organizing the files.

O

occlusal – the chewing surface of the posterior teeth.

occlusal plane – a horizontal line at the point where the upper and lower teeth come together

occlusion – relationship between the upper and lower teeth as they close together.

occupational exposure – an exposure incident that involves accidental contact with blood or OPIMs that directly results from the performance of an employee's duties.

Occupational Safety and Health Administration (OSHA) – a government agency that enforces guidelines for protection of workers; OSHA has federal, regional, and state offices.

offer letter – a formal proposal of employment outlining the job with details of compensation including benefits.

One-Write system – manual accounting system that uses a peg board to assist in alignment; system enables the user to enter information payments and charges once.

online – connected to the Internet by an Internet Service Provider (ISP); having access to individuals and organizations via email addresses or website addresses.

operating system – a system software program that coordinates the hardware capabilities of the computer.

operatory – the treatment room where dental procedures are performed; preferred term is *treatment room*.

oral maxillofacial surgery – a specialty dealing with diagnosis and treatment of injuries, diseases, and defects of the face and jaws.

oral and maxillofacial radiology – specialty dealing with the exposure and interpretation of traditional and digital radiographs to evaluate the oral-facial structures and determine health or disease.

oral pathologist – a dental specialist who studies diseases and conducts research related to the oral cavity.

oral and maxillofacial pathology – the field of diagnosis and treatment of oral disease that may affect the entire body.

oral surgeon – a dental specialist who extracts teeth, removes diseased tissue, surgically exposes impacted teeth, wires fractured jaws, and places dental implants; a maxillofacial surgeon may also treat victims of automobile accidents or disease (for example, cancer), who require reconstruction of facial features and tissues; also performs orthognathic surgery.

oral surgery – the field of diagnosis and treatment of diseases and malformations of the oral cavity and surrounding structures.

Organization for Safety and Asepsis Procedures (OSAP) – a national organization of teachers, practitioners, dental health care workers and manufacturers/distributors of dental equipment and products; it focuses on developing and communicating standards and information on aseptic technology to dental practices and educational institutions.

orthodontics – specialty that involves the repositioning of teeth to create a functional bite that will improve the appearance of the smile and make the teeth last longer by reducing abnormal biting stresses.

Other Potentially Infectious Material (OPIM) – substances in addition to blood that have the potential to cause contamination in the dental office.

output device(s) – the equipment that translates the information from the CPU into a format that can be read by the user; may be a *monitor* (screen), a *printer*, or *speaker(s)*.

overhead – the operating expenses associated with running the dental practice.

overtime pay – awarded to hourly wage earners who work beyond the standard 40 hours per week or the weekly hours determined by the practice and communicated to the employees.

P

packing slip – a piece of paper identical to the original order and subsequent invoice for payment due; the packing slip is shipped with the merchandise.

paid leave – compensated time away from the office, including holidays, vacation, sick time, and other days as determined by the dental practice.

palliative – treatment offered to relieve immediate discomfort only.

panoramic x-ray – an extra-oral radiograph that includes a wide view of the maxilla and mandible. Sometimes this film is referred to as a pano.

Palmer system – the tooth numbering system that designates teeth by quadrant; the adult (permanent) dentition starts with #1 as the central incisor and continues through the third molar, which is #8; the primary (deciduous) dentition starts with letter A as the central incisor through the second deciduous molar, which is letter E. Specific quadrants are indicated by brackets.

patient attributes – specific information about a patient; date of birth, hobbies, names of family members, and so on.

patient base – the total number of active patients in the practice.

patient education brochures – describe oral conditions and the need for preventive, restorative, postoperative, or corrective treatment.

patient flow – the progression of patients seen throughout the day in a dental practice.

patient profile – a list of characteristics, attributes, or information about a patient.

pediatric dentistry – the field of dentistry especially dedicated to treating children.

pegboard system – a method for recording activities of the day on a ledger sheet. The One-Write is an example of a pegboard system.

performance review – a review by the dentist-employer (or in large practices the office manager) of an employee's employment performance; usually conducted annually.

periodontal – the area around the tooth.

periodontal charting – recording the measurement of the pocket created as the tooth and the gingiva come together; the depth of this pocket is a diagnostic tool for periodontal disease. Measurements are made with a calibrated instrument called a periodontal probe.

periodontal ligament – acts as a shock absorber to cushion the tooth in the socket and provides attachment to the jawbone.

periodontics – the field of preserving natural tooth structures through prevention of disease and treatment of the supporting bone and soft tissue around the teeth.

periodontist – a dental specialist whose practice involves diagnosis, treatment and prevention of the diseases affecting the supporting and surrounding tissues of the tooth.

periodontium – a collective term for tissue surrounding the tooth.

permanent/secondary/succedaneous dentition – the second or adult set of teeth; a full complement comprises 32 teeth.

personal protective equipment (PPE) – a minimum of four items, (gloves, gown, eye protection, and mask) that must be worn by chairside personnel, who have a reasonable potential to come into contact with infectious diseases.

petty cash voucher – a tangible receipt as proof of cash monies paid for office expenses.

pharmaceutical prescription – an order for a drug or medication the patient requires and can't be purchased over the counter.

phobia – subject to or suffering from irrational fear.

Pinboard – the area of Dentrix G4 software where an appointment can be kept to quickly schedule it in the future.

plaque – an accumulation of sticky bacterial film that can be brushed away with a toothbrush by the patient.

porcelain-fused-to-metal crown – a single crown or multiunit bridge that is made with porcelain on the outside and metal on the inside.

posterior – toward the back.

practice brochure – the written document with a description of the practice to provide patients, prospective patients or other practices with information about the doctor and practice philosophy.

practice goals – an extension of the practice philosophy and mission statement; may be broken down into written, measurable outcomes.

practice mission statement – a succinct declaration of the practice philosophy, usually formulated into one or two sentences.

practice philosophy – the theme that drives the practice on a daily basis.

practice survey – a survey designed to solicit feedback from patients for improvement of services and office amenities.

predetermination – an estimate of how much of a proposed treatment will be covered under the subscriber's dental plan, also called a pretreatment estimate. It is not a guarantee of coverage.

preferred provider organization (PPO) – a type of third-party payment plan that allows requires patients receive dental care from a defined list of dentists.

premolar/bicuspid – a permanent tooth having two cusps. The adult dentition contains a first and second premolar/bicuspid in each quadrant. *Premolar* is the more contemporary term.

primary carrier – the insurance company that is billed first when a person has coverage with more than one company.

primary dentition – see deciduous dentition.

primary insurance – the insurance that is billed first when a patient has dual coverage.

probe systems – calibrated devices used to automatically calculate periodontal pocket depths and record this information into a computer database.

probing depth – the size of the periodontal pocket measured in millimeters.

production – the amount of dentistry being done by the practice; directly tied to its profitability.

production scheduling – a philosophy and system of scheduling for maximum productivity.

prognoses – anticipated or expected treatment outcomes; *prognosis* is the singular form.

prophylaxis – the removal of stains and hard deposits from the teeth by the dentist or dental hygienist.

prostheses – artificial teeth or appliances that replace or repair existing natural teeth.

prosthodontics – the field of dentistry dedicated to the restoration and maintenance of normal dentition and its functions through replacement with artificial teeth.

prosthodontist – a dentist who has received additional postgraduate training following completion of dental school to replace lost natural teeth with fixed or removable prostheses.

protocol – from the same root as in "prototype," protocol refers to an accepted form or format, usually for behavior in a specified professional or social situation; protocol in a dental practice refers to the accepted and standard way of doing things.

provider – the person or entity providing direct patient care and to whom third-payment is released; the dentist or in some cases the hygienist.

provisional employment – temporary employment, usually for 90 days, that implies permanent employment upon completion of a satisfactory trial period.

public health dentistry – the field of study, prevention, and treatment of dental diseases through community, county, state, and federal programs and agencies.

proximal – the tooth surface that is adjacent to another tooth.

proximate cause – a directly contributing action that results in an undesirable outcome.

public health dentist – a dental specialist who provides dental services to a variety of population groups under the sponsorship of a community- or government-sponsored agency or program.

pulp – provides the blood and nutritional supply from the body to the tooth; the pulp enters each tooth through the apical foramen.

purchase order – a specific document used for supply purchases and repair requisitions.

purchase order number – a specific number assigned to each purchase or repair requisition.

Q

quadrant – one quarter of the mouth; the deciduous quadrant comprises five teeth; the secondary quadrant comprises eight teeth.

quantity discounts – ordering dental supplies in bulk to save money.

Quick Launch – method of starting Dentrix that allows access to the time clock.

R

rate of use – the rate of consumption of items and supplies commonly used in the office.

recall card – a printed reminder of a return visit for preventive dental care, usually issued every six months.

recall program – once a patient has completed current necessary treatment he or she will be "recalled" to the practice at some time in the future for an oral examination, prophylaxis, and any subsequently required radiographs or treatment; the most common recall interval is six months.

recare/recall/recurring care – regularly scheduled appointments for preventive care; referred to as recurring or recall care.

reception area – the area of the office in which patients are received and await treatment and care.

references – names of people who could provide a job recommendation; these are usually former employers.

referral – a recommendation made by one person to another; a recommendation for professional treatment.

refill – the part of the prescription where the dentist indicates the number of refills (if any) allowed.

Registered Dental Assistant (RDA) – a state specific credential awarded upon satisfactory completion of the testing and licensing requirements.

Registered Dental Hygienist (RDH) – the credential awarded upon satisfactory completion of the testing and licensing requirements.

release – the document signed by the patient giving permissions for the transfer of records.

reorder point – a predetermined minimum quantity of a specific supply left in inventory; when the item reaches the minimum quantity additional units are to be ordered to avoid running out.

responsible party – the person who accepts the financial responsibility for paying a dental fee. If this person is not the patient, it is usually a parent, guardian, or a spouse. For insurance purposes, the patient must be a covered claimant on the responsible person's policy, but if there will not be any insurance participation in the fee, there are no restrictions. Anyone can sign an agreement to pay for the patient's care. These exceptions are typically a companion other than a spouse, or an older sibling who is not actually the legal guardian of a minor patient.

restoration – the repair of a tooth diseased by caries or damaged by trauma.

restrictive endorsement – special conditions or restrictions limiting the receiver of the check concerning use that can be made of the check.

résumé – a review of the employment candidate's credentials that states his or her qualifications for employment; it contains the candidate's biographical information, type of employment sought, and education and previous work experience pertinent to desired employment.

risk management – strategies taken by the dentist and staff to prevent or reduce the likelihood of a patient bringing legal action.

S

salutation – the part of a letter that acts as a greeting.

scanner – a device that can digitize documents or photos so they can be stored electronically.

secondary carrier – the insurance company that is billed after the primary carrier has paid their portion of the dental fee for a patient with duel coverage.

secondary insurance – the insurance company designated to pay a benefit after the primary insurance company has made their payment

severance pay – an allowance based upon the length of service, or award unused vacation pay at termination of employment.

sextant – a division of the mouth into six sections based on anatomy and including teeth with similar functions.

shelf life – the amount of time a product is guaranteed fresh; a product should be used before the shelf life expires or it should be discarded.

signature – part of the prescription the provides directions to the patient.

Signature on File – the insured's signature kept on file by the office manager to facilitate processing of claims.

social networking – online sites that focus on building social connections or relationships among people that share interests. Increasingly used to promote products and services to these groups of individuals.

software – the instructions that direct the CPU to process information.

solo practice – an office run and owned by one dentist.

specialty practice – a practice that limits its treatment to one faucet of dentistry; for example, oral surgery.

standard of care – the treatment guidelines that a dentist with the same knowledge, skill, and care in the same community would provide; there are no absolutes in standard of care.

standard precautions – an expanded version of universal precautions that includes not just blood but more body fluids.

State Board of Dental Examiners – the regulatory body that maintains and enforces the rules and regulations of the State Dental Practice Act and issues dental licenses; it is charged with protecting the health, safety, and welfare of the public.

State Dental Practice Act – a written set of rules and regulations governing the legal conduct of dental licensees within each state.

statement – the primary means by which a practice receives compensation from patients for services provided.

study models – stone or plaster casts of the patient's teeth and supporting structures.

subscriber – the holder of the insurance policy holder.

subscription – the portion of the prescription that contains the amount of the drug and directions for preparation of the drug for dispensing.

succedaneous dentition – the secondary dentition, which succeeds the primary dentition.

superscription – the portion of a pharmaceutical prescription that contains the date of the prescription, the patient's name, address, age, and gender.

supplier – a company through whom the dental office orders supply items used in the office.

suppuration – generating pus; important for documentation of periodontal disease.

system unit – the electronic circuitry housed within the computer cabinet; it performs the memory and processing functions of computer processing.

T

target audience – a segmented, predetermined group of people, based upon specific criteria or attributes.

target mailing – a promotional mailing piece directed toward a specific group of people called a target audience.

template – a pattern or design that is used for communication such as letters.

temporomandibular joint (TMJ) – the only joint in the head; it connects the mandible to the cranium.

termination – discontinuation of employment or dismissal of a patient.

tone of service – the projected attitude of the staff and surroundings

toolbar – a group of icons that allow quick access to specific part of a computer program.

treatment code – a specific number assigned to each scheduled procedure.

treatment plan – A complete diagnosis, including recommended treatment and sequence of scheduled visits.

U

unit – amount of time designated to perform specific treatments for the purpose of scheduling; most commonly 10 or 15 minutes in length.

universal precautions – treating all patients as if they have a potentially infectious disease; part of standard precautions.

universal system – a tooth numbering system adopted by the American Dental Association in which the teeth of the permanent dentition comprise #1 and continuing through #32; the teeth of the primary dentition is comprised of letters A through T.

unpaid leave – time away from the office for which the employee is not compensated.

unprofessional conduct – any act or deed that fails to uphold the State Dental Practice Act.

User's Guide – detailed instructions for use of computer software.

usual, customary, and reasonable fees (UCR) – the amount (the fee) typically charged by a dentist for procedures performed and the average charged by other dentists in the area for the same procedure.

V

variable expenses – the overhead expenses associated with the practice that change from month to month.

voice-activated dental charting – a computerized system of dental charting whereby the operator verbally dictates the clinical findings of the exam into the practice's data base.

voice mail – a recorded message service that intercepts the line after a set number of rings and asks the caller to leave a message.

voice messaging – a telephone answering system that automatically answers the call with a recorded message; it provides further instructions for the caller to leave a message or stay on the line for operator assistance.

W–Z

walk-out statement – a statement of the individual patient's services and charges, amount paid (if any), and remaining balance (if any) provided before the patient leaves the office following the appointment.

wait list – a group of patients with appointments that would like to change the date or time of an appointment if another time becomes available.

warranty – period of time during which a product is guaranteed to work or it will be repaired or replaced.

will call – a group of patients that need treatment but did not schedule an appointment at the time of diagnosis and are not currently scheduled.

wireless – the ability to connect to the Internet from a digital or electronic product without being hard wired into a system.

working interview – a part of the interview where the prospective employee works in the office with the current staff. An opportunity for the job candidate to demonstrate expertise.

work practice controls – changing the way procedures are currently performed to ensure a higher degree of safety or protection from accidental exposure.